Small Animal Paediatric Medicine and Surgery

Giselle Hosgood BVSc, MS
Johnny D. Hoskins DVM, PhD

with
Jacqueline R. Davidson DVM, MS
and
Julie A. Smith DVM

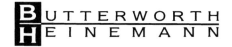
BUTTERWORTH
HEINEMANN

Butterworth-Heinemann
225 Wildwood Avenue, Woburn, MA 01801-2041
Linacre House, Jordan Hill, Oxford OX2 8DP
A division of Reed Educational and Professional Publishing Ltd

 A member of the Reed Elsevier plc group

OXFORD   BOSTON   JOHANNESBURG
MELBOURNE   NEW DELHI   SINGAPORE

First published 1998

British Library Cataloguing in Publication Data
A catalogue record for this book is available from the British Library

Library of Congress Cataloguing in Publication Data
A catalogue record for this book is available from the Library of Congress

ISBN 0 7506 3599 1

Typeset by BC Typesetting, Bristol BS31 1NZ
Printed and bound in Great Britain by The Bath Press, Somerset

Contents

1

Physical examination and related diagnostic procedures

Puppies and kittens arrive into this world in a care-dependent state. The fact that their eyes and ears are sealed reflects their incompletely developed nervous system. They are born with little spontaneous movement and must be stimulated by the mother's licking to begin breathing, irregularly at first (Hoskins, 1995a; 1995b). Because of an inability to maintain body heat, puppies and kittens must stay close to their mother and littermates. A puppy or kitten will orient itself towards the source of licking directed at its head and dorsum. This natural rooting reflex encourages the puppy and kitten to turn and push towards any warm object near its head. Since warm objects would most likely be its mother or littermates, the reflex is important in establishing the puppy's and kitten's initial bonding with the mother. The reflex begins to disappear at 4 days. Puppies and kittens suckle every 1–2 h for the first week of life; after each feeding the mother stimulates urination and defecation by licking the anal and genital areas.

Physical examination

Most healthy puppies are first examined by veterinarians at 6–8 weeks of age when they receive their first vaccines. Puppies younger than 4 weeks of age should be examined with the mother present to keep them calm. Puppies younger than 5 weeks should be examined on a warm surface and by an individual with warm hands. Warm the surface with a warm-water heating blanket or use a small cardboard box lined with blankets containing hot water bottles.

Before handling the puppy, first observe its reaction to the environment. Take note of the puppy's general physical condition, mentation, posture, locomotion and breathing pattern. Next, record the puppy's weight in grams or kilograms and obtain vital signs – rectal temperature, heart rate and character and respiratory rate. The normal rectal temperature for newborn puppies is 35.6–36.1° C (96–97° F). After 1–2 weeks the rectal temperature gradually increases until it reaches 37.8° C (100° F) by 4 weeks of age. The heart rate should be rapid and strong; breathing should be regular and unlaboured (Table 1.1).

Body weight is an important parameter in determining the health of very young puppies. Weight loss or failure to gain weight is one of the first signs of illness. Having the owner keep an accurate daily record of each puppy's weight for the first 3 weeks of life and every 2 weeks thereafter is helpful in detecting a health-related problem. Puppies should gain 2–4 g/day per kg of expected adult weight daily or double their birth weight within 2 weeks. For example, to achieve an adult weight of 25 kg, a puppy should gain 50–75 g of weight daily.

Assessment of the physical condition of a puppy that is still developing requires knowledge of normal developmental stages (Table 1.1). The physical examination should be conducted in a systematic manner. Although the examination may be easier to complete by proceeding from the puppy's head to tail, it is advisable to examine and record observations according to various body systems – digestive, urinary, circulatory, nervous, respiratory and musculoskeletal. All puppies should have functional hearing by 6 weeks of age and older.

Table 1.1 Age-related developmental stages in puppies

Body system	Age	Developmental stages
Eyes	Birth–13 days	Eyelids are closed, but puppies respond to a bright light with a blink reflex. This reflex disappears at 21 days, probably due to development of accurate pupil control. Palpebral reflex is present at 3 days, becoming adult-like by 9 days
	5–14 days	Menace reflex is present, but slow. Eyelids separate into upper and lower lids. Pupillary light responses are present within 24 h after eyelids separate. Reflex lacrimation begins when eyelids separate. Corneal reflex is present after eyelids separate
	3–4 weeks	Vision should be normal
Ears	Birth–5 days	External ear canals are closed. Hearing is poor
	10–14 days	External ear canals open (should be completely open by 17 days). For the first week after the ear canals are completely opened there is an abundance of desquamated cells, which is normal as the ear canals remodel to the external environment
Teeth	4–6 weeks	Deciduous incisors erupt, followed by deciduous canines
	4–8 weeks	Deciduous premolars erupt
Circulatory	Birth–4 weeks	Lower blood pressure, stroke volume and peripheral vascular resistance present. Increased heart rate (> 220 beats/min), cardiac output and central venous pressure present. Heart rhythm is regular sinus rhythm
Respiratory	Birth–4 weeks	Respiratory rate is 15–35 breaths/min
Neuromuscular	Birth	Flexor dominance is present at birth, with extensor dominance starting as early as 1 day. Seal posture reflex can last up to 19 days. Sucking reflex is present, but disappears by 23 days. Anogenital reflex disappears between 23 and 39 days. Cutaneous pain perception is present, but withdrawal reflex is noticeable at about 7 days. Tonic neck reflexes are present until 3 weeks of age. Can raise head. Righting response is present. Myotactic reflexes are present at birth, but difficult to elicit in newborns. Panniculus reflex is present at birth
	5 days	Nystagmus associated with rotatory stimulation appears at the end of the first week. Cross-extensor reflex ends between 2 and 17 days – persistence of this reflex indicates upper motor neuron disease. Direct forelimb support of body weight
	14–16 days	Puppies are crawling. Rear-limb support of body weight
	20 days	Puppies can sit and have reasonable control of distal phalanges
	22 days	Puppies are walking normally. Vestibular nystagmus becomes adult-like
	23–40 days	Puppies are climbing and have a righting response
	3–4 weeks	Hemi-walking response present, but may not be fully developed in rear limbs until 6 weeks old
	6–8 weeks	Postural reactions are fully developed

The umbilical cord usually falls off 2–3 days after birth. The testicles should descend by 4–6 weeks of age. If both testes have not descended by 7–14 weeks, cryptorchidism should be suspected.

Most healthy kittens are first examined by veterinarians at 6–9 weeks of age, when they receive their first vaccines. As in puppies, body weight is an important parameter in gauging the health of very young kittens. Weight loss or failure to gain weight is one of the first signs of illness. Having the owner keep an accurate daily record of each kitten's weight for the first 3 weeks of life and every week thereafter is helpful in detecting a health-related problem. The kitten at birth should weigh 80–140 g (most weigh around 100–120 g) and gain 50–100 g weekly. To assess the physical condition of a kitten that is still developing after birth requires knowledge of normal developmental stages (Table 1.2).

Table 1.2 Physical examination of kittens

Body system	Characteristic findings
Head and oral cavity	Check for malformations of the skull, cleft lip, stenotic nares or cleft palate. Brachycephalic cat breeds are predisposed to these malformations.
	Mucous membranes should be light pink and moist.
	The teeth, if present, should be examined for early occlusion.
Ears	External ear canals open between 6 and 14 days after birth and should be completely open by 17 days. When ear canals first open, cytological examination shows an abundance of desquamative cells and some oil droplets. A thorough otoscopic examination can be made in kittens older than 4 weeks of age.
	Functional hearing is present after 6 weeks of age; blue-eyed, white cat breeds have a higher incidence of congenital unilateral or bilateral deafness.
Eyes and eyelids	The eyelids separate into upper and lower eyelids at 5–14 days after birth.
	Menace reflex may not appear until 3–4 weeks of life.
	Reflex lacrimation begins when the eyelids separate, therefore evaluation of tear production by Schirmer's tear test can be done thereafter.
	Pupillary light responses are present after the eyelids open but may not be evident until 21 days of age.
Nose	Check appearance and patency of the nostrils and the presence of fluids (mucus, pus, blood, milk, clear discharges).
Thorax	Check the thoracic wall, whether symmetrical or deformed and auscultate the thorax using a stethoscope with a paediatric chest piece (2-cm bell; 3-cm diaphragm).
	The heart rate approximates 220 beats/min, and the respiratory rate is from 15–35 breaths/min during the first 4 weeks of life and then becomes similar to adults thereafter. The normal heart rhythm of kittens is a regular sinus rhythm. Heart sounds are localized to the left cardiac apex (left fifth to sixth intercostal space, ventral third of thorax), the left cardiac base (left third to fourth intercostal space above the costochondral junction) or the right cardiac apex (right fourth to fifth intercostal space opposite the mitral valve area).
	Absence of lung sounds or audible asymmetry may indicate abnormalities within the thorax and/or lungs.
Abdomen	Unless the liver margins extend beyond the ribs, the liver is not enlarged.
	The spleen normally is not palpable unless it is enlarged.
	Both kidneys are palpable in all kittens.
	The stomach may feel like a large, fluid-filled sac if it is full.
	The intestines palpate as soft, slightly fluid or gas-filled structures that are freely movable and non-painful.
	The urinary bladder can be gently squeezed to determine resistance to urine outflow.
Skin and umbilicus	The skin should be inspected for wounds, state of hydration and condition of foot pads. The skin and haircoat should also be examined for evidence of bacterial infection, external parasites or dermatophytosis.
	The umbilicus should be carefully inspected for evidence of inflammation and infection or abnormalities of the abdominal wall. The umbilical cord normally drops off by 2–3 days of age.

Table 1.2 (continued)

Body system	Characteristic findings
Limbs, tail, anus and genitalia	Check the limbs for deformities or absence of long bones, number and position of toes and pads, position of limbs at rest and during movement, presence of soft tissue injuries (bruises, swelling, wounds) and condition of joints (deformities, range of mobility).
	The tail is inspected for length, mobility and deformities.
	The anus should be evaluated for patency, redness and signs of diarrhoea; the genitalia should be checked for position and appearance.
	The testes are fully descended into the scrotum at birth.
	Despite their normal descent into the scrotum, they may move up and down in the inguinal canal and do not remain permanently in the scrotum until 10–14 weeks of age. If both testes have not descended by 14 weeks, cryptorchidism should be suspected.
Nervous system	Sucking reflex is present at birth and disappears by 3 weeks of life. Eliminative behaviours are controlled for the first 3–4 weeks of life by anogenital reflex.

Diagnostic evaluation

Laboratory tests

A puppy's and kitten's serum chemistry and haematological values are different from adults' (Tables 1.3–1.6). Reference laboratories may provide their normal value ranges for puppies and kittens for their tests. Collecting adequate blood samples from external jugular veins of puppies and kittens younger than 4 weeks of age can be difficult. It is advisable to perform at least simple in-house tests, i.e. obtaining the packed cell volume (PCV) from a microhaematocrit, blood cell morphology from microscopic examination of a stained blood smear, blood glucose and blood urea nitrogen (BUN) determinations by reagent strips for whole blood, urine evaluation by reagent strip and a urine sediment microscopic examination, and total plasma solids and urine-specific gravity determinations by refractometer. Even knowing the results of these few tests may be sufficient information to confirm the cause of the puppy's or kitten's illness or to assist in the management of the illness.

Radiography

Puppies and kittens are frequently a challenge to perform quality radiographic studies. They are often more mobile than adults and generally non-responsive to voice commands that may calm or help immobilize them. Because of their small size, most radiographic studies are performed using table-top techniques (Greco and Partington, 1994). It is important that puppies and kittens for radiographic studies are properly positioned and radiographic film is correctly exposed and developed. Holding on to puppy or kitten extremities while wearing lead gloves is nearly impossible; therefore, using slip-knot gauze-tie extenders on the limbs for positioning of radiographic studies is helpful (Greco and Partington, 1994). The gauze ties allow personnel to immobilize the limbs while keeping lead-gloved hands out of the primary X-ray beam. Soft sponge wedges can also be used to hold down the head and other mobile areas to extend the distance between the gloved fingers and the area of X-ray exposure. The use of X-ray beam collimation to cover just the area of interest is important. Close collimation decreases scatter radiation, which will improve radiograph image quality and decrease radiation exposure to personnel.

Manual restraint is the preferred form of restraint used for radiographic positioning in puppies and kittens younger than 3 weeks of age. However, some puppies and kittens resist restraint so strongly that diagnostic radiography cannot be obtained without injury, excessive stress or exposure of personnel to the primary

Table 1.3 Haematological values (means and ranges) of growing healthy puppies (Anderson & Gee, 1958; Earl *et al.*, 1973)

Test	Age (weeks)				
	Birth	1	3	6	12
Packed cell volume (%)	47.5 45.0–52.5	40.5 33.0–52.0	31.7 27.0–37.0	32.5 26.5–35.5	40.9
Red blood cell count ($\times 10^6/\mu l$)	5.1 4.7–5.6	4.6 3.6–5.9	3.8 3.5–4.3	4.7 4.3–5.1	6.3
Haemoglobin (g/dl)	15.2 14.0–17.0	12.9 10.4–17.5	9.7 8.6–11.6	10.2 8.5–11.3	14.3
Mean corpuscle volume (fl)	93	89	83	69	64.6
Mean corpuscle concentration (pg)	32	32	31	31.5	35.3
Reticulocytes (%)	6.5 4.5–9.2	6.9 3.8–15.2	6.9 5.0–9.0	4.5 2.6–6.2	NA
Total white blood cell count ($\times 10^3/\mu l$)	12.0 6.8–18.4	14.1 9.0–23.0	11.2 6.7–15.1	16.3 12.6–26.7	17.1
Band neutrophils ($\times 10^3/\mu l$)	0.23 0–1.5	0.50 0–4.8	0.09 0–0.5	0.05 0–0.3	0.08
Segmented neutrophils ($\times 10^3/\mu l$)	8.6 4.4–15.8	7.4 3.8–15.2	5.1 1.4–9.4	9.0 4.2–17.6	9.8
Lymphocytes ($\times 10^3/\mu l$)	1.9 0.5–4.2	4.3 1.3–9.4	5.0 2.1–10.1	5.7 2.8–16.6	5.7
Monocytes ($\times 10^3/\mu l$)	0.9 0.2–2.2	1.1 0.3–2.5	0.7 0.1–1.4	1.1 0.5–2.7	0.9
Eosinophils ($\times 10^3/\mu l$)	0.4 0–1.3	0.8 0.2–2.8	0.3 0.07–0.9	0.5 0.1–1.9	0.4
Basophils ($\times 10^3/\mu l$)	0	0.01 (0–0.02)	0	0	0

X-ray beam. For those animals and for animals requiring skull, spine or contrast studies, chemical sedation is necessary to stop motion artefacts and achieve good positioning.

A fine-tuned technique chart is necessary if good-quality radiographs are to be produced for all body parts of puppies and kittens (Morgan and Silverman, 1987). Seldom can a technique chart designed for one X-ray machine be used on another X-ray machine with any degree of success. A technique chart that works well for adult dogs and cats is required first; then quality radiographs of young puppies and kittens can be produced with the same X-ray machine.

Kilovoltage should be greatly reduced for radiography of a young puppy and kitten because of decreased absorption of X-rays by undermineralized bones and thin body parts (Morgan and Silverman, 1987). A general guideline for reducing kilovoltage is to reduce the radiographic exposure to about one-half of that used for adult dogs and cats of the same thickness. Extrapolations to thinner dogs and cats can be made based on the fact that each centimetre of soft tissue is the equivalent of 2 kVp at settings equal to or less than 80 kVp. Most radiography of young puppies and kittens will be performed in the 40–60 kVp range; therefore, a change of 4–6 kVp doubles or halves the film exposure.

Thoracic radiography

Thoracic radiographs are indicated for evaluation of oesophageal, cardiovascular and pulmonary diseases. Most thoracic exposure settings in puppies and kittens will have the same peak kilovoltage as used for the equivalent abdomen thickness, and one-half the abdominal milliamps setting (Greco and Partington, 1994). Puppies and kittens 2 weeks or younger have one-third the alveolar surface area of an adult. As a result, younger animals have an increased respiratory rate to increase their minute

Table 1.4 Haematological values (mean and ranges) of growing healthy kittens (Meyers-Wallen *et al.*, 1984)

Test	Age (weeks)				
	0–2	*2–4*	*4–6*	*6–8*	*12–13*
Packed cell volume (%)	35.3 (1.7)	26.5 (0.8)	27.1 (0.8)	29.8 (1.3)	33.1 (1.6)
Red blood cell count ($\times 10^6/\mu l$)	5.29 (0.24)	4.67 (0.10)	5.89 (0.23)	6.57 (0.26)	7.43 (0.23)
Haemoglobin (g/dl)	12.1 (0.6)	8.7 (0.2)	8.6 (0.3)	9.1 (0.3)	10.1 (0.3)
Mean corpuscle volume (fl)	67.4 (1.9)	53.9 (1.2)	45.6 (1.3)	45.6 (1.0)	44.5 (1.8)
Mean corpuscle haemoglobin concentration (pg)	34.5 (0.8)	33.0 (0.5)	31.9 (0.6)	30.9 (0.5)	31.3 (0.9)
Total white blood cell count ($\times 10^3/\mu l$)	9.67 (0.57)	15.31 (1.21)	17.45 (1.37)	18.07 (1.94)	23.2 (3.36)
Band neutrophils ($\times 10^3/\mu l$)	0.06 (0.020	0.11 (0.04)	0.20 (0.06)	0.22 (0.08)	0.15 (0.07)
Segmented neutrophils ($\times 10^3/\mu l$)	5.96 (0.52)	6.92 (0.59)	6.41 (0.77)	9.59 (1.57)	10.46 (2.61)
Monocytes ($\times 10^3/\mu l$)	0.01 (0.01)	0.02 (0.02)	0	0.01 (0.01)	0
Eosinophils ($\times 10^3/\mu l$)	0.96 (0.43)	1.40 (0.16)	1.47 (0.25)	1.08 (0.20)	1.55 (0.35)
Basophils ($\times 10^3/\mu l$)	0.02 (0.01)	0	0	0.02 (0.02)	rare

volume. The rapid respiratory rate combined with their greater thoracic wall motion increases the difficulty of obtaining thoracic radiographs without motion. It is important to time the radiographic exposure for the slight pause at the end of peak inspiration.

Thoracic radiographs have a generalized increased interstitial opacity owing to the decreased alveolar air volume present. The veterinarian should avoid overinterpretation of a mildly increased interstitial opacity as a sign of disease, as seen in viral pneumonia. It may be helpful to have a series of normal (healthy) thoracic radiographs using the equipment in the practice for comparison with radiographs of ill puppies and kittens. Keeping a separate radiograph log of puppies and kittens at different ages will help establish a comparison file (Greco and Partington, 1994).

A technique which helps in interpreting pulmonary disease is to place the affected lung uppermost. If the kitten or puppy has abnormal respiratory noise on one side of the thorax, the opposite side should be laid against the radiograph cassette during exposure. By placing the affected side up, one increases the inflation of the diseased hemithorax and increases the contrast between affected and unaffected lung. The cranial mediastinum normally will appear thicker and more opaque in the puppy and kitten, and the thymus may appear as an opaque triangle (sail sign) in the cranial left hemithorax in the dorsoventral and ventrodorsal view.

When taking thoracic radiographs for the evaluation of a congenital heart defect, it is important to position the puppy or kitten in a perfectly straight line. Because of the decreased alveolar volume in the puppy's or kitten's lungs, the heart appears larger within the thoracic cavity (Greco and Partington, 1994). With growth, the heart will gradually assume its normal heart-to-thorax size relationship. Slight obliquity on the dorsoventral, ventrodorsal or lateral exposure may cause misinterpretation of cardiac abnormalities. On the oblique view, the dilation of the proximal descending aorta (ductus bump) and enlarged pul-

Table 1.5 Serum chemistry values (means and ranges) of growing healthy puppies (Chandler, 1992)

Test	Age (weeks)				
	0.5–1 (n = 10)	3 (n = 12)	5 (n = 18)	8–12 (n = 10)	12–24 (n = 200)
Glucose (mg/dl)	123 (104–132)	126 (109–140)	131 (110–146)	114 (88–131)	111 (85–133)
Blood urea nitrogen (mg/dl)	30 (22–37)	23 (15–23)	15 (10–21)	24 (21–30)	13 (7–19)
Creatinine (mg/dl)	0.5 (0.4–0.6)	0.4 (0.3–0.5)	0.4 (0.3–0.5)	0.5 (0.5–0.6)	0.6 (0.3–0.9)
Total protein (g/dl)	4.2 (3.8–4.7)	4.1 (3.6–4.6)	4.7 (3.9–5.3)	4.6 (3.9–5.0)	5.1 (4.6–5.8)
Albumin (g/dl)	2.6 (2.3–2.9)	2.7 (2.1–3.2)	3.3 (2.4–4.3)	2.9 (2.0–3.3)	2.8 (2.4–3.1)
Total bilirubin (mg/dl)	1.0 (0.5–1.8)	0.4 (0.2–0.5)	0.5 (0.2–0.7)	0.2 (0.1–0.5)	0.4 (0.2–0.9)
Alkaline phosphatase (IU/l)	706 (371–1297)	378 (249–512)	355 (150–539)	569 (411–705)	117 (77–199)
Alamine aminotransferase (IU/l)	45 (25–82)	18 (10–24)	24 (6–61)	38 (26–56)	19 (9–30)
Calcium (mg/dl)	12.4 (11.9–13.1)	11.4 (10.7–12.3)	11.1 (10.3–12.6)	11.5 (10.5–12.1)	11.0 (9.8–12.4)
Phosphorus (mg/dl)	10.4 (8.7–11.8)	9.1 (7.8–10.1)	8.8 (7.0–9.8)	10.5 (10.1–11.3)	9.0 (7.2–10.1)
Sodium (mEq/l)	144 (143–145)	144 (142–148)	142 (138–145)	149 (146–153)	152 (138–160)
Potassium (mEq/l)	5.6 (5.1–6.5)	4.8 (4.2–5.5)	5.7 (4.0–6.8)	5.5 (5.2–6.6)	5.3 (4.3–6.2)
Chloride (mEq/l)	102 (99–105)	105 (102–108)	108 (102–117)	106 (104–109)	105 (103–114)

monary artery trunk are not visible, whereas they are clearly seen on properly positioned radiographs.

It is wise to evaluate the pulmonary vascularity as the first step when interpreting thoracic radiographs of a possible congenital heart defect (Greco and Partington, 1994). Check the size of the pulmonary artery and vein and see if the vein is larger than the artery (as seen with venous congestion), both artery and vein are small (evidence of pulmonary undercirculation) or both artery and vein are large (evidence of pulmonary overcirculation). Once the circulatory status of the lungs is determined, then look at the cardiac silhouette to determine chamber size alterations.

Abdominal radiography

Positioning for abdominal radiographs in the puppy and kitten is the same as for the adult (Greco and Partington, 1994). The cranial margin of the lateral view is midway between the dorsal portion of the last rib and the xiphoid. The caudal margin should include the ischiatic tuberosities. Ventrodorsal views should be made during expiration for maximum expansion of the abdominal cavity. Radiographic techniques for abdominal radiography can be extrapolated from the adult technique chart, using table-top techniques until the abdomen exceeds 10 cm in width (Greco and Partington, 1994). Above 10 cm, a grid is used on top of the cassette or the cassette is placed beneath the table in a sliding grid tray.

The major problem with abdominal radiography in the puppy or kitten is the poor abdominal detail (Greco and Partington, 1994). This lack of radiographic detail is attributed to the lack of intra-abdominal fat, a slightly increased amount of peritoneal fluid and a

Table 1.6 Serum chemistry values (means and ranges) of growing healthy kittens (Chandler, 1992)

Test	Age (weeks)				
	0.2	2–4	4–6	7–12	12–20
Glucose (mg/dl)	117 (76–129)	110 (99–112)	NA	NA	82 (59–102)
Blood urea nitrogen (mg/dl)	39 (22–54)	23 (17–30)	25 (15–36)	31 (25–38)	26 (19–34)
Creatinine (mg/dl)	0.4 (0.2–0.6)	0.4 (0.3–0.5)	0.7 (0.2–1.2)	0.6 (0.4–1.0)	0.7 (0.4–0.9)
Total protein (g/dl)	4.1 (3.5–4.7)	4.4 (4.1–4.7)	5.0 (4.1–5.9)	5.4 (5.1–5.7)	6.0 (5.4–6.8)
Albumin (g/dl)	2.1 (2.0–2.4)	2.3 (2.2–2.4)	NA	NA	3.1 (2.5–3.6)
Total bilirubin (mg/dl)	0.3 (0.1–1.0)	0.2 (0.1–0.2)	NA	NA	0.7 (0.4–1.2)
Alkaline phosphatase (IU/l)	123 (68–269)	111 (90–135)	NA	NA	71 (39–124)
Alanine aminotransferasae (IU/l)	21 (10–38)	14 (10–18)	25 (9–41)	36 (23–50)	33 (18–58)
Calcium (mg/dl)	NA	NA	9.7 (8.4–11.0)	9.9 (8.8–11.2)	9.9 (8.9–10.9)
Phosphorus (mg/dl)	8.0 (6.9–9.3)	8.5 (7.5–9.5)	8.7 (7.6–9.8)	8.6 (7.7–9.5)	8.2 (6.9–10.9)
Sodium (mEq/l)	140 (134–145)	145 (142–148)	147 (143–151)	150 (147–152)	156 (143–162)
Potassium (mEq/l)	4.7 (4.0–5.4)	5.4 (4.7–6.1)	5.3 (4.7–5.9)	5.6 (5.0–6.2)	5.0 (4.1–5.9)
Chloride (mEq/l)	NA	NA	122 (118–127)	122 (113–128)	115 (107–121)

higher proportion of total body water (80% of body weight is water in puppies and kittens versus 60% in adults). The poor abdominal detail decreases the value of abdominal radiographs for routine evaluation of abdominal organ size, shape and position. One therefore depends on the presence of gas/air and heterogeneous ingesta to aid in the evaluation of the gastrointestinal tract. Radiopaque foreign bodies and complete intestinal obstruction are still identifiable, even with the lack of abdominal detail.

The liver is comparatively larger in the puppy and kitten and occupies a large portion of the abdominal cavity (Greco and Partington, 1994). The ratio of liver weight to body weight decreases with age – the liver weighs 40–50 g/kg body weight versus 20 g/kg in the adult. Even with poor abdominal detail, the liver size can be estimated by the position of the stomach. If the pylorus is displaced dorsally and caudally, the liver is enlarged. If the pylorus is displaced cranially towards the diaphragm, the liver is small, as is commonly seen with congenital portosystemic shunts.

Because of the inherent lack of abdominal detail, contrast agents may be used to evaluate further the gastrointestinal and urogenital systems (Greco and Partington, 1994). Barium sulphate suspensions can be given for examination of the upper gastrointestinal tract. Barium sulphate is inert and non-irritating. If precautions are taken to prevent constipation, there should be no side-effects with barium sulphate given orally. A 30% micropulverized suspension given via orogastric tube at a dose of 7–10 ml/kg can be given. For evaluation of rectal anomalies, a 15% barium sulphate suspension can be gently injected into the rectum via a soft-tipped catheter. Do not use barium sulphate powder mixed with water. The powder will not go into suspension well, and it quickly precipitates out along the gastrointestinal tract.

Oral organic iodine solutions should not be used in puppies or kittens younger than 4 weeks of age (Greco and Partington, 1994). Oral iodine solutions are irritating to the mucous membranes and are hyperosmotic. The hyperosmolality causes fluid to accumulate in the intestinal lumen, resulting in diarrhoea and dehydration. Because puppies and kittens have less intracellular fluid reserves and a high water turnover rate, oral iodine solutions may put them at greater risk. If perforation in the oesophagus or intestine is suspected in a puppy or kitten, oral non-ionic contrast such as iohexol or iopamidol (concentrated contrast solution is diluted 1 : 3 with warm water before administration and administered at 10 ml/kg body weight by orogastric tube) may be used. Instilling contrast agents into the urethra or urinary bladder for evaluation of the lower urinary tract should be relatively safe at any age (Greco and Partington, 1994).

Intravenous and intra-arterial contrast agents for excretory urography, portography and angiocardiography should be safe for puppies and kittens after 6 weeks of age. Unnecessary or excessive use of intravascular contrast agents should be avoided owing to the puppy's or kitten's immature renal function and inability to conserve fluids. Recommended maximum intravascular iodine solution dosage is 750 mg iodine per kg body weight (Greco and Partington, 1994) but up to 1500 mg per kg body weight can be used for some procedures. Most special contrast procedures are postponed until 6 weeks of age or older to increase animal size for easier vascular access and decreased problems with anaesthesia.

Skeletal radiography

The most common radiographic procedure done in puppies and kittens is evaluation of extremities. Puppies and kittens differ from adults because their bones have generalized decreased mineralization, flared metaphyseal growth areas, open physes, thick articular cartilage and secondary centres of ossification which can mimic disease to the untrained observer (Greco and Partington, 1994). The bones of the puppy or kitten (younger than 8 weeks of age) have a non-lamellated structure. The flared irregular metaphysis is an area of active remodelling where the wide distal metaphysis decreases in diameter to form tubular bone.

This area is called the cutback zone and has a rough and irregular periosteal surface.

Open physes begin as wide radiolucent bands between the metaphysis and epiphysis and can mimic fracture lines and joint spaces (Greco and Partington, 1994). The physes narrow as the puppy or kitten grows and finally the metaphysis and epiphysis fuse to form a radiopaque physeal scar in the adult. Joint spaces artefactually appear wide because cartilage is the same soft-tissue opacity as a joint fluid, synovium and joint capsule. The pseudo-widened joint spaces are formed from the cartilage model of the epiphysis and cuboidal bones.

Because of incomplete bone mineralization, technique charts for extremities will have peak kilovoltage ranges 5–7% lower than the corresponding adult extremity chart (Greco and Partington, 1994). This adjustment will prevent overexposure and increase visualization of soft-tissue structures. Identifying an area of soft-tissue swelling on a radiograph often indicates trauma or associated pathology. Just because there is no radiographic evidence of bone lesions does not indicate that lesions are not present. Early septic arthritis and osteomyelitis may first present as increased soft-tissue opacity from joint effusion or soft-tissue swelling (Greco and Partington, 1994). When in doubt, radiograph the opposite limb for age-matched comparison.

A technique that is useful in small puppies and kittens is magnification radiology (Morgan and Silverman, 1987). If the distance between the X-ray tube and film remains constant, the size of the body part will increase as the part is moved away from the radiographic film and closer to the X-ray tube. If the body part is placed halfway between the X-ray tube and film cassette, the body part will be twice as large as actual size. Exposure techniques do not change if the radiographic film, intensifying screen, focal film distance and film developing remain the same. The standard focal film distance is 100 cm so the X-ray tube is lowered to 50 cm from the table and the cassette is placed 50 cm below the table. The body part is positioned in halfway between the X-ray tube and cassette. Magnification radiology will only assist in the diagnosis if the original image is too small to be seen clearly; it does not increase detail or image sharpness. Magnified radiographs need to be made with an X-ray tube focal spot of 0.3 mm or less, and the puppy or kitten must be completely motionless.

Ultrasonography

Real-time, grey-scale ultrasonography is the newest diagnostic tool used in puppies and kittens for identifying abdominal and cardiac diseases (Greco and Partington, 1994). Ultrasonography is usually well-tolerated and safer for personnel than diagnostic radiography. For ultrasonography in puppies and kittens, at least a 5 MHz ultrasound transducer or, better, a 7.5 MHz transducer, is preferred. The higher the transducer frequency, the better the image resolution but the greater the ultrasound beam attenuation in soft tissue (Herring, 1985). The increased attenuation decreases the depth of ultrasound beam penetration; but because of the small animal size, attenuation is rarely important. The contact area of the transducer should be as small as possible to allow for better intercostal access for cardiac imaging and subcostal access for cranial abdominal imaging. Linear array transducers used transrectally for reproductive examination are inadequate for imaging puppies and kittens.

Ultrasonography is useful for abdominal examination of puppies and kittens. Gently restrain the puppy or kitten in dorsal recumbency on a soft-padded warm surface. It is important to clip all hair completely on the ventral abdomen, especially the short down coat present even in the young animal. Hair traps air and prevents the ultrasound beam from penetrating into the abdomen. Transducers have a specific focal zone, or distance from the transducer surface where the image is sharpest. In small puppies and kittens, the focal zone may be deeper than the animal is wide, decreasing the image quality of the ultrasound. In addition, the bright band at the top of the ultrasound image or near-field artefact may obscure superficial structures. The use of an ultrasound stand-off pad may help with these problems (Biller and Meyer, 1988). An ultrasound stand-off pad is a gelatin-like disc or cube that has the ultrasound characteristics of soft tissue. Ultrasound gel is placed on both sides of the stand-off pad, and the pad is placed between the transducer and the animal. This will place the near-field artefact in the stand-off pad and place the animal deeper into the transducer's focal zone.

Abdominal ultrasonography can be used to identify peritoneal fluid, intestinal obstructions (e.g. lodged foreign objects, intussusceptions), soft-tissue masses (e.g. tumours, abscesses), organ diseases (e.g. liver, spleen, kidney, urinary bladder) and congenital vascular defects such as portosystemic shunts (Ackerman, 1991; Pennick et al., 1990). Because ultrasonography is non-invasive and does not require the use of contrast agents to identify internal organ architecture, it is less stressful to the puppy or kitten than contrast radiography.

Another common use of ultrasonography in the puppy or kitten is evaluation for congenital heart defects (Bright and Holmberg, 1990). Most echocardiography is performed in puppies and kittens that are 6 weeks of age and older. For echocardiography in puppies and kittens, a 7.5 MHz transducer is preferred. Heart lesions readily identified with M-mode or two-dimensional echocardiography include pericardial effusion, valvular vegetations, chamber size, myocardial hypertrophy and abnormal cardiac motion (Bright and Holmberg, 1990). Although specific cardiac lesions cannot always be directly imaged, echocardiography usually demonstrates the secondary effects of a lesion on the heart (i.e. dilation, hypertrophy, hyperkinesis). Contrast echocardiography may be helpful in confirming a right-to-left shunting lesion (Bright and Holmberg, 1990). Doppler ultrasonography is becoming increasingly available as a non-invasive means of assessing and quantitating the direction and velocity of blood flow within the heart and blood vessels. Doppler imaging of high-velocity, retrograde or turbulent flow through valves or intracardiac communications provides useful diagnostic and prognostic information in puppies and kittens with congenital heart defects (Bright and Holmberg, 1990).

Interpretation of echocardiography from puppies and kittens requires an awareness of the growth pattern and developmental anatomy of the heart during the first year of life (Bright and Holmberg, 1990). After birth, there is a decrease in right ventricular mass relative to the left ventricle and to body weight; this occurs by the third week of life in puppies. Sequential M-mode echocardiographic measurements obtained during growth have been studied in healthy English Pointers (Sisson and Schaeffer, 1991). These measurements reveal that, at least in this breed, the linear dimensions of the growing English Pointer heart can be expressed as exponential functions of body weight. Echocardiographic measurements of healthy, growing kittens have not been done.

Ultrasonography can also be used for intra-cranial examination through an open fontanelle (Hudson, 1990). A liberal volume of coupling gel is placed on top of the puppy's head, and the transducer is placed on top of the head with the centre of the transducer placed directly over the skull depression of the open fontanelle. Hydrocephalus is diagnosed by a lateral ventri-cular height greater than 3.5 mm.

Electrocardiography

Electrocardiography can be used to diagnose arrhythmias and conduction disturbances in puppies and kittens; however, electrocardio-graphic identification of right- or left-sided chamber enlargement or hypertrophy and alterations in mean electrical axis (MEA) usually are not attempted. Any electrocardio-graphic lead with easily recognizable P waves and QRS complexes can be used to identify arrhythmias (Bright and Holmberg, 1990).

Electrodiagnostic procedures

The development of computer equipment that can average electrical signals by extracting low-amplitude, time-locked potentials from random background electrical activity has pro-vided procedures for non-invasive evaluation of the auditory and visual system. Recording of the brainstem auditory-evoked response (BAER) is the best objective procedure for assessment of hearing in puppies and kittens (Strain, 1991). The electrical potential from the cochlea, cochlear nerve and brainstem in response to an auditory stimulus is recorded. The BAER approximates functional maturity by 4–6 weeks of age. If there is no response at all in puppies and kittens older than 6 weeks of age, the cochlea is not functioning, as may occur with congenital deafness. Dog breeds that are currently recognized to have congenital deafness are presented in Chapter 10 (Strain, 1991).

Electroretinography (ERG) is the electrical recording of retinal response to light. The ERG approximates functional maturity by 5–10 weeks of age. If there is no response at all after 10 weeks of age, the retina is not function-ing, as may occur in retinal blindness due to con-genital or acquired causes. The visual-evoked response (VER) provides an objective evalua-tion of the central visual pathways. The VER is the cortical electrical activity that occurs in response to a light stimulus administered to the eye. The VER approximates functional maturity by 6 weeks of age. If there is an altered VER after 10 weeks of age, central visual path-ways may not be functioning, as may occur in central blindness due to congenital or acquired causes (Strain, 1991).

References

Ackerman, N. (1991) *Radiology and Ultrasound of Uro-genital Diseases in the Dog and Cat.* Ames: Iowa City Press.

Anderson, A.C. and Gee, W. (1958) Normal blood values in the beagle. *Veterinary Medicine*, **53**, 135.

Biller, D.S. and Meyer, W. (1988) Ultrasound scanning of superficial structures using an ultrasound standoff pad. *Veterinary Radiology*, **29**, 138–142.

Bright, J.M. and Holmberg, D.L. (1990) The cardiovascular system. In: Hoskins, J.D. (ed.) *Veterinary Pediatrics: Dogs and Cats From Birth to Six Months*, vol. 1, pp. 43–70. Philadelphia: WB Saunders.

Chandler, M.L. (1992) Pediatric normal blood values. In: Kirk, R.W. and Bonagura, J.D. (eds) *Current Veterin-ary Therapy XI*, vol. 1, pp. 981–984. Philadelphia: WB Saunders.

Earl, F.L., Melvegar, B.A. and Wilson, R.L. (1973) The hemogram and bone marrow profile of normal neonatal and weanling beagle dogs. *Laboratory Animal Science*, **23**, 690–695.

Greco, D.S. and Partington, B.P. (1994) The physical examination and diagnostic imaging techniques. In: Hoskins, J.D. (ed.) *Veterinary Pediatrics: Dogs and Cats From Birth to Six Months*, vol. 1, pp. 1–21. Philadelphia: WB Saunders.

Herring, D.S. (1985) Physics, facts, and artifacts of diag-nostic ultrasound. *Veterinary Clinics of North America [Small Animal Practice]*, **15**, 1107–1122.

Hoskins, J.D. (1995a) The world of a kitten. *Perspectives*, **March/April**, 47–56.

Hoskins, J.D. (1995b) The world of a puppy. *Perspectives*, **January/February**, 41–46.

Hudson, J. (1990) Ultrasound diagnosis of hydrocephalus in the dog. *Veterinary Radiology*, **31**, 50–58.

Meyers-Wallen, V.N., Haskins, M.E. and Patterson, D.F. (1984) Hematologic values in healthy neonatal, weanling, and juvenile kittens. *American Journal of Veterinary Research*, **45**, 1322–1327.

Morgan, J.P. and Silverman, S. (1987) *Techniques of Veterinary Radiography*. Ames: Iowa State University Press.

Pennick, D.G., Nyland, T.G., Kerr, L.Y. and Fisher, P.E. (1990) Ultrasonographic evaluation of gastrointestinal diseases in small animals. *Veterinary Radiology*, **31**, 134–141.

Sisson, D. and Schaeffer, D. (1991) Changes in linear dimensions of the heart, relative to body weight, as measured by M-mode echocardiography in growing dogs. *American Journal of Veterinary Research*, **52**, 1591–1596.

Strain, G.M. (1991) Congenital deafness in dogs and cats. *Compendium of Continuing Education for the Practicing Veterinarian*, **13**, 245–253.

2
Preventive care

Preventive care is an integral part of providing for the general health needs of young puppies and kittens. Regularly scheduled vaccinations alone do not represent comprehensive preventive care. However, they are an important part of the preventive care and should reward the puppy or kitten by preventing life-threatening infectious diseases peculiar to the growing puppy and kitten (Hoskins, 1995). The veterinarian should ensure that the vaccination programme is being met.

Before a puppy or kitten is vaccinated, a complete physical examination and recording of body weight should always be done. In addition to recording the rectal temperature, respiratory and heart rates and capillary refill time on the health record, the thorax should be thoroughly auscultated and the abdomen palpated for evidence of physical abnormalities (see Chapter 1). Recording the body weight is extremely important. First, the weight provides information needed for dispensing medication; and second, it is an immediate indicator of the nutritional status of the animal. A steady increase in the body weight of a growing puppy or kitten at each vaccination time is an indication that it is receiving adequate nutrition and is likely to be free of life-threatening congenital defects.

Vaccinations for puppies

Puppies are very susceptible to certain infectious diseases, especially canine distemper, infectious canine hepatitis, parvovirus, coronavirus, parainfluenza, leptospirosis, bordetellosis and rabies (Hoskins, 1992). Puppies receive antibodies from the dam via colostrum, which usually protects them from these diseases for 6–8 weeks. Once the puppies lose their maternal antibody protection, they are at high risk of contracting these diseases if exposed to an infected animal. Since the duration of protection provided by maternal antibodies can vary (the range is 3–20 weeks), it is recommended that puppies be vaccinated on a repeat basis until 4 months of age. Once the vaccination series is completed, annual boosters are recommended to maintain protective antibody levels.

The initial vaccination series consists of one injection of a multivalent vaccine given at 6–8 weeks of age and two boosters given at 9–12 weeks of age and 14–16 weeks of age (Table 2.1; Hoskins, 1995). Puppies whose immune status is uncertain may receive additional injections of multivalent vaccine as early as 2 weeks of age. Where appropriate, the rabies injection is given at 3 months of age or older.

In addition to regularly scheduled canine distemper, infectious canine hepatitis, parvovirus, coronavirus, parainfluenza, leptospirosis and rabies vaccinations, other vaccines may be incorporated into the vaccination programme, as detailed below (Hoskins, 1995).

Infectious tracheobronchitis vaccine

Vaccination can be an effective means for preventing, or at least reducing, the occurrence of infectious tracheobronchitis (i.e. bordetellosis or kennel cough) in dogs of all ages (Appel, 1981; Wagnener *et al.*, 1984). Intranasal vaccination, in particular, provides rapid, long-term protection against *Bordetella bronchiseptica*

Table 2.1 A vaccination protocol for puppies (Hoskins, 1995)

Age	Disease
6 weeks	Canine distemper
	Infectious canine hepatitis
	Parvovirus
	Coronavirus
	Parainfluenza
	Leptospirosis
	Bordetellosis
9 weeks	Canine distemper
	Infectious canine hepatitis
	Parvovirus
	Coronavirus
	Parainfluenza
	Leptospirosis
	Bordetellosis
12 weeks	Canine distemper
	Infectious canine hepatitis
	Parvovirus
	Coronavirus
	Parainfluenza
	Leptospirosis
	Bordetellosis
	Rabies†
15–16 weeks	Immunity check*
Annually thereafter	Canine distemper
	Infectious canine hepatitis
	Parvovirus
	Coronavirus
	Parainfluenza
	Leptospirosis
	Bordetellosis
	Rabies†

* Immunity check means determining serum antibody titre response for any component in the multivalent vaccine administered. This is especially important for canine parvovirus response in high-risk breeds such as the Rottweiler and Dobermann Pinscher.
† Rabies vaccinations are given annually or triennially, depending on the vaccine used and local statutes, some countries have restrictive measures.

infection and disease. Puppies can be vaccinated intranasally as early as 2–4 weeks of age without interference from maternal antibody, or they can be vaccinated when they receive their initial multivalent vaccine. One dose is effective for 1 year. Adults can receive a one-dose intranasal vaccination at the same time as their puppies or at the time they receive their annual vaccinations. Puppies being prepared for shipment or entering a boarding kennel or veterinary hospital should be vaccinated at least 1–2 weeks before admission or shipping. Other infectious tracheobronchitis vaccines available include inactivated *Bordetella bronchiseptica* parenteral vaccine administered as two doses 2–4 weeks apart. When puppies younger than 4 months of age are being vaccinated, they should be revaccinated after reaching the age of 4 months. Initial vaccination of puppies with parenteral vaccines is recommended at or about 6–8 weeks of age.

Canine Lyme borreliosis vaccine

Canine *Borrelia burgdorferi* vaccine provides protection against canine Lyme disease (Wagnener *et al.*, 1984). According to the manufacturers currently marketing canine *Borrelia burgdorferi* vaccines, puppies 12 weeks of age or older should receive two doses administered intramuscularly at 2 to 3 week intervals. Annual revaccination with a single dose is recommended.

Vaccinations for kittens

Kittens should be vaccinated regularly to protect them from life-threatening infectious diseases. These include the upper respiratory diseases, viral rhinotracheitis and feline calicivirus; feline panleukopenia (cat distemper); rabies and feline leukaemia virus (FeLV) diseases (Hoskins, 1995). Kittens become susceptible to infectious diseases, if exposed, once they begin to lose the protection provided by the queen's colostrum. The length of this protection varies individually and can range from 3 to 15 weeks.

The initial vaccination series consists of a combination injection given at 9–10 weeks and a booster given at 12–13 weeks (Table 2.2; Hoskins, 1995). Testing for FeLV infection is generally performed before vaccination, especially if the queen's FeLV status is unknown. Feline leukaemia virus vaccinations can be given as early as 9 weeks with a booster at 3 weeks after the initial injection. Some veterinarians prefer not to administer other vaccinations at the same time as the FeLV vaccine because some kittens react with a mild fever, depression, lethargy or inappetence for a few days. A feline pneumonitis vaccine may also be given to kittens living in catteries or multiple-cat households where *Chlamydia*-induced upper respiratory infections and conjunctivitis are a problem.

In addition to regularly scheduled viral rhinotracheitis, feline calicivirus, feline panleuko-

Table 2.2 A vaccination schedule for kittens (Hoskins, 1995)†

Age	Disease
9 weeks	Feline viral rhinotracheitis Feline calicivirus Cat distemper Feline leukaemia virus Pneumonitis (optional)
12 weeks	Feline viral rhinotracheitis Feline calicivirus Cat distemper Feline leukaemia virus Rabies*
16 weeks	Feline infectious peritonitis (optional) – booster 3–4 weeks later
12 months and annually thereafter	Feline viral rhinotracheitis Feline calicivirus Cat distemper Feline leukaemia virus Rabies* Pneumonitis (optional) Feline infectious peritonitis (optional)

†Note that recommendations for the site and frequency of vaccination administration are indefinite at present due to investigation into vaccine-related fibrosarcoma in the cat. Veterinarians should consult with their national Veterinary Association for current recommendations.
*Rabies vaccinations are given annually or triennially, depending on the vaccine used and local statutes, some countries have restrictive measures.

penia and rabies vaccinations, other vaccines may be incorporated into the vaccination programme, as detailed below (Hoskins, 1995).

Feline Chlamydia vaccine

Although feline chlamydiosis is not as common as feline viral rhinotracheitis or feline calicivirus infections, it is evident that in some cat populations chlamydial infection is contributing to persistent conjunctivitis and upper respiratory tract disease (Scott, 1983). The vaccines currently available apparently produce effective protection only against *Chlamydia psittaci* infections. As with other vaccines for respiratory ailments, complete protection is not afforded; however, signs of conjunctivitis or upper respiratory tract disease, if they do occur, can be restricted to short courses and are mild. Vaccines for feline chlamydiosis can be obtained from several manufacturers in various combinations with the more traditional feline vaccine components.

Feline leukaemia virus vaccine

Several FeLV vaccines are currently available to protect cats of all ages against FeLV infection. The vaccines are administered subcutaneously in healthy kittens or older cats as two doses, with the second dose given 3 or 4 weeks after the first. Annual revaccination with a single dose is recommended. According to the manufacturers, the vaccines cause no interference with simultaneous vaccinations against rabies, panleukopenia and upper respiratory viruses. The vaccines do not cause a positive FeLV test results in kittens vaccinated at any age.

Feline infectious peritonitis (FIP) vaccine

A temperature-sensitive FIP virus (TS-FIPV) vaccine that affords protection against FIP is available. This TS-FIPV vaccine contains attenuated whole coronavirus and is recommended by the manufacturer to be administered intranasally to healthy cats (Hoskins, 1993). Primary vaccination with two doses should be given at 16 weeks and older, with the second dose administered 3–4 weeks after the first. Annual revaccination with a single dose is recommended.

Feline fungal vaccine

A *Microsporum canis* killed fungal vaccine that affords protection against ringworm-induced skin lesions is available. The vaccine is used in cats 4 months of age and older as an aid in the prevention and treatment of clinical signs of disease caused by *M. canis*. Vaccination has not been demonstrated to eliminate *M. canis* organisms from infected cats. Primary vaccination with two doses should be given, with the second dose administered 3–4 weeks after the first, and revaccination with a single dose every 6 months is recommended.

Parasite control

Puppies should be checked for gastrointestinal parasites and dewormed at 3 weeks of age and older. They also require faecal re-examinations and dewormings when they return for their routine vaccinations. Gastrointestinal parasites can cause serious disorders in puppies, including life-threatening anaemia, diarrhoea, weakness from hypoglycaemia and weight loss. The most common parasites of puppies are hookworms, roundworms (ascarids), whipworms, tapeworms, *Giardia* and coccidia (Zimmer, 1986). The method of infection varies with the type of worm, but includes transplacental transfer, infection via milk while suckling, skin penetration and ingestion. Treatment includes immediate therapy with appropriate deworming medications, follow-up therapy 2–4 weeks later to kill migrating stages of the parasite and environmental clean-up to prevent reinfection.

Puppies should be checked for worms on a regular basis: at 3 weeks of age, 6–8 weeks of age, 10–12 weeks of age and 14–16 weeks of age in puppies; and on an annual basis (minimum) as adults. The test requires a small sample of fresh faeces, flotation solution (sodium nitrate solution prepared to a specific gravity of 1.36 works well) and a good microscope. The faecal sample is suspended in flotation solution, topped with a coverslip and allowed to stand undisturbed for 5–10 minutes. The coverslip is then placed on a glass slide and examined for parasite ova. Tapeworm infections are rarely diagnosed by faecal examinations because the eggs are contained within segments of the tapeworm (proglottids), which crawl out of the puppy's anus and fall to the ground. Commercially produced test kits can also be obtained to identify parasite ova in faeces.

Heartworm-preventive medication should be started at 6–8 weeks of age in areas where heartworms are endemic. Heartworm infection can be prevented by administering oral medications to heartworm-negative dogs on a regular basis. Duration of administration will vary depending on the mosquito season in the particular geographic area. In areas where the heartworm is endemic, prophylactic medication should be administered year-round.

A puppy is usually started on heartworm prophylaxis, using diethylcarbamazine, ivermectin or milbemycin oxime (Hribernik, 1989). Heartworm products that contain diethylcarbamazine are available for oral administration as a chewable tablet, standard tablet and syrup from a variety of manufacturers and should be given once a day at a dose rate of 6.6 mg/kg body weight (3 mg/lb body weight). The ivermectin product should be administered orally at the recommended minimum dose level of 6.0 μg/kg of body weight at monthly dosing intervals. The heartworm product that contains milbemycin oxime should be administered orally at the recommended minimum dose level of 0.5 mg/kg of body weight at monthly dosing intervals. Heartworm-preventive products of any type should be started in heartworm-infested areas 1 month before the beginning of the mosquito season and for about 2 months thereafter. Dogs should be given a heartworm examination after 6 months of age and annually thereafter to ensure they remain free of heartworms.

Kittens should be checked and dewormed for gastrointestinal parasites on a regular basis. At 3 weeks of age and older and annually in adults, a faecal flotation test should be performed. The signs of parasitism vary with the type and number of worms present and may be particularly severe in young kittens. Anaemia, vomiting, diarrhoea, cough, unthriftiness, dull haircoat, a pot-bellied appearance and the presence of rice grain-like organisms around the anus may indicate parasitism. The most common parasites found in kittens are tapeworms (carried by fleas or rodents), roundworms, hookworms and coccidia (Zimmer, 1986). The method of infection varies with the type of worm but includes transfer through the queen's milk, skin penetration and ingestion.

The deworming procedure for parasitism includes immediate therapy with appropriate anthelminthics and follow-up therapy 2–4 weeks later to kill the migrating stages of the parasite.

Dental care (see Chapter 6)

Feeding

Nutritional requirements, feeding and care of puppies and kittens after birth are substantially different during their different stages of growth. Proper nutrition consists of supplying all necessary nutrients in adequate amounts and in proper proportions. Growth is a demanding time in any puppy's or kitten's life (Lewis *et al.*, 1987). Puppies and kittens will fail to grow to the size determined by their hereditary factors unless they consume sufficient food of adequate quality. If poor-quality, unbalanced, commercially prepared diets or home-made diets of single food items or indiscriminate mixtures of single food items are fed during growth, nutrition-related disorders often occur. Proper nutrition, therefore, is crucial to the general health and performance of puppies and kittens after birth (see Chapter 4).

References

Appel, M. (1981) Canine infectious tracheobronchitis (kennel cough): a status report. *Compendium of Continuing Education for the Practicing Veterinarian*, **3**, 70–79.

Hoskins, J.D. (1992) Practices in modern vaccination. *Veterinary Technician*, **13**, 51–55.

Hoskins, J.D. (1993) Coronavirus infection in cats. *Veterinary Clinics of North America [Small Animal Practice]*, **23**, 1–16.

Hoskins, J.D. (1995) The preventative health program. In: Hoskins, J.D. (ed.) *Veterinary Pediatrics: Dogs and Cats From Birth to Six Months*, pp. 65–70. Philadelphia: WB Saunders.

Hribernik, T.N. (1989) Canine and feline heartworm disease. In: Kirk, R.W. (ed.) *Current Veterinary Therapy X*, pp. 263–270. Philadelphia: WB Saunders.

Lewis, L.D., Morris, M.L.J. and Hand, M.S. (1987) *Small Animal Clinical Nutrition III*. Topeka, KS: Mark Morris Associates.

Scott, F.W. (1983) Feline immunization. In: Kirk, R.W. (ed.) *Current Veterinary Therapy VIII*, pp. 1127–1129. Philadelphia: WB Saunders.

Wagnener, J.S., Sobonya, R., Minnich, L. and Taussig, L.M. (1984) Role of canine parainfluenza virus and *Bordetella bronchiseptica* in kennel cough. *American Journal of Veterinary Research*, **45**, 1862–1869.

Zimmer, J.F. (1986) Intestinal parasites of dogs and cats. *Kal Kan Forum*, **5**, 12–18.

3

Anaesthesia and pain management

Puppies and kittens may require surgery for correction of life-threatening congenital anomalies and for institution of an early spay and castration programme. In addition to the obvious challenge of performing surgery on an often very small animal, most body systems in puppies and kittens are not fully developed compared with adult dogs and cats, especially during the first few weeks of life. Although there are no specific contraindications for anaesthesia in puppies and kittens, it is important to dose anaesthetic agents carefully, based on consideration of age-related physiological differences. The development of an anaesthetic plan is also influenced by the procedure, patient status and drugs and equipment available.

Table 3.1 Normal parameters in puppies and kittens

Parameter	Normal value
Heart rate (beats/minute)	200 + beats/minute
Respiratory rate (breaths/minute)	15–35 breaths/minute (2–3 times adult rate)
Blood pressure (mmHg)	70/45 (60) mmHg systolic/ diastolic (mean)
Body temperature < 2 weeks of age > 4 weeks of age	35.5–36° C (96–97° F) 37.7° C (100° F)
Haemoglobin concentration; packed cell volume At birth 3–4 weeks of age	11–12 g/dl; 35–45% 8.4 g/dl; 25–30% (increase to near adult values by 20 weeks)

Preoperative considerations

Physical examination

All animals should have a thorough physical examination prior to anaesthesia, paying particular attention to the cardiovascular and respiratory systems. It should be noted that the range of normal values for vital parameters in young animals differs from adult values (Table 3.1).

Hydration status may influence fluid therapy during the perioperative period. Because skin turgor is not a useful assessment of hydration in puppies and kittens less than 6 weeks of age, hydration status is estimated by evaluation of moistness of mucous membranes, position of eyes in their orbits, heart rate, character of peripheral pulses and capillary refill time. Urine output is an excellent indicator of hydration status in animals less than 12 weeks of age and should be at least 0.5 ml/h.

Activated clotting time and buccal mucosal bleeding time are useful clinical tests for preoperative coagulation screening. Any coagulation disorder should be pretreated prior to surgery. The necessity of elective procedures should be evaluated in light of the risks associated with a clotting disorder.

Physiological differences relevant to anaesthesia and surgery

During the first 6–12 weeks after birth, many organ systems are functionally immature. Age-related physiological differences in the autonomic, cardiovascular, respiratory, hepatorenal and thermoregulatory systems are important considerations in anaesthetic and surgical planning. These differences have a profound effect on the ability of a young animal to maintain homeostasis during surgery and recovery (Table 3.2).

Cardiovascular system

Compared with adult animals, puppies and kittens have higher heart rates, cardiac outputs, plasma volumes and central venous pressures, but lower blood pressures, stroke volumes and peripheral vascular resistance. The paediatric heart has less contractile myocardial mass and low ventricular compliance, resulting in a fixed stroke volume and low cardiac reserve. Consequently, cardiac output is primarily dependent on heart rate and there is poor tolerance to volume loading and increased afterload. Blood pressure increases after 6 weeks of age and approaches adult values within several months (Arango and Rowe, 1971).

The paediatric heart has mature parasympathetic innervation, but immature sympathetic innervation (Friedman, 1972). Many anaesthetic agents enhance parasympathetic effects and can lead to the development of serious bradycardia (< 150 beats/minute). Since cardiac output is dependent on heart rate, hypotension can occur fairly readily. In addition, young animals have immature baroreceptor reflexes which, when further depressed by anaesthetic agents, are unable to respond effectively to hypotension with an increase in heart rate. Therefore, puppies and kittens are also less

Table 3.2 Physiological differences in puppies and kittens

Organ system	Physiological characteristics of puppies and kittens
Cardiovascular system	Cardiac output is heart-rate-dependent Poor tolerance to volume loading Low myocardial contractile mass Low ventricular compliance Low cardiac reserve
Respiratory system	Oxygen demand 2–3 times adult demand High respiratory rate Small airways = increased resistance and work of breathing Small alveoli = minimal respiratory reserve High closing volume Increased susceptibility to hypoxia
Hepatorenal system	Immature hepatic microsomal enzyme systems Lower albumin levels = low protein binding of drugs Limited glycogen stores = tendency to hypoglycaemia Immature renal function Decreased glomerular filtration rate
Thermoregulatory system	Immature thermoregulatory system Large surface area to body weight ratio = increased heat loss Reduced subcutaneous fat and insulation Inability to shiver
Nervous systems	Dominant parasympathetic nervous system = predisposition to bradycardia Immature sympathetic nervous system Permeable blood–brain barrier Poor vasomotor control

able to compensate for even small amounts (5–10 ml/kg) of blood loss. Every effort should be made to prevent the development of bradycardia during anaesthesia and to be prepared to treat it if it occurs.

Respiratory system

The oxygen demand of puppies and kittens is two to three times that of adult animals. In order to meet this demand, the respiratory rate is also greater (Table 3.1). Due to a number of anatomical differences, the respiratory system of young animals is less efficient than that of adults. Small-diameter, less rigid airways increase both resistance to air flow and the work of breathing, and there is a greater risk of airway obstruction. Smaller alveoli, with less functional residual capacity (FRC), together with a highly compliant, poorly supported chest wall, result in poor maintenance of negative intrathoracic pressure and functional airway closure. The respiratory-depressant effects of anaesthetic agents may make it difficult to overcome the critical opening pressure necessary to expand collapsed alveoli and lead to hypoventilation and atelectasis. Animals less than 8 weeks of age are especially susceptible to hypoxia during apnoea or airway obstruction because of their high oxygen consumption, high closing volume and low FRC (Thurmon *et al.*, 1969). Providing respiratory support with intermittent positive-pressure ventilation (IPPV) will help prevent hypoventilation and hypoxaemia and maintain respiratory rate. Increased alveolar ventilation will enhance gas exchange in the lungs and result in faster induction and recovery from inhalation anaesthesia. When using IPPV in young animals, it is vital to avoid excessive airway pressures (not to exceed 20 cm H_2O) which may cause barotrauma and possible pneumothorax.

Hepatorenal system

Hepatic enzyme systems are functionally immature at birth. As puppies grow and hepatic blood flow increases, enzymatic systems mature and reach mature activity by 5–8 weeks of age, around the time of weaning (Kawalek and El Said, 1990). The clinical effects of anaesthetic agents that require hepatic degradation for termination of action may last longer and be more intense in animals less than 8 weeks of age, and reduced dosages should be used.

Serum concentrations of albumin and other proteins necessary for drug binding are lower in puppies younger than 4 weeks of age than in adult dogs; mature concentrations are reached by 8 weeks of age (Center *et al.*, 1995). An increased sensitivity to highly protein-bound anaesthetic agents may be seen in animals less than 8 weeks of age due to a greater fraction of unbound active drug.

Hepatic glycogen stores are minimal in puppies and kittens and decline rapidly during fasting. When hepatic glycogen stores are depleted, hepatic gluconeogenesis maintains normoglycaemia. However, the ability to regulate blood glucose levels in puppies and kittens is difficult because of a lack of adequate feedback mechanisms between blood glucose levels and the liver. In order to ensure normoglycaemia in puppies and kittens, fasting should be minimal, if at all, and perioperative fluids should contain glucose (see Chapter 4).

Renal function is diminished in animals less than 8 weeks of age due to low perfusion pressure and immature glomerular and tubular function. Therefore, neonatal animals do not tolerate fluid loading and are more susceptible to fluid and electrolyte derangements. Glomerular filtration does not reach adult levels until 2–3 weeks of age, and tubular secretion matures between 4–8 weeks of age (Horster *et al.*, 1971; Kleinman and Lubbe, 1972; Aschinberg *et al.*, 1975). Renal clearance of drugs and their metabolites is limited in animals less than 8 weeks of age, and may lead to increased duration of action.

Thermoregulatory system

Paediatric animals are predisposed to hypothermia due to an immature thermoregulatory system, less ability to shiver and minimal subcutaneous fat. Heat loss can occur by several mechanisms (Table 3.3). Small size relative to a large body surface area further predisposes young animals to hypothermia. Low body temperature may cause a decrease in heart rate, cardiac output and blood pressure. Anaesthetic agents depress metabolic rate and decrease muscle activity, further exacerbating hypothermia. These effects, in turn, may prolong

Table 3.3 Four mechanisms of heat loss

Category	Effects
Conduction	Heat lost due to contact with cold surfaces – cold table or cold blankets
Convection	Cooling due to air flowing over body – increases with increased air flow
Radiation	Greatest cause of heat loss (60%) – loss from hairless areas, incision and open body cavity
Evaporation	Accounts for 25% total heat loss from airways and open body cavity

drug elimination and recovery from anaesthesia. It is critical to take precautions in order to minimize heat loss and prevent hypothermia during anaesthesia and surgery (Table 3.4).

Drug distribution

The intensity and duration of drug effects are altered by volume of distribution, protein binding, functional maturity of the liver and kidneys, amount of fat and muscle, distribution of cardiac output and permeability of the blood–brain barrier. In puppies and kittens, variation in these factors results in an increased sensitivity to many drugs (Table 3.5). Total body water of

newborns comprises 75–80% of body weight, compared to 50–60% in the adult. A greater percentage of the total body water is extracellular, leading to a larger volume of distribution and a smaller intracellular water reserve. Young animals have less muscle mass and decreased fat deposits, resulting in a higher distribution of cardiac output to the vessel-rich organs, most importantly the brain and heart.

Anaesthetic selection and management

Preanaesthetic fasting

It is usually unnecessary to withhold food from suckling puppies and kittens before anaesthesia. Animals between 6 weeks and 6 months of age should not be fasted for prolonged periods, but rather 2–3 hours, and access to water should not be restricted. An exception to this would be animals that have delayed gastric emptying or a similar ailment. These animals may require preoperative fluid support.

Preanaesthetic agents

In many instances, the administration of premedications to animals less than 12 weeks of

Table 3.4 Factors contributing to hypothermia in paediatric animals during anaesthesia and surgery, and precautions to minimize hypothermia

Factor	Precautions
Predisposing Large surface area to body mass ratio Immature thermoregulatory system Reduced subcutaneous fat Reduced ability to shiver	Maintain a warm ambient temperature in the surgical suite Use infrared heat lamps to increase ambient temperature; do not shine directly on animal
Perioperative Conduction heat loss to cold table Evaporative heat loss due to cold prep solutions and excessive wetness Evaporative heat loss due to open body cavity Radiation heat loss into a cool environment	Insulate the animal from cold surfaces Use circulating warm-water heating blankets Keep the animal covered whenever possible Warm the intravenous fluids Minimize the amount of hair clipped Avoid using alcohol or alcohol-containing skin-disinfectants
Effects of anaesthesia Depressed thermoregulatory system Reduced metabolic activity Reduced muscular activity Inhalation of cold dry gases	Warm the prep solutions Keep the animal as dry as possible Minimize the surgery time Use warm lavage fluids Heat-humidify inhaled gases Use clear plastic drapes

Table 3.5 Factors affecting drug distribution in puppies and kittens

Factor	Effect
Larger percentage of total body water	Larger volume of distribution so that water-soluble drugs may require larger initial dose to achieve desired effect
Low total protein (albumin) concentration	Highly protein-bound drugs have greater unbound (active) fraction
Immature hepatic enzyme systems	Increased intensity and duration of effects due to decreased metabolism in animals < 8 weeks of age
Reduced glomerular filtration rate and renal excretion	Prolonged drug effects due to reduced clearance
High distribution of cardiac output to vessel-rich organs	Increased drug sensitivity
Low body fat	Drugs that redistribute to fat will have longer duration of effect
Reduced muscle mass	Drugs that redistribute to muscle will have longer duration of effect; muscle-relaxant dose requirement is reduced
Increased blood–brain barrier permeability	Increased drug sensitivity, especially lipid-soluble drugs

age may not be necessary or desirable. Administration of a tranquilizer or analgesic preoperatively can reduce stress and smooth induction, maintenance and recovery, as well as reduce the dose of the more haemodynamically depressing induction and maintenance agents. The decision to use preanaesthetic medication is based on the agents available, and the experience and preference of the veterinarian. Consideration should be given to the animal's age, breed, temperament and underlying medical condition, as well as the length and type of surgery. Preanaesthetics available for use include anticholinergics, tranquilizers/sedatives, analgesics and dissociatives.

Anticholinergics

The potentially high vagal tone, due to a dominant parasympathetic nervous system, predisposes puppies and kittens to bradycardia. Because cardiac output is dependent on heart rate, the administration of an anticholinergic (atropine or glycopyrrolate) is recommended whenever anaesthetic agents are used. Anticholinergics may not be effective in animals younger than 14 days of age due to their immature autonomic nervous system (Robinson, 1983). Both atropine and glycopyrrolate have the additional benefit of decreasing respiratory tract secretions, which reduces the potential for airway obstruction. Compared with atropine, glycopyrrolate takes longer to exert its effects, yet lasts longer (2–3 vs 1–1.5 hours), is less likely to produce sinus tachycardia, and does not cross the

blood–brain barrier. Either agent can be given, intravenously to effect, during anaesthesia to treat sinus bradycardia.

Tranquilizers/sedatives

Benzodiazepines (diazepam and midazolam) are the sedatives of choice in puppies and kittens. These agents are mild, non-analgesic, short-acting sedatives; however, duration may be prolonged in those animals less than 8 weeks of age due to immature hepatic mechanisms. Benzodiazepines produce good muscle relaxation with minimal central nervous system and cardiovascular depression. Midazolam is more potent yet shorter-acting than diazepam. Both diazepam and midazolam are dose-dependent respiratory depressants and may cause hypoventilation or apnoea.

Careful monitoring of the respiratory system is recommended when using benzodiazepines, especially if they are administered with other potentially depressing agents. Due to its propylene glycol carrier, diazepam cannot be mixed in the same syringe with any other agents except ketamine and has unpredictable absorption from intramuscular sites. In contrast, the water-soluble midazolam readily combines with other agents and is absorbed from subcutaneous or intramuscular sites. Both agents are commonly used in combination with narcotics or dissociative agents for premedication, induction of anaesthesia or alone for short non-painful procedures (Table 3.6). Zolazapam is a benzodiazepine combined with the dissociative

Table 3.6 Anaesthetic and analgesic agents and suggested doses for use in puppies and kittens*

Agent	Dosage	Comments
Anticholinergics		
Atropine	0.02–0.04 mg/kg IV, IM, SC	Recommended to offset dominant parasympathetic effects and maintain heart rate, cardiac output and blood pressure. Also decrease airway secretions
Glycopyrrolate	0.01 mg/kg IV, IM	Glycopyrrolate does not cross the blood–brain barrier, takes longer to onset of action and has increased duration compared with atropine
Tranquillizers/sedatives		
Diazepam	0.2–0.4 mg/kg IV, IM	Propylene glycol carrier makes uptake unpredictable from IM site. Will not mix in same syringe with any drug, except ketamine
Midazolam	0.1–0.2 mg/kg IV, IM, SC	Water-soluble. More potent and shorter-acting than diazepam. Mixes with other agents. May cause excitement on recovery in some cats
Acepromazine	0.025–0.05 mg/kg IM, SC 2 mg maximum	Avoid in animals less than 8 weeks of age. Requires hepatic degradation. Potentiates hypotension and hypothermia. Does not provide analgesia and is not reversible. Best to dilute to 1 mg/ml solution for accurate dosing
α_2 *-Agonists*		
Xylazine	1–2 mg/kg IM	Avoid in animals less than 12 weeks of age. Requires hepatic degradation and causes marked bradycardia and decreased cardiac output. May cause vomiting. Always use with an anticholinergic.
Medetomidine	20–30 μg/kg IM	Medetomidine is more potent and longer-acting than xylazine. Both agents are reversible (see Table 3.7)
Opioids		
Meperidine	1–2 mg/kg IM Epidural: 0.5–1.5 mg/kg	Mild analgesia. May cause histamine release if injected IV. Reversible
Morphine	0.2–1.0 mg/kg IM, SC Epidural: 0.1 mg/kg in 0.5 ml/kg volume of NaCl	Analgesia with sedation and cardiopulmonary depression. Administer with an anticholinergic. Potentiates hypothermia. Most common agent used for epidural analgesia. Reversible
Oxymorphone	0.05–0.2 mg/kg IV, IM, SC Epidural: 0.1 mg/kg in 0.5 ml/kg volume of NaCl 4 mg maximum Reversible	Analgesia with sedation. Causes panting. Administer with an anticholinergic. Commonly combined with acepromazine in animals > 12 weeks of age for neuroleptanalgesia. Can be used for epidural analgesia.
Fentanyl	2–4 μg/kg IV CRI: 2–4 g/kg per hour IV Transdermal patch: 2.5–10 kg: 25-μg patch (all or part) 10–20 kg: 50-μg patch 20–30 kg: 75-μg patch Epidural: 1–10 μg/kg in 0.5 ml/kg volume of NaCl	Very potent analgesic. Rapid onset and short duration of action. Minimal cardiopulmonary effects. Can be delivered by a variety of routes, including epidural. Reversible (see Table 3.7)
Buprenorphine	0.01–0.02 mg/kg IV, IM, SC	30–45 minutes to onset. Long duration due to slow rate of dissociation from receptor. Unpredictible reversal with opioid antagonists
Butorphanol	0.2–0.4 mg/kg IV, IM, SC CRI: 0.2–0.4 mg/kg/hour IV	Agonist–antagonist. Minimal cardiopulmonary depression. Good visceral analgesia. Used to reverse agonist adverse effects and preserve analgesia

Table 3.6 (continued)

Agent	Dosage	Comments
Intravenous anaesthetics		
Thiopentone	4–6 mg/kg IV, to effect	Ultrashort-acting thiobarbiturate. Termination of action depends on redistribution and hepatic degradation. May be dysrhythmic. Respiratory depression common; be prepared to intubate and ventilate
Methohexitone	4–6 mg/kg IV, to effect	Ultrashort-acting oxybarbiturate. Terminated by redistribution with minimal hepatic metabolism. May cause excitement on induction and recovery. Be prepared to intubate and ventilate
Propofol	2–6 mg/kg IV, to effect CRI: 10–12 mg/kg per hour IV	Alkyl phenol. Do not bolus – give slowly, over several minutes. Ultrashort-acting – rapid onset, rapid recovery. Non-cumulative, can be used as CRI without prolonged recovery. Be prepared to intubate and ventilate
Etomidate	1–2 mg/kg IV CRI: 2–4 mg/kg per hour IV	Non-barbiturate. No cardiopulmonary effects. May cause nausea, vomiting, myoclonus, excitement on induction and recovery. Non-cumulative, can be used as CRI
Ketamine	1–2 mg/kg IV 11–22 mg/kg IM	Dissociative anaesthetic. Excessive salivation controlled with anticholinergics. Increases intracranial and intraocular pressures. May cause seizures. Elimination depends on renal and hepatic function
Telazol	1–2 mg/kg IV 5–13 mg/kg IM	Contains 50 : 50 tiletamine, a dissociative anaesthetic, and zolazepam, a benzodiazepine. Tiletamine is more potent and longer-lasting than ketamine. Zolazepam effects may be prolonged in some cats and cause rough recovery

* Use low end of opioid dose for kittens. Opioids are best used in combination protocols for kittens.
IV = Intravenous; IM = intramuscular; SC = subcutaneous; CRI = continuous-rate infusion.

anaesthetic tiletamine in Telazol. Both midazolam and zolazapam have been reported to cause prolonged excitement in adult cats. This excitement can be alleviated by administration of the specific benzodiazapine antagonist flumazenil (Table 3.7) or the administration of another tranquillizer.

Acepromazine, a commonly used tranquilizer in adult animals, can be used safely in young animals if reduced doses are used (Table 3.6). However, it is not recommended for use in animals that are compromised or less than 8 weeks of age. The current availability of less depressing, reversible tranquillizers/sedatives makes acepromazine a less desirable choice for animals less than 6 months of age. Acepromazine does not provide analgesia and can cause pronounced and prolonged central nervous system depression in young animals with immature hepatic function. A peripheral vasodilator, acepromazine causes hypotension and potentiates hypothermia. The commercially prepared concentration (10 mg/ml) makes it difficult to measure small doses accurately, therefore a dilute solution (1 mg/ml) can be made by combining nine parts of sterile water with one part of acepromazine.

α_2-Agonists (xylazine and medetomidine) provide sedation, analgesia and muscle relaxation, while profoundly depressing both heart rate and decreasing minute ventilation, even at low doses. These agents undergo extensive hepatic degradation and are not recommended in animals that are compromised or less than 8 weeks of age. Concurrent use of an anticholinergic is imperative. Specific antagonists are available (Table 3.7).

Opioids

Opioids provide analgesia and sedation and are well-tolerated even by critically ill paediatric animals. Their effects are due to activation of one or more endogenous opioid receptors. The degree of analgesia and potential for side-effects are related to their individual receptor affinity (Table 3.8).

Table 3.7 Specific antagonists and suggested dosages

Agent	Antagonistic effects	Dose	Comments
Flumazenil	Benzodiazepines	0.1 mg/kg IV to effect	Duration short – 1 hour in adults. May have agonist effects at high dose
Yohimbine	α_2-receptors	0.25–0.5 mg/kg IM 0.15 mg/kg IV to effect	May cause excitement when given IV
Atipamazole	α_2-receptors	0.2–0.4 mg/kg IM	Most effective reversal agent
Tolazoline	α_1- and α_2-receptors	0.3 mg/kg IV to effect	
Naloxone	Pure narcotic antagonist	0.04–0.4 mg IV to effect	Short duration – 0.5–1.5 hours. Animals may renarcotize
Naltrexone	Pure narcotic antagonist	0.04 mg/kg IV	8–12 hour duration. Most effective for reversal of central effects relative to epidural opioid administration
Nalmefene	Pure narcotic antagonist	0.1–0.2 mg/kg IV or IM	8–10 hour duration. New agent
Butorphanol	Narcotic agonist–antagonist	0.2 mg/kg IV, IM, SC	Used to reverse bradycardia and respiratory depression of agonists, while maintaining analgesia
Nalbuphine	Narcotic agonist–antagonist	0.5–2.0 mg/kg IV, IM, SC	Lasts 2–4 hours Less potent analgesic than butorphanol

IV = Intravenous; IM = intramuscular; SC = subcutaneous.

Bradycardia, a potentially serious, dose-related side-effect of opioids, can be avoided by co-administration of an anticholinergic. Any reduction in heart rate, and resultant drop in cardiac output, is poorly tolerated in neonatal and paediatric animals. Respiratory depression is another potentially serious dose-related effect, due to the limited respiratory reserve of paediatric animals. Concurrent administration of other anaesthetic agents may potentiate the cardiopulmonary depressant effects. Agents classified as partial agonists or agonist–antagonists provide moderate analgesia with the least cardiopulmonary depression (Table 3.6). Premedication with an opioid can decrease the amount of inhalation agent necessary. Thus, the use of a well-balanced anaesthetic regimen can provide the desired level of anaesthesia and analgesia without significantly depressing the myocardium and maintain haemodynamics. Whenever opioids are used, careful cardiopulmonary monitoring is prudent. Antagonists are available if reversal is desired (Table 3.7). Reversal with a pure antagonist (naloxone, naltrexone) will reverse analgesia along with any adverse effects. In order to preserve analgesia,

Table 3.8 Comparative activity and potency of opioids

Agent	Schedule	Receptor activity Mu	Kappa	Potency	Duration of action
Morphine	II	+ +	+	1	4 hours
Meperidine	II	+	+	0.5	1–2 hours
Oxymorphone	II	+ +	+	5–10	4–6 hours
Fentanyl	II	+ + +	+	100	15–30 minutes
Buprenorphine	V	P	?	5	8–12 hours
Butorphanol	not controlled*	—	+ +	3–5	4–6 hours

+ = Agonist; — = antagonist; P = partial agonist.
Mu = Supraspinal analgesia, respiratory depression, bradycardia, sedation, miosis, hypothermia, euphoria, physical dependence.
Kappa = Spinal analgesia, mild respiratory depression, sedation.
* Some states in America have begun to Schedule butorphanol as a Class IV agent.

reversal of agonists with partial antagonists, like butorphanol, is recommended. Opioids can be effectively administered by a variety of routes: parenteral, oral, nasal, rectal, transdermal, epidural, spinal and intra-articular. Short-acting, highly potent opioid agonists, like fentanyl, can be delivered through a transdermal patch or as a continuous rate infusion intravenously or epidurally. Local application of these agents (epidurally or intra-articularly) provides prolonged analgesia without systemic side-effects.

Induction to general anaesthesia

Mask induction with isoflurane or halothane in oxygen is often the method of choice in animals that are less than 8 weeks of age or weigh less than 2.5 kg. Since catheter placement can be difficult in small, uncooperative animals, it is often less stressful and more expedient to induce by mask, or in a chamber, and intubate before an intravenous catheter is placed. Mask and chamber inductions greatly increase the risk of exposure of personnel to elevated concentrations of waste anaesthetic gases, and should be done in a well-ventilated area. Rapid induction with an intravenous anaesthetic is preferred for animals in respiratory distress (respiratory disease, diaphragmatic hernia, etc.) or when there is risk of aspiration, in order to gain rapid control of the airway and provide ventilatory support.

Injectable anaesthetics

A rapid and reliable induction to general anaesthesia can be accomplished with several injectable anaesthetic drugs. Young animals have a higher percentage of total body water than adults and a larger volume of distribution, which may necessitate higher doses of water-soluble agents to achieve desired effects. However, duration of action and side-effects may then be prolonged due to decreased muscle and fat for redistribution, immature hepatic enzyme systems and delayed excretion. Several of the intravenous induction agents cause respiratory depression and apnoea after injection. This is of particular importance in young animals with little or no respiratory reserve. Always be prepared to intubate and provide oxygen after the administration of these agents.

Thiopentone

Thiopentone is an ultrashort-acting barbiturate that can be used for intravenous induction to general anaesthesia in healthy puppies and kittens greater than 8 weeks of age. Thiopentone is highly protein-bound in plasma, therefore in puppies and kittens that have lower albumin concentrations than adults, there is a greater percentage of active circulating drug available to cross the blood–brain barrier. This results in a lower dose requirement for induction. Dose-dependent respiratory depression makes it important to obtain an accurate weight in order to ensure proper dosing. The use of a dilute 1–2% solution will increase the total volume injected and facilitate titration of small doses. Termination of anaesthetic effect is due to redistribution to fat and muscle as well as hepatic degradation. In puppies and kittens, after induction additional doses of thiopentone should be avoided. As limited fat and muscle deposits become saturated, immature hepatic enzyme systems become overwhelmed and recovery will be prolonged. Thiopentone may precipitate cardiac arrhythmias, does not provide analgesia and is irritating to tissues if injected perivascularly.

Methohexitone

Methohexitone is another ultrashort-acting barbiturate with similar effects to thiopentone, but a shorter elimination half-life, resulting in a faster recovery. In human infants weighing less than 20 kg, methohexitone provides a safe and reliable induction to general anaesthesia when administered rectally (Cote, 1990). However, methohexitone may cause seizures, and dysphoria is often seen on induction and recovery in unpremedicated animals.

Propofol

Propofol is an ultrashort-acting intravenous anaesthetic agent that can be used for induction or maintenance of general anaesthesia in puppies and kittens. Two major dose-related side-effects of propofol administration are respiratory depression and hypotension. Propofol should be used with care in animals less than 8 weeks of age due to their lack of respiratory reserve and unreliable baroreceptor reflexes. Occurrence and severity of depressant effects are also influenced by the rate of injection. Propofol should be administered slowly, over 1–2 minutes until the desired effect is achieved. A slow injection rate allows the use of a lower total induction dose and avoids cardiopulmonary depression. Termination of effects is due to redistribution and hepatic metabolism. Extrahepatic mechanisms, that are not fully understood, contribute to metabolism. Therefore, repeat doses or a continuous-rate infusion of propofol can be administered without accumulation and a prolonged recovery. Propofol does not provide analgesia and should not be used as the sole anaesthetic for painful procedures. It is formulated in a 1% emulsion similar to parenteral lipid formulations and packaged in vials designed for single use that contain no preservatives or bacteriostatic agents. Since each vial contains much more than a single dose, to prevent waste, the remainder can be carefully transferred into empty 10 ml sterile, multiuse vials. This emulsion is a perfect culture medium, so great care must be taken to avoid contamination during transfer to and withdrawal from the multiuse vial. Use each vial as quickly as possible.

Etomidate

Although proven safe in adult animals, the suitability of Etomidate in puppies and kittens has not been documented. It is an ultrashort-acting non-barbiturate intravenous anaesthetic agent that can be used for induction or maintenance of general anaesthesia. Etomidate does not depress respiratory or cardiac function. Duration is determined by rate of redistribution to well perfused tissues and hepatic metabolism. Etomidate's anaesthetic effects are non-cumulative, and anaesthesia can be maintained by continuous rate infusion. Etomidate does not provide analgesia and administration is associated with several adverse effects, including pain on injection, vomiting and dysphoria during induction and recovery. These effects can be prevented by premedication.

Ketamine

Ketamine is a dissociative anaesthetic that can be safely used alone, or in combination with a tranquilizer/sedative, for induction or maintenance of general anaesthesia in puppies and kittens (Tables 3.6 and 3.9). At recommended dosages, ketamine does not compromise cardiopulmonary function. Because termination of effects depends on renal elimination in cats and hepatic degradation in dogs, dissociative agents must be used with caution in animals less than 8 weeks old due to their reduced hepatic metabolism and renal clearance abilities. Additional doses should be avoided due to accumulation and prolonged recovery. The level of analgesia provided by ketamine is a matter of controversy. Ketamine interferes with the perception of pain by depressing spinal cord transmission of pain impulses and functionally disorganizing specific midbrain and thalamic pathways. There may also be some activity at opioid receptors. The degree of analgesia provided by ketamine alone is sufficient for some minor procedures, but supplementation with opioids and/or inhalation agents is necessary for invasive surgical procedures. Copious salivation is a common side-effect that can be controlled by the co-administration of atropine or glycopyrrolate. Pharyngeal reflexes remain intact during dissociative anaesthesia, but aspiration can still occur.

Endotracheal intubation is highly recommended after the administration of ketamine. Both intraocular and intracranial pressures are increased by ketamine, therefore it is contraindicated in animals with head trauma or injury to the globe. Seizures have also been reported after its administration. There is not an antagonist available for ketamine. Ketamine is the principal agent in many popular drug combinations used for anaesthetic induction and general anaesthesia in puppies and kittens (Table 3.9).

Telazol

Telazol is a commercial preparation composed of a dissociative anaesthetic, tiletamine, and a benzodiazepine, zolazepam. Tiletamine is similar in activity to ketamine except that it is more potent and has a longer duration. This combination provides smooth anaesthetic induction and recovery. The same precautions should be taken as with ketamine. Recovery may be prolonged in cats due to the effects of zolazepam, which outlast the effects of tiletamine. In contrast, dogs may have rough recoveries due to the effects of tiletamine, which outlasts the zolazepam in this species.

Table 3.9 Anaesthetic combinations for use in puppies and kittens 6–14 weeks of age (Fagella and Arohnson, 1993; and 1994)

Agents	Dose	Comments
Kittens		
{ Midazolam	0.22 mg/kg IM	Most effective combination for
{ Ketamine	11–22 mg/kg IM	ovariohysterectomy in kittens when
		followed by inhalation anaesthesia
		Provides insufficient analgesia as a sole
		protocol for castration of kittens
{ Atropine	0.04 mg/kg IM	Not recommended as sole protocol
{ Midazolam	0.22 mg/kg IM	Supplement with inhalation anaesthesia
{ Ketamine	11 mg/kg IM	
{ Butorphanol	0.44 mg/kg IM	
{ Atropine	0.04 mg/kg IM	Not recommended as sole protocol
{ Midazolam	0.11 mg/kg IM	Supplement with inhalation anaesthesia
{ Ketamine	11 mg/kg IM	May cause hyperexcitement during recovery
{ Oxymorphone	0.07 mg/kg IM	
Telazol	11 mg/kg IM	Most effective protocol for castration of
		kittens
		Provides good analgesia
		May be necessary to supplement with
		inhalation anaesthesia
Puppies		
{ Atropine	0.04 mg/kg IM	Not recommended
{ Midazolam	0.22 mg/kg IM	Unsatisfactory protocol for castration of
{ Butorphanol	0.44 mg/kg IM	puppies
{ Xylazine	1.1 mg/kg IM	Significant respiratory depression
{ Atropine	0.04 mg/kg IM	Not recommended
{ Midazolam	0.22 mg/kg IM	Unsatisfactory protocol for castration of
{ Oxymorphone	0.22 mg/kg IM	puppies
{ Xylazine	1.1 mg/kg IM	Significant respiratory depression
{ Atropine	0.04 mg/kg IM	Provides best quality anaesthesia for
{ Oxymorphone	0.22 mg/kg IM	castration of puppies
{ followed by	followed by	Provides best-quality anaesthesia for
{ Propofol	3.5 mg/kg IV	ovariohysterectomy of puppies when
		followed by inhalation anaesthesia
		Transient apnoea following Propofol
		administration
{ Midazolam	0.22 mg/kg IM	Provides little sedation prior to Propofol
{ Butorphanol	0.44 mg/kg IM	injection but provides good operative
{ followed by	followed by	analgesia
{ Propofol	3.5 mg/kg IV	Transient apnoea following Propofol
		administration
		Administer Propofol to effect over
		1–2 minutes to avoid apnoea
{ Atropine	0.04 mg/kg IM	
{ Midazolam	0.22 mg/kg IM	
{ Oxymorphone	0.22 mg/kg IM	
{ Midazolam	0.22 mg/kg IM	Suitable premedication prior to inhalation
{ Butorphanol	0.44 mg/kg IM	induction of anaesthesia
Telazol	13.2 mg/kg IM	Unsatisfactory protocol for castration of
		puppies
		Causes hypersalivation

IV = Intravenous; IM = intramuscular; SC = subcutaneous.

Inhalation anaesthetics

Anaesthetic induction with inhalation agents occurs quickly in paediatric animals because of decreased Functional Residual Capacity (FRC), increased alveolar ventilation and centralized circulation. The speed of induction is also affected by hydration status, type of breathing circuit used and oxygen flow rate. These factors make it easier to rapidly reach excessive depths in a paediatric animal, but they also make an overdose easier to reverse.

All inhalation agents depress cardiopulmonary function in a dose-dependent manner. Premedication will decrease the amount of inhalation agent required and reduce depressant effects. Isoflurane and halothane are the agents of choice. Isoflurane is potentially more hypotensive than halothane, but maintains heart rate better, undergoes minimal hepatic metabolism and lowers cerebral oxygen needs. Halothane is less irritating to airways, but is dysrhythmogenic and undergoes greater hepatic metabolism. Sevoflurane, a new inhalation agent similar to isoflurane, is gaining popularity for use in human infants because it provides an even faster induction and recovery without airway irritation. Nitrous oxide can be used at a 50:50 ratio with oxygen to invoke the second-gas effect and accelerate induction. Animals less than 12 weeks of age are particularly sensitive to apnoea and hypoxia and nitrous oxide should not be used during maintenance without the support of an oxygen analyser to ensure adequate oxygen delivery. Waste anaesthetic gases from anaesthetic machines must be scavenged and removed from the workplace to eliminate danger to personnel.

Intubation and ventilation

Intubation

Whenever possible, puppies and kittens should be intubated during general anaesthesia. Endotracheal tubes should be of clear plastic with a low-pressure cuff. Intubation with the largest-diameter tube possible will reduce resistance to breathing and decrease the possibility of obstruction from airway secretions. The pharyngeal and laryngeal tissues of puppies and kittens are delicate and great care must be taken during insertion of the endotracheal tube. A difficult or traumatic intubation may result in laryngeal oedema and postoperative airway obstruction. An anti-inflammatory dose of dexamethasone or prednisolone should be administered prior to extubation if there is concern about laryngeal swelling. The smallest endotracheal tube commercially available is 2.0 mm internal diameter. If a smaller tube is required, an adaptor can be attached to a piece of silicone tubing or an intravenous, over-the-needle catheter with the stylet removed (Fig. 3.1).

Small-diameter endotracheal tubes are easily dislodged, kinked or obstructed by secretions and should be closely monitored. Obstructed tubes should be suctioned or replaced. An endotracheal tube that is too long will increase resistance to and work of breathing, and may cause significant rebreathing of exhaled gases. Tubes should be measured along the outside of the neck and cut to appropriate size. They should reach from the nose to the thoracic inlet. If intubation is not possible, inhalation anaesthesia can be delivered by mask. A small, clear, tight-fitting mask will minimize dead space, prevent gas leakage into the immediate environment and allow visualization of mucous membrane colour.

Ventilation

Neonatal and paediatric animals have a high metabolic need and oxygen consumption. Their respiratory rate is two to three times that of adults in order to meet this need (Table 3.1). The administration of anaesthetic agents depresses respiratory function. This is particularly critical in young animals with little or no respiratory reserve who are prone to hypoventilation and hypoxaemia. In order to guarantee

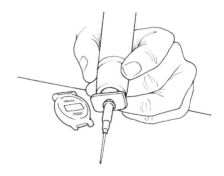

Figure 3.1 Endotracheal tube constructed from a 20-gauge over-the-needle intravenous Teflon catheter with a special adaptor to connect it to the anaesthetic delivery system.

adequate ventilation and oxygenation during anaesthesia, ventilation should be assisted or controlled. Ventilation can be assisted manually or with a mechanical ventilator. The tidal volume for animals less than 12 weeks of age is 2.5–3 ml/kg; older animals have a tidal volume of 5 ml/kg. Airway pressures should not exceed 15–20 cmH$_2$O. Specific paediatric ventilators are available or adult ventilators can be fitted with a paediatric bellows system.

Anaesthetic breathing circuit

The selection of an anaesthetic delivery circuit depends on body weight. Non-rebreathing systems (Ayre's T-piece, Norman elbow, Bain circuit) are used in animals weighing less than 4.5 kg to reduce resistance and work of breathing. The fresh gas flow should be 200 ml/kg per minute to prevent rebreathing of exhaled gases. The fresh gas enters directly at the airway in these systems and response to vaporizer adjustments is much faster. The high gas flows of non-rebreathing systems contribute to hypothermia and insensible fluid loss, and use more oxygen and inhalation agent. For animals weighing 4.5–10 kg, either a non-rebreathing or paediatric circle system can be used. A paediatric circle system is similar to the adult system, except that the delivery hoses are shorter and smaller in diameter (15 vs 22 mm). Some systems are equipped with smaller carbon dioxide absorber canisters. These systems should be used with oxygen flow rates of 30 ml/kg per min. An adult circle system can be used for animals weighing more than 10 kg.

Intraoperative support

Fluid support

During anaesthesia an intravenous fluid rate of 4–10 ml/kg per hour should be maintained to off-set the hypotension and replace limited blood loss and insensible water losses. Although puppies and kittens have high requirements for fluids, they cannot accommodate large volumes within a short period and fluid therapy should be administered carefully (Table 3.10).

An accurate body weight is important for calculation of rate, and administration should be precisely controlled by using a paediatric mini-drip fluid administration set (60 drops/ml), an inline fluid regulator (Fig. 3.2), an inline reservoir or a syringe infusion pump. If none of these control devices is available, the hourly requirement can be divided into microboluses that can be given every 5–10 minutes.

The maintenance fluid of choice in young animals is 2.5–5% dextrose in a balanced electrolyte solution. In the case of a septic or hypoglycaemic animal, 10% dextrose or higher may be indicated. During prolonged anaesthetic periods, glucose should be checked periodically and the dextrose concentration of the fluid adjusted as necessary. When there is measurable blood loss during surgery, replacement is 3 ml of the balanced electrolyte maintenance fluid being used for every 1 ml of blood. However, if blood loss exceeds 15–20% of blood volume, it should be replaced with an equal volume of a blood product.

Intravenous catheterization of the jugular or cephalic vein is best for administration of intra-

Table 3.10 Factors affecting fluid requirements of puppies and kittens

Factors	Effect
Higher metabolic rate and fluid requirements than adults	Increased risk of dehydration after water restriction
Larger ratio of body surface area to weight than adults	Greater insensible fluid loss
Decreased renal perfusion and glomerular filtration rate; less able to handle a solute load	Cannot accommodate rapid administration of large volumes of fluids Fluid therapy must be administered with care Unable to excrete large amounts of excess water or electrolytes

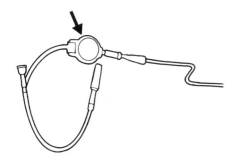

Figure 3.2 Inline fluid regulator used to prevent overhydration of small animals (arrow). The fluid regulator encircles the fluid line and the degree of fluid line compression can be adjusted. This device is inexpensive and reusable.

operative fluids, electrolytes, drugs or blood products. Carefully purge all air from the administration set before connection, as even a small amount may be significant in an animal weighing less than 5 kg. Drugs administered intravenously during fluid administration should be given as closely to the catheter as possible to avoid having to give a fluid bolus.

When intravenous catheterization cannot be performed, fluids can be administered by intraosseous or subcutaneous routes. Intraosseous cannulation of the humerus, femur or tibia can be performed readily without any special equipment or training. This route can be used for rapid administration of fluids, blood and many different drugs. Fluid flow rates of up to 11 ml/minute can be achieved with gravity.

Subcutaneous fluid administration is less reliable than intravenous or intraosseous fluid and the amount of fluid that can be administered is limited by the animal's size. Small volumes should be administered through multiple sites. Only isotonic fluids with less than 5% dextrose fluids should be used.

Intravenous catheter or intraosseous cannula placement can be facilitated by applying a local anaesthetic cream on the skin before puncture. EMLA cream (ASTRA Pharmaceutical Products, Inc., Westborough, MA, USA) is a eutectic mixture of local anaesthetics, lignocaine and prilocaine, specifically prepared for application to the skin. The area must be shaved and cleaned before application, and the cream must stay in contact with the skin, under a bandage, for at least 1 hour for best results. However, although it is certain that puppies and kittens do not like the pain associated with vene-

puncture, it is often the resistance to restraint that is more difficult to control.

Intraoperative monitoring

The level of monitoring for puppies and kittens should be consistent with the seriousness of the underlying disease and the surgical procedure. Puppies and kittens, especially those less than 12 weeks of age, decompensate rapidly due to minimal cardiopulmonary reserves. Therefore, diligent monitoring of all systems is critical to their well-being. Physiological monitoring can be accomplished by invasive or non-invasive methods, through simple observation or with the use of specialized equipment (Table 3.11).

Non-invasive methods are generally easy and inexpensive. Depending on the method used, the information may be accurate and reliable or only an indication of trends. Direct observation during surgery is facilitated by the use of a clear plastic drape. Invasive methods require the placement of instrumentation inside the body. These methods are more accurate, but often require more expensive equipment and special techniques and may pose a potential risk to the animal if there are complications.

Young animals weighing less than 2.5 kg present a unique monitoring challenge. It is imperative that instrumentation be done as rapidly as possible and not take longer than the planned procedure! This is a critical period during which hypothermia may become significant. Monitoring methods that provide the most information with the least fuss are preferred. Accurate interpretation and integration of information obtained by individual monitoring methods are imperative if it is to be of value. There is, however, no monitor yet available that is superior to the eyes, ears and touch of an observant anaesthetist.

Cardiovascular system

Basic cardiac monitoring includes the constant evaluation of heart rate and rhythm, pulse quality, capillary refill time and mucous membrane colour, all of which can be determined by simple auscultation and palpation. Direct contact with a small patient undergoing surgery, however, may be difficult.

The oesophageal stethoscope provides a remote, non-invasive and simple way to monitor

Table 3.11 Intraoperative monitors for use in puppies and kittens

Monitor	Parameter	Comments
Oesophageal stethoscope $US 17–300	Heart and respiratory rate and rhythm	Inexpensive, user-friendly, accurate. It can be used with earpieces or an amplifier
Respiratory monitor $US 115–300	Respiratory air movement and apnoea monitor	Inexpensive, sensitivity depends on monitor. It can be used with a mask. Pressure on thorax can produce false respiratory sounds. Use of adaptor adds dead space
Ultrasonic Doppler unit $US 500–700	Pulse rate, rhythm and quality; estimates systolic blood pressure	Relatively inexpensive, versatile and accurate. Small probes are available. Use with cuff and manometer to measure systolic blood pressures, inaccurate at low blood pressure
Oscillometric blood pressure $US 2500	Heart rate, systolic, diastolic and mean blood pressures	Easy to use. Accuracy depends on cuff size. Is inaccurate at low blood pressure and in small animals. Provides useful reflection of trends
Pulse oximeter $US 1200–2000	Pulse rate and functional oxygen saturation of haemoglobin	Non-invasive. Various style probes available. Valuable in animals less than 8 weeks of age which have rapid desaturation. Accuracy affected by hypotension and hypothermia
Electrocardiograph $US 2700–5995	Heart rate, identification of rhythm	Expensive. Various style leads available; electrical activity can continue without mechanical activity
Capnometer/capnograph $US 2695	Inspired or expired carbon dioxide concentration, respiratory rate	Non-invasive. Assesses ventilation and rebreathing. Use adds dead space and maybe less accurate with non-rebreathing circuits
Invasive blood pressure $US 2700–5995	Heart rate, direct arterial systolic, diastolic and mean blood pressures, pulse pressure wave	Requires placement of arterial catheter. Is the most accurate method. Pulse wave reflects inotropic function, stroke volume, volume status and peripheral vascular resistance. A transducer is necessary between catheter and monitor. Samples from arterial catheter can be used for blood-gas determination

continuously both cardiac and respiratory sounds (Table 3.11). The electrocardiograph (ECG) provides a non-invasive continuous evaluation of heart rate and rhythm (Table 3.11). However, the ECG records only myocardial electrical activity and provides no information about myocardial function. Lead placement is not critical for monitoring intraoperatively. What is important is the recognition of any changes in the appearance of the complexes or rhythm during the anaesthetic period. An ultrasonic Doppler crystal, placed over a peripheral artery, detects blood flow and provides an audible signal that allows continuous evaluation of pulse rate, rhythm and strength (Table 3.11). In small animals the crystal can be placed on the thorax, directly over the heart. The Doppler can be used to measure systolic blood pressure by placing an occlusive cuff connected to an aneroid manometer proximal to the Doppler crystal on a limb or at the base of the tail. The cuff is inflated until the pulse is no longer detected. The pressure is then slowly released

until the pulse can be detected again. The pressure at which the first sound is detected is systolic blood pressure.

Systolic, diastolic and mean arterial blood pressure, as well as heart rate, can be obtained intermittently using an automatic oscillometric blood pressure monitor (Table 3.11). The oscillations caused by varying pulse pressures are measured during gradual deflation of an air-filled cuff. The measurements are then interpreted and electronically displayed. Accuracy, for both Doppler and oscillometric methods, depends on the use of the appropriate-sized cuff. The width of the cuff should be approximately 40% of the circumference of that part of the limb to which it is applied. Indirect blood pressure determinations are difficult to obtain consistently in animals less than 4.5 kg and accuracy is decreased at low blood pressures. However, knowledge of blood pressure trends provides important information about cardiovascular status.

Direct measurement of arterial blood pressure requires catheterization of a peripheral artery. The arterial catheter is then connected to a measuring device. Fluid-filled extension tubing connected to an aneroid manometer is an inexpensive way of determining mean arterial blood pressure. Connection of the arterial catheter to a commercially available transducer and recording system provides a continuous, accurate, quantitative measurement of heart rate and systolic, diastolic and mean blood pressures (Table 3.11). A pulse pressure wave display is also generated and provides insight with regard to myocardial inotropic function, stroke volume, volume status and peripheral vascular resistance.

The arteries most accessible for catheterization in puppies and kittens are the dorsal pedal, femoral and lingual. The area over the artery is surgically prepared and the appropriate-sized catheter is inserted. Complications associated with arterial catheterization include haematoma formation, air embolization, infection and arterial thrombosis.

Respiratory system

Basic monitoring of the respiratory system consists of constant evaluation of respiratory rate, pattern, effort of breathing, changes in tidal volume and mucous membrane colour through simple observation and auscultation. Observation of thoracic excursions or movement of the rebreathing bag is a reliable method for determination of rate and rhythm. However, in animals less than 4.5 kg it may be difficult to visualize chest movement once they are draped in for surgery, and movement of the reservoir bag on a non-rebreathing system is often hard to detect and less reliable than that of a circle system.

The oesophageal stethoscope provides a remote, non-invasive and simple way to monitor continuously both respiratory and cardiac sounds (Table 3.11). Simple breath monitors attached to the end of the endotracheal tube beep with each breath, or sound an alarm if no breaths are detected within a specified time (Table 3.11). The movement of air or change in temperature is detected by a sensor located within the connector on the end of the endotracheal tube.

The high sensitivity of these monitors may result in false breaths being registered during surgical manipulation of viscera, whenever the thorax is touched or when the animal is moved. False breath sounds may also be heard when the oesophagus is mistakenly intubated, delaying recognition of a problem. The endotracheal tube connector increases dead space in the breathing circuit, which could be significant in animals weighing less than 2 kg.

Respiratory frequency and rhythm, however, do not reflect ventilatory effectiveness. Direct measurement of arterial partial pressure of carbon dioxide (Pa_{CO_2}) is the most accurate and representative way of determining if ventilation is normal. This requires the collection of an arterial blood sample. The measurement of expired or end-tidal carbon dioxide concentrations ($ETCO_2$) is an easy and reliable method of approximating Pa_{CO_2}. A capnometer or capnograph uses infrared technology to measure continuously P_{CO_2} in expired respiratory gases, as well as respiratory rate (Table 3.11). Two types of sample analysis are available: mainstream and sidestream. With mainstream evaluation, the sensor is located on a connector attached to the endotracheal tube and readings are instantaneous. In sidestream analysis, gases are aspirated from the breathing system via a sampling line attached to a T-connector placed at the end of the endotracheal tube. Samples are drawn into the monitor for evaluation and there is a slight delay. The $ETCO_2$ is typically less than the actual Pa_{CO_2}; a 1–10 mmHg gradient is normal in dogs and cats. The endotracheal tube connector increases dead space and rebreathing of expired gases, which may be significant in animals weighing less than 2 kg. Capnography is an important tool that can be used for detection of airway obstruction or disconnection, bronchospasm, severe cardiovascular disturbances, increased metabolic rate, malignant hyperthermia and hypothermia.

Oxygenating efficiency of the lungs is best determined by analysis of the arterial partial pressure of oxygen (Pa_{O_2}), requiring an arterial blood sample. A pulse oximeter is a non-invasive method of continuously monitoring pulse rate and functional haemoglobin oxygen saturation (Table 3.11). Haemoglobin saturation is related to the Pa_{O_2} by a sigmoid curve. A specially designed probe transmits red and near infrared light through tissues, senses the movement of a pulsating arteriolar bed, interprets colour absorption in the moving tissue and relates it to oxygen saturation (Sa_{O_2} or Sp_{O_2}). A variety of probe configurations are available.

The most useful sites for probe placement include tongue, cheek, gums, pinna, toe or toe web and skin folds. Hair and highly pigmented skin will interfere with the ability to obtain an accurate and consistent reading. A reflectance-type probe for oesophageal or rectal placement is also available. Accuracy is affected by changes in cardiopulmonary status, peripheral vasoconstriction, hypothermia, dyshaemoglobinaemias, shivering and interference from fluorescent or red heat lights. Puppies and kittens are highly susceptible to the development of hypoxaemia, and pulse oximetry is a valuable tool for the early detection of haemoglobin desaturation and hypoxaemia.

As stated above, the most accurate way of evaluating ventilation and oxygenation is by the analysis of carbon dioxide and oxygen concentrations in an arterial blood sample. This requires the collection of an arterial blood sample and the availability of a blood-gas analyser. There are several portable blood analysers currently available that make determination of arterial blood-gas concentrations more affordable and practical. However, arterial samples may be difficult to obtain in puppies and kittens and analysis can only be done intermittently rather than on a continuous basis.

Temperature

It is difficult to maintain normothermia in puppies and kittens. Therefore it is imperative that precautions be taken to prevent heat loss throughout the perioperative period (Table 3.11). Heat lamps and bottles or gloves filled with hot water should be used with caution, as thermal injury can occur. Temperature monitoring can be done continuously with an oesophageal or rectal probe attached to a temperature monitor, or intermittently with a thermometer. Some oesophageal temperature probes are also oesophageal stethoscopes and can be used to monitor heart and lung sounds. Aural temperatures are used if other sites are inaccessible. Aural temperatures are usually about 1°F less than rectal.

Postoperative considerations

It is important to recover puppies and kittens in a quiet, warm environment. Heart rate, respiratory rate and body temperature should be monitored closely during the immediate postoperative period. When appropriate, fluid therapy can be discontinued after the animal has recovered sufficiently to eat and drink. Body temperature should be returned to normal slowly. Do not remove thermal support and blankets as soon as temperature returns to normal, as young animals may have difficulty maintaining normothermia. It is desirable to return puppies and kittens to normal function as soon as possible.

Analgesia

All animals, regardless of age or size, are capable of feeling pain. Postoperative pain management in animals less than 8 weeks of age can be a unique challenge, especially with the concerns about bradycardia and respiratory depression. Whenever possible, analgesics should be administered before the painful event in a pre-emptive fashion. This approach to pain management reduces the analgesic dose necessary and alleviates the stress on the animal. Analgesics can be administered as preanaesthetics or intraoperatively. Parenterally administered agents, like butorphanol or buprenorphine, that cause minimal cardiopulmonary depression are recommended (Table 3.6). Fentanyl is a potent analgesic that has minimal sedative and cardiopulmonary effects when delivered via transdermal patch at the appropriate dose (Table 3.6). However, it takes at least 12 hours for effective drug levels to be reached and the patch configuration makes it difficult to dose and regulate in animals that weigh less than 2 kg. Fentanyl can also be administered by continuous-rate infusion, providing excellent analgesia with minimal side-effects (Table 3.6). This may require an additional intravenous catheter and is best done with the aid of a syringe infusion pump. Due to fentanyl's short duration of action, effects are terminated within 15 minutes of stopping the infusion.

Table 3.12 Epidural anaesthesia/analgesia

Indications	Postoperative analgesia (opioids) without cardiopulmonary depression Total regional anaesthesia (locals) Decreased requirement for general anaesthesia
Procedures	Hindlimb fractures, amputation, etc. Caudal abdominal surgeries Surgery of the perineum Tail amputation or surgery Thoracotomy
Contraindications	Hypovolaemia (local anaesthetics) Hypotension (local anaesthetics) Coagulopathy Localized pyoderma at site of needle placement Septicaemia Neurological disorder Anatomical abnormalities Clipping hair on dorsum undesirable to owner

Regional techniques provide postoperative analgesia without the potentially serious cardiopulmonary side-effects of parenterally administered medications (Skarda, 1996). Most local techniques used in adult dogs and cats can be used in puppies and kittens (Table 3.12).

Close attention to dose and technique is essential to avoid complications. A lumbosacral epidural or spinal (subarachnoid) using a local anaesthetic, an opioid or both is an acceptable technique for providing intraoperative and postoperative analgesia for many procedures (Table 3.12). Epidural placement is associated with less risk of spinal cord damage and decreased incidence of side-effects compared with spinal administration. The selection of an agent or combination of agents depends on the condition of the animal, the type of surgery and the desired effect (Krechel, 1990). Local anaesthetics provide a total sensory and motor blockade from 1 to 6 hours, depending on the agent used (Table 3.13).

This blockade allows many caudal surgical procedures to be done with the animal sedated or at a very light plane of general anaesthesia, thus preserving cardiopulmonary status. However, the depression of sympathetic tone in the area of the local block results in vasodilation and may lead to profound hypotension and contribute to hypothermia. If the block should ascend to the level of C7, C6 and C5, the phrenic nerve, which innervates the diaphragm will be paralysed, resulting in respiratory arrest. Local anaesthetics interfere with the transmission of pain impulses along nerve fibres and must come in direct contact with the nerves to be

Table 3.13 Comparison of epidural anaesthesia and analgesia

	Local anaesthetics	*Opioids*
Agents used	Lignocaine 2%* Procaine 2%* Carbocaine 2%* Bupivicaine 0.5%* Etidocaine 1%*	Morphine Oxymorphone Meperidine Fentanyl
Effects	Sensory blockade Motor blockade Sympathetic tone blockade	Long-duration visceral and somatic analgesia without systemic effects Does not cause a nerve block
Complications	Hypotension Hypothermia Respiratory depression Respiratory arrest Accidental IV or subarachnoid injection Incomplete nerve block Sepsis due to non-sterile technique	Pruritus Delayed-onset respiratory depression Delayed-onset sedation Delayed-onset bradycardia Urinary retention Reduced gastrointestinal motility Accidental IV or subarachnoid injection Sepsis due to non-sterile technique

* With or without adrenaline.
IV = intravenous

effective. Hence, immediately after administration of a local anaesthetic into the epidural space, the animal must be placed with the affected limb down or in sternal recumbency to ensure contact with the nerves that innervate the area to be blocked.

Opioids provide analgesia through their effects on the opioid receptors in the dorsal horn of the spinal cord. After injection into the epidural space, these agents are slowly absorbed into the cerebrospinal fluid and the spinal cord, and do not require direct contact with nerve fibres. Doses much lower than those recommended for parenteral use, when administered epidurally or subarachnoid, provide analgesia for as long as 24 hours with minimal physiological effects. Analgesia is maintained without blocking motor function or depressing sympathetic vasomotor activity. The occurrence of sedation, bradycardia and respiratory depression is rare, but may be observed several hours after injection (Table 3.6). If delayed depression occurs it can be reversed by the administration of a narcotic antagonist (Table 3.7) without diminishing the degree of analgesia. A combination of local anaesthetic and opioid injected epidurally provides sensory and motor blockade during surgery with a gradual return to function and residual analgesia for the postoperative period. If desired, an epidural catheter can be inserted for continuous or intermittent administration of local anaesthetic or opioid. The epidural or spinal deposition of drugs may be contraindicated in some animals (Table 3.12).

Epidurals can be done in a sedated or anaesthetized animal. When part of the anaesthetic protocol, they are best done immediately after induction, before the surgical procedure, but may be done at the termination of the surgery prior to recovery. The animal is placed in lateral or sternal recumbency with the hind legs pulled forwards to increase the size of the lumbosacral space. The major landmarks are the craniodorsal wings of the ileum and the dorsal processes of L6, L7 and S1, S2 (Fig. 3.3). The area directly over the lumbosacral space is clipped and surgically prepared. Sterile surgical gloves should be worn. A 22- to 20-gauge, 1.5–2.5-inch spinal needle is inserted into the lumbosacral space, between L7 and S1, on the midline, parallel to the spine, at a 90° angle with the skin. The needle is advanced slowly until a pop is felt as it penetrates the ligamentum flavum or it contacts bone on the bottom of the canal. A distinc-

tive pop may not be appreciated in animals less than 6 months of age or when using a sharp, disposable spinal needle. The stylet is removed and the hub of the needle carefully inspected for cerebrospinal fluid or blood. The presence of cerebrospinal fluid indicates subarachnoid puncture. If this occurs, the needle can be withdrawn slightly or one-half of the dose injected into the subarachnoid space.

The subarachnoid space of cats normally extends to or beyond the lumbosacral area, but in adult dogs it ends before L7. This subarachnoid space often extends further caudally, in young and small dogs, making the risk of dural puncture high in puppies and kittens less than 6 months of age. If blood is encountered after initial placement of the spinal needle, the needle should be removed, flushed and another attempt made to place it in the epidural space. Lack of resistance to injection of 1 ml of air or saline is the best way to identify the epidural space. All agents should be injected slowly, over 1–2 minutes, to avoid pain and provide even distribution. The placement of an epidural catheter enables continuous epidural anaesthesia/analgesia to be administered.

A specifically designed epidural catheter is introduced through a Huber-point (Tuohy) or Crawford needle. If an epidural catheter is not available, a jugular catheter or sterile tubing can be used. The technique is the same as described above. Although placement is not difficult, epidural catheters are not commonly used in dogs and cats due to technical and management concerns.

Intra-articular injection of local anaesthetics and opioids has been shown to provide effective postoperative analgesia in adult dogs. For best results, the joint capsule should be closed before drugs are introduced into the joint space. Either 0.5% bupivacaine at 0.5 ml/kg or morphine at 0.1 mg/kg diluted in saline to a volume of 0.5 ml/kg will reduce pain related to intra-articular surgery (Sammarco *et al.*, 1996). These agents can be combined, using bupivacaine as the diluent for the morphine.

A thoracotomy is a common surgical approach for correction of congenital cardiac anomalies, and is associated with significant postoperative pain. Intercostal nerve blocks provide analgesia during and after thoracotomy. Local anaesthetic is deposited on the nerves of two adjacent intercostal spaces both cranial and caudal to the incision. A long-acting local

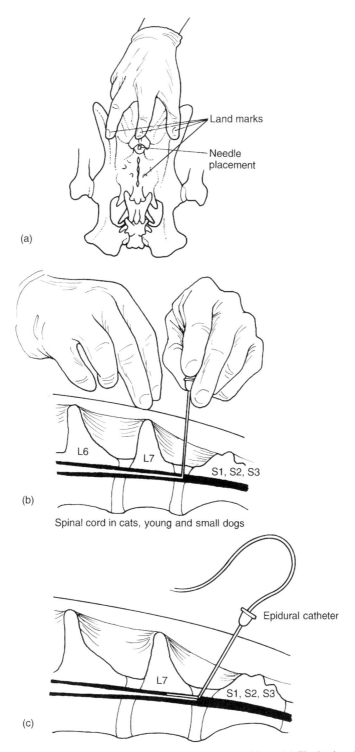

Figure 3.3 Needle and catheter placement for epidural analgesia in a puppy or kitten. (a) The landmarks – the craniodorsal wings of the ileum and the dorsal processes of L6, L7 and sacral dorsal processes are located and (b) the spinal needle is inserted into the lumbosacral space, between L7 and S1, on midline, parallel to the spine, at 90° angle with the skin. (c) For placement of a catheter, oblique placement is necessary to facilitate feeding of the catheter.

anaesthetic is injected caudal to the dorsal angle of the rib. A dose of 0.25–1.0 ml of 0.25% or 0.5% bupivacaine, with or without adrenaline, will provide 3–6 hours of analgesia without respiratory compromise. Care should be taken not to exceed a total dose of 3 mg/kg.

Pain originating from the thoracic or upper abdominal area can be controlled by intra-pleural administration of local anaesthetics (Thompson and Johnson, 1991). This technique requires the placement of a chest tube, which can be done percutaneously or before closure of a thoracotomy. Bupivacaine, 1–2 mg/kg, injected slowly over 1–2 minutes and flushed through with saline, will provide analgesia for 3–12 hours. Local anaesthetics must have contact with the target nerves, therefore the animal must be placed with the incision down for best effect. Possible complications include pneumothorax, trauma to the lung or inappropriate catheter position. The presence of fluid within the thorax, such as pleural effusion, blood, pus or lymph, will interfere with the ability of the local anaesthetic to provide an effective block. Cardiopulmonary function is not compromised by this technique.

Complications and cardiopulmonary resuscitation

Close monitoring is imperative to the early detection and correction of complications (Table 3.14). Cardiopulmonary resuscitation in puppies and kittens is similar to that of adults. Success is directly related to early recognition of and rapid response to the arrest. All anaesthetics should be discontinued and the patency and placement of the endotracheal tube evaluated. If the animal is not already intubated, this should be accomplished immediately. Ventilation should be controlled at a rate of

Table 3.14 Complications associated with anaesthesia in puppies and kittens

Complication	Possible cause	Response
Tachypnoea		
	Pulmonary oedema from volume overload	Discontinue IV fluids Furosemide 0.5–1.0 mg/kg IV
	Insufficient depth of anaesthesia or pain	Increase depth of anaesthesia/administer analgesic
	Hyperthermia	Remove heating pads, turn off heat lamps, remove cover, etc.
	Hypercapnoea/acidosis	Increase ventilation
	Hypoxaemia	Increase oxygen concentration, evaluate perfusion
Respiratory distress while intubated		
	Airway obstruction; mucus plug, kinked tube	Clear or replace tube; reposition tube
Respiratory distress after extubation		
	Pneumothorax, barotrauma, underlying disease	Chest tube or trochar
	Laryngeal oedema or spasm	Dexamethasone 0.25–0.5 mg/kg IV
	Traumatic or difficult intubation Prolonged surgery	May need to reintubate or perform tracheostomy
Bradypnoea		
	Excessive anaesthetic depth	Decrease depth of anaesthesia. Support ventilation
	Opioid administration	Complete or partial opioid reversal. Support ventilation
	Hypothermia	Increase body temperature
	Cerebral oedema from hypoventilation or volume overload	Increase ventilation. Administer furosemide 0.5–1.0 mg/kg IV; mannitol 0.5–1.0 g/kg IV slowly
Hypoxaemia/cyanosis		
	All of the above	See above
	Disconnection from circuit/ventilator	Reattach to oxygen source/ventilator

Table 3.14 (continued)

Complication	Possible cause	Response
Hypercapnoea	Hypoventilation	Increase ventilation respiratory rate and/or tidal volume. Check airway. Decrease anaesthesia
	Rebreathing exhaled gases (CO_2)	Increase oxygen flow or change to non-rebreathing circuit
Bradycardia	Increased vagal tone, opioid administration, excessive depth of anaesthesia, surgical manipulation	Complete or partial opioid reversal. Decrease depth of anaesthesia. Gentle tissue handling. Glycopyrrolate or atropine is administered
	Hypothermia	Increase body temperature
Hypotension	Bradycardia	See above
	Excessive anaesthetic depth	Decrease anaesthetic depth. Complete or partial opioid reversal
	Hypovolaemia	Balanced electrolyte solution or blood component therapy. Do not to exceed 10 ml/kg per hour
	Depressed/immature sympathetic nervous system	Dopamine infusion 2–10 μg/kg per minute
Tachycardia	Insufficient anaesthetic depth	Increase anaesthetic depth
	Pain	Administer analgesic
	Hypotension	Conservative fluid therapy. Vasopressors are administered
Hypothermia	See Table 3.4	See Table 4.10
Hyperthermia	Fever or underlying disease	Treat with antipyretic if appropriate
	Excessive supplemental heat	Remove heating pads, turn off heat lamps, remove cover, etc.
Hypoglycaemia	Fasting, preoperative conditioning, prolonged surgical procedure, prolonged recovery, stress	Balanced electrolyte fluids spiked with glucose IV. Alternatively, administer 50% glucose orally
Difficult IV access	Animal too small, hypovolaemia. Animal difficult to restrain	Place interosseous catheter, or give fluids subcutaneously. Fluids may be administered intraperitoneally as last resort; use tranquilizers
Vocalization or excitement	Emergence delirium	Comfort for several minutes until dysphoria passes. Administer tranquilizer or opioid if dysphoria persists.
	Discomfort	
	Pain	Administer opioid analgesic, either systemic or regional
	Fear	
Cardiopulmonary arrest	Excessive anaesthetic depth	Airway – make sure airway is open. Check tube placement and patency
	Respiratory arrest – opioids	
	Hypothermia	Breathing – ventilate on pure oxygen 20–30 breaths/minute (discontinue all inhalation anaesthetics)
	Hypotension	Circulation – external chest compressions as fast as you can: 60/minute or faster
	Hypoglycaemia	Drugs and arrhythmia control are the same as for adults
		Do not overhydrate

IV = Intravenous.

20–30 breaths/minute, and supplemental oxygen should be administered. The thoracic wall of puppies and kittens is extremely pliable, and external chest compressions should be done gently so as not to damage the heart and lungs. Compressions should be in excess of 60/minute, making sure to allow the chest to expand and the heart to fill between compressions.

The cardiac status should be evaluated by ECG and the dysrhythmia identified and treated accordingly. The indications for and dosing of first-line drugs like adrenaline, lignocaine and atropine are similar to that of adults. These drugs can be administered intravenously, intraosseously, intratracheally or, as a last resort, intracardiac. Fluid therapy should be started and closely monitored to avoid fluid overload by rapid administration of shock volumes.

References

Arango, A. and Rowe, M.I. (1971) The neonatal puppy as an experimental subject. *Biology Neonates*, **18**, 173–179.

Aschinberg, L.C., Goldsmith, D.O., Olbing, H. *et al.* (1975) Neonatal changes in renal blood flow distribution in puppies. *American Journal Physiology*, **228**, 1453–1461.

Center, S.A., Hornbuckle, W.E. and Hoskins, J.D. (1995) The liver and pancreas. In: Hoskins, J.D. (ed.) *Veterinary Pediatrics: Dogs and Cats from Birth to Six Months*, pp. 189–226. Philadelphia: WB Saunders.

Cote, C. (1990) Pediatric anesthesia. In: Miller, R.D. (ed.) *Anesthesia*, pp. 1897–1926. New York: Churchill Livingstone.

Fagella, A.M. and Arohnson, M.G. (1993) Anesthesia techniques for neutering 6 to 14-week-old kittens. *Journal of American Veterinary Association*, **202**, 56–62.

Fagella, A.M. and Aronsohn, M.G. (1994) Evaluation of anesthetic protocols for neutering 6 to 14-week-old pups. *Journal of American Veterinary Medical Association*, **205**, 308–314.

Friedman, W.F. (1972) The intrinsic physiological properties of the developing heart. *Progress in Cardiovascular Disease*, **15**, 87–111.

Horster, M., Kember, B. and Valtin, H. (1971) Intracortical distribution of number and volume of glomeruli during postnatal maturation in the dog. *Journal of Clinical Investigation*, **50**, 796–800.

Kawalek, J.C. and El Said, K.R. (1990) Maturational development of drug-metabolizing enzymes in dogs. *American Journal of Veterinary Research*, **51**, 1742–1745.

Kleinman, L.I. and Lubbe, R.J. (1972) Factors affecting the maturation of glomerular filtration rate and renal plasma flow in the newborn dog. *Journal Physiology*, **223**, 395–409.

Krechel, S.W. (1990) Spinal opiates in pediatric anesthesia practice. *Progress in Anesthesiology*, **IV**, 78–86.

Robinson, E.P. (1983) Anesthesia of pediatric patients. *Compendium of Continuing Education for the Practicing Veterinarian*, **12**, 1004–1011.

Sammarco, J.L., Conzemius, M.G., Perkowski, S.Z. *et al.* (1996) Postoperative analgesia for stifle surgery: a comparison of intra-articular bupivacaine, morphine, or saline. *Veterinary Surgery*, **25**, 59–69.

Skarda, R.T. (1996) Local and regional anesthetic and analgesic techniques A: dogs. In: Thurmon, J.C., Tranquilli, W.J. and Benson, G.J. (eds) *Lumb and Jones Veterinary Anesthesia*, pp. 426–447. Baltimore: Williams & Wilkins.

Thompson, S.E. and Johnson, J.M. (1991) Analgesia in dogs after intercostal thoracotomy. A comparison of morphine, selective intercostal nerve block, and interpleural regional analgesia with bupivicaine. *Veterinary Surgery*, **20**, 73–77.

Thurmon, J.C., Tranquilli, W.J. and Benson, G.J. (1996) Anesthesia for special patients D: neonatal and geriatric patients. In: Thurmon, J.C., Tranquilli, W.J. and Benson, G.J. (eds) *Lumb and Jones Veterinary Anesthesia*, pp. 812–848. Baltimore: Williams & Wilkins.

4

Intensive care

Nutrition

Feeding puppies and kittens from birth to adulthood is substantially different during the different life stages. Growth is an extremely demanding time in a puppy's or kitten's life. Most puppies and kittens will fail to grow (or thrive) to the size determined by their hereditary factors unless they consume sufficient food of adequate quality. If poor-quality commercially prepared diets or home-made diets of single food items or indiscriminate mixtures of single food items are fed during growth, nutrition-related disorders often occur. Proper nutrition is crucial to the general health and performance of puppies and kittens.

Feeding the growing puppy

Puppies during their first 2–3 weeks of life should just eat and sleep. Suckling should be vigorous and active. If the bitch is healthy and well-nourished, the puppy's nutritional needs for its first 3–4 weeks of life should be handled completely by her. Indications that the puppy is not receiving adequate milk are shown by constant crying, extreme inactivity and/or failure to achieve weight gains in accordance with the general guidelines that a puppy should gain 2–4 g/day per kg of anticipated adult weight (Lewis

et al., 1987). For example, if the adult dog is expected to weigh 10 kg, as a puppy it should gain 20–40 g/day during its first 5 months of life.

The transition from bitch's milk to a growth diet should be a gradual process beginning at about 3 weeks of age (4 weeks of age for most toy breeds); however, if necessary, supplemental feeding of the growth diet may be started as soon as the puppy fails to show adequate weight gain. The puppy can then be offered a mixture of a growth diet and water as a thick gruel (a mixture of one part dry food blended with three parts water or two parts canned food blended with one part water). To get the puppy eating, the gruel is placed in a shallow food bowl or given orally by using a dosing syringe. Once the puppy is eating the gruel well, gradually reduce the amount of water in the gruel until the water is omitted. The puppy may be permanently separated from the bitch as soon as it learns to eat readily and drink satisfactorily. Most puppies are completely weaned at 5–7 weeks of age, depending somewhat on the dog breed.

The food fed solely to the weaned puppy should be one specifically formulated for growth. Because the puppy's eating habits are still in the formative stage, it remains important that a good-quality growth puppy food be fed daily at regular intervals until adulthood and fresh water in a clean bowl is available at all times. Feeding the weaned puppy should always be directed to attaining the average growth rate for the dog breed (Lewis *et al.*, 1987). Overfeeding for maximal weight gain is not recommended. Instead of making food available to the puppy at all times (free-choice feeding), time-limited meal feeding is recommended. At each feeding, give the puppy 20 minutes to eat all it wants and then remove the remaining food. From weaning to 6 months of age (12 months for giant breeds), puppies are best fed at least three times a day at regular intervals.

Feeding the growing kitten

Kittens during their first 4 weeks of life should suckle vigorously and actively. If the queen is healthy and well-nourished, the nutritional needs of the kittens for the first 4 weeks of life should be provided completely by her. Kittens not receiving adequate milk cry constantly, are restless or extremely inactive and/or fail to achieve the normal weight gains of 10–15 g/day for the first 5 months of life.

Kittens should be encouraged to begin eating a growth diet at 4 weeks of age. At this time, the kitten can be offered a mixture of a growth diet and milk or water as a thick gruel (a mixture of one part dry food blended with three parts milk or two parts canned food blended with one part milk). The gruel is placed in a shallow bowl or given orally by using a dosing syringe. Once the kitten is eating the gruel well, gradually reduce the amount of milk or water in the gruel until the kitten is consuming only the growth diet. Most kittens are completely weaned at 6–8 weeks of age. Cow's milk is often fed to kittens after weaning and is a good food provided that it does not cause diarrhoea. However, milk should never be fed in place of fresh water.

Kittens should be fed all the food they will consume (Lewis *et al.*, 1987). Excessive caloric intake and excessively rapid growth rate are seldom problems in growing kittens. Most kittens nibble at their food frequently. Kittens fed unlimited amounts of food (free-choice feeding), regardless of the form of food (dry or canned), will eat every few hours. Free-choice feeding, or at least three-times-a-day feeding, is preferred during growth.

Feeding orphaned puppies and kittens

Successful rearing of orphaned puppies and kittens requires the provision of a suitable environment; the correct quantities and quality of nutrients for different life stages; a regular schedule of feeding, sleeping, grooming and exercise; and the stimulus that provokes micturition and defecation during the first 18–21 days of life (Sheffy, 1978).

Newborn puppies and kittens are unable to control their body temperature effectively (Bjorck, 1982). They gradually change from being largely poikilothermic to being homeothermic during their first 4 weeks of life. That is, for the first week of life their body temperature is directly related to the environmental temperature, and a steady ambient temperature of 30–32° C (86–90° F) is needed. Over the next 3 weeks, the ambient temperature can be gradually lowered to 24° C (75° F). Humidity should be maintained at 55–60%. It is equally important that sudden changes of environmental conditions be avoided and that disturbances are minimized outside socialization, exercise and hygiene activities.

Feeding orphaned puppies and kittens that still require mother's milk can be rewarding. The most obvious alternative to a mother rearing her own young is for another lactating mother to act as a foster mother. If a foster mother is not available, then hand-feeding the puppies or kittens a replacement food that is a prototype of nutritive substance formulated to meet the optimum requirements of the puppy or kitten is needed (Sheffy, 1978). Various modifications of home-made and commercially prepared formulas simulating mother's milk are available (Baines, 1981; Bjorck, 1982; Remillard *et al.*, 1993, Tables 4.1 and 4.2). Most commercially prepared formulas generally provide 1–1.24 kcal of metabolizable energy per millilitre of formula. Caloric needs for most puppies and kittens is 22–26 kcal per 100 g of body weight for

Table 4.1 Home-made formula for orphaned kittens

Formula
90 ml condensed milk
90 ml water
120 ml plain yogurt (not low-fat yogurt)
Three large or four small egg yolks

Table 4.2 Commercial milk replacement formulas for nursing-age puppies and kittens

Product	Manufacturer recommended	Species
Esbilac powder	Pet-Ag	Puppies
Esbilac liquid	Pet-Ag	Puppies
Havolac-Plus	Bayer	Puppies and kittens
KMR liquid	Pet-Ag	Kittens
KMR powder	Pet-Ag	Kittens
Nurturall liquid	Veterinary Products Lab	Puppies and kittens
Unilact powder	Veterinary Products Lab	Puppies and kittens
Veta-Lac powder	Vet-A-Mix	Puppies and kittens

the first 3 months of life. The amount of formula should be fed in equal portions three or four times daily. Before each feeding, the formula should be warmed to about 100°F (37.8°C) or near their body temperature for the first 3 weeks of life.

When a formula is first fed, less than the prescribed amount should be given per feeding for the first feedings. The amount is then gradually increased to the recommended feeding amount by the second or third day. The amount of formula is increased accordingly as the puppy or kitten gains weight and a favourable response to feeding occurs. Puppies should gain 2–4 g/day per kg of anticipated adult weight for the first 5 months of their lives. The kitten at birth should weigh 80–140 g (most weigh around 100–120 g) and gain 50–100 g weekly (Lewis *et al.*, 1987).

When preparing the formula, always follow the manufacturer's directions on the label for its proper preparation, and keep all feeding equipment scrupulously clean. A good way of handling prepared formula is to prepare only a 48-hour supply of formula at a time and divide this supply into portions required for each feeding (Sheffy, 1978). Once formula is prepared, it is best stored in the refrigerator at 4°C.

The easiest and safest ways of feeding commercially prepared formula to puppies and kittens is by nipple bottle feeding, dosing syringe feeding or by tube feeding (Lewis *et al.*, 1987; Sheffy, 1978). Nipple bottles made especially for feeding orphan puppies or kittens or bottles equipped with premature infant nipples are preferred. When feeding with a nipple bottle, hold the bottle so that the puppy or kitten does not ingest air. The hole in the nipple should be such that when the bottle is inverted, milk slowly oozes from the nipple. When feeding, squeeze a drop of milk on to the tip of the nipple and then insert the nipple into the puppy's or kitten's mouth. Never squeeze milk out of the bottle while the nipple is in the mouth; doing so may result in laryngotracheal aspiration of the milk into the lungs. In addition, prepared formula should never be fed to a puppy or kitten that is hypothermic or does not have a strong sucking reflex. Only when the sucking reflex is present should feeding be attempted.

Dosing syringe feeding and tube feeding are the fastest ways to feed orphaned puppies or kittens. The dosing syringe is a regular plastic syringe that comes in various sizes and has a larger nipple portion at its administration end. A number 5 French infant feeding tube for puppies or kittens weighing less than 300 g, a number 8–10 French infant feeding tube for puppies or kittens weighing over 300 g, or an appropriately sized, soft male urethral catheter can be used. Once weekly, mark the feeding tube to be used clearly to indicate the depth of insertion to ensure gastric delivery (the distance from the last rib to the tip of the nose can be measured and marked off on the feeding tube as a guide).

When tube feeding, fill a syringe with warm commercially prepared or home-made formula and fit it to the feeding tube, making sure to expel any air in the tube or syringe. Open the mouth slightly, and with the head held in the normal suckling position, gently pass the feeding tube to the marked area. If an obstruction is felt or coughing occurs before reaching the mark, the tube is in the trachea. If this is not the case, slowly administer the prepared formula over a 2-minute period to allow sufficient time for slow filling of the stomach. Regurgitation of formula rarely occurs, but if it does, withdraw the feeding tube and interrupt feeding until the next scheduled meal.

After puppies and kittens have fed, a vital aspect of tending orphaned puppies and kittens is to stimulate reflex micturition and defecation. These reflexes can be achieved by swabbing the anogenital area with moistened cotton or soft tissue paper to stimulate the reflex elimination manually. It is often possible to effect the same response simply by running a forefinger along the abdominal wall. This stimulation should be done after each feeding. After about 3 weeks of age, puppies and kittens are usually able to relieve themselves without simulated stimulation.

Most puppies and kittens benefit from gentle handling before feeding to allow for some exercise and to promote muscular and circulatory development. In addition, at least weekly the orphaned puppy or kitten should be washed gently with a soft moistened cloth for general cleansing of the skin, simulating mother's cleansing licks with her tongue.

As previously mentioned, the orphaned puppy or kitten should be encouraged to begin eating a growth diet gruel at 3–4 weeks of age.

Fluid therapy

The purpose of fluid therapy is to re-establish a positive fluid balance (DiBartola, 1992). Effective fluid therapy for most puppies and kittens depends on an accurate assessment of the animal's state of dehydration. The hydration status of mature dogs or cats is estimated by evaluation of the history, physical examination findings and the results of a few simple laboratory tests (packed cell volume, total plasma protein concentration and urine specific gravity). Similar principles apply for effective fluid therapy in puppies and kittens.

Historical information about diminished fluid intake and volume, and route of fluid loss may suggest the puppy's or kitten's immediate fluid needs as related to hydration deficit and electrolyte and acid–base imbalances. The physical examination findings associated with fluid deficits of 5–15% of body weight vary from no clinically detectable changes (5%) to signs of hypovolaemic shock and impending death (15%). The hydration deficit in puppies and kittens older than 6 weeks can be estimated by evaluating skin turgor or pliability, moistness of the

mucous membranes, position of the eyes in their orbits, heart rate, character of peripheral pulses, capillary refill time and extent of peripheral venous distension (DiBartola, 1992). In puppies and kittens younger than 6 weeks of age, skin turgor, and probably the percentage estimation of hydration deficit (5–15%), does not apply. A more accurate estimation of dehydration is by evaluating the moistness of mucous membranes and the volume and colour of urine. The normal urine colour of euhydrated puppies and kittens younger than 6 weeks of age is clear or colourless. Normal urine production is 0.5–1.0 ml/kg body weight per hour.

Fluid preparations used in fluid therapy may be either crystalloids or colloids (Table 4.3). Crystalloid solutions should be stored at room temperature or preferably warmed to body temperature in a 37° C (98.6° F) water bath or warm incubator before use. This warming procedure eliminates any decrease in core body temperature that otherwise may occur during administration.

The choice of fluid to administer depends on the nature of the disease process and the composition of the fluid lost. The rate of fluid administration is dictated by the magnitude and rapidity of the fluid loss (Table 4.4).

The intravenous route of fluid administration is preferred in critically ill puppies and kittens that have had severe fluid loss or when fluid loss has been acute. The intravenous route requires close monitoring during fluid administration to avoid complications, such as overhydration, infection, thrombosis, phlebitis, embolism and impaired fluid delivery (obstruction of venous line by changes in animal's position). The peripheral veins available for venous access in puppies and kittens younger than 6 weeks of age are generally the external jugular and cephalic veins. The external jugular vein is preferred because it allows uniform delivery of fluids in small uncooperative animals with small veins.

The intraosseous route can be life-saving in those critically ill puppies and kittens in which venous access is difficult or impossible. The intraosseous route provides quick venous access via bone marrow sinusoids and medullary venous channels and allows rapid dispersion of fluid solutions. Sites that can be used for intraosseous administration of fluids include the tibial tuberosity, trochanteric fossa of the

Table 4.3 Crystalloid and colloid fluid preparations

Fluid type	Comments
Crystalloids	Contain electrolyte and non-electrolyte solutes capable of entering all body fluid compartments
	Indicated for replacement or maintenance of fluid and electrolyte requirements, e.g. dehydration and electrolyte depletion due to anorexia, vomiting and diarrhoea
	Avoid crystalloid solutions with antimicrobial preservatives (benzoic acid derivatives such as benzyl alcohol, ethylparaben, methylparaben, propylparaben)
	Complications such as behavioural changes, hypersalivation, ataxia, muscle fasciculations, seizures, dilated non-responsive pupils, coma and death have been reported in kittens (Cullison *et al.*, 1983)
Maintenance crystalloid solutions	Contain less sodium (40–60 mEq/l) and more potassium (15–30 mEq/l) than replacement fluids
Replacement crystalloid solutions, e.g. lactated Ringer's solution, Ringer's solution	Composition resembles that of extracellular fluid
Dextrose solutions e.g. 5% dextrose in water, 2.5% dextrose/0.45% saline	Indicated for treatment and prevention of hypoglycaemia
	Half-strength saline/dextrose can be used as a maintenance solution but may require potassium supplementation
Colloids e.g. plasma, dextrans, hydroxyethyl starch (hetastarch)	Large-molecular-weight substances that remain in the plasma compartment
	Use in the treatment of severe hypoproteinaemia and hypoalbuminaemia

femur, wing of the ilium and greater tubercle of the humerus (Otto *et al.*, 1989). In most puppies and kittens younger than 6 weeks of age, the trochanteric fossa of the femur and greater tubercle of the humerus are the preferred sites for intraosseous administration of warm replacement or maintenance fluid solutions.

For intraosseous administration of fluid solutions into the femur, an 18- or 20-gauge spinal needle (the gauge of needle depends on the size of the puppy or kitten) is aseptically inserted parallel to the long axis of the femur; the stylet is removed from the needle immediately before fluid infusion (Otto *et al.*, 1989). Fluid flow rates up to 11 ml/minute can be achieved with gravity flow. The needle is then secured to the skin. Routine needle care is required; intraosseous needles can be left in place for up to 72 hours. The potential risks include needle-induced osteomyelitis and pain observed during the administration of fluid solutions. Pain generally results from injecting too cold a fluid solution or an irritating solution, placing too much weight on the needle inserted into the marrow cavity, or administering too large a fluid volume at a time.

Repeated assessment of the puppy and kitten by observation of clinical signs and determination of body weight is mandatory in making appropriate readjustments of fluid therapy. Reasons for failure to achieve satisfactory hydration include underestimation of the amount of fluid needs, losses greater than first appreciated (vomiting, diarrhoea) and infusion of fluids at an excessive, rapid rate with obligatory urinary loss of fluid and electrolytes (DiBartola, 1992). Failure to achieve satisfactory hydration is an indication to increase the volume of fluids administered if cardiopulmonary and renal function are adequate. As a general guide, the daily fluid volume may be increased by an amount equivalent to 5% of body weight if the initial infusion fails to restore hydration. It is important to remember that the hydration deficit is an estimate based on an animal's history and physical examination findings, and fluid therapy should be tailored to physical examination findings (maintenance of body weight, moistness of mucous membranes and clearness of urine) over the first 12 hours to few days of fluid therapy.

When an intravenous or intraosseous route is chosen for fluid administration, the veterinarian has made an obligation to careful, aseptic catheter placement and proper maintenance. The puppy or kitten should be checked periodically for cleanliness of the catheter site, local pain or swelling, or fever. If any of these signs occur,

Table 4.4 Fluid therapy in critically ill puppies and kittens

---

Intravenous or intraosseous fluid administration

---

1. Replace losses with a fluid that is similar in volume and electrolyte composition to that which has been lost from the body

2. Use multiple electrolyte solution (Ringer's solution, lactated Ringer's solution) supplemented with 5% dextrose solution

3. In puppies and kittens < 6 weeks of age, Ringer's solution is preferred over lactated Ringer's since puppies and kittens at this age may be ineffective in metabolizing the lactate to bicarbonate and, therefore, receive limited benefit from the lactate

4. Supplement the fluids with potassium chloride solution if plasma potassium concentration is less than 2.5 mEq/l

5. Administer warm fluids slowly by intravenous or intraosseous route.
   Maintenance: 40–50 ml/kg per day administered over a 24-hour period
   Moderate dehydration: rapid replacement of hydration deficit unnecessary in chronic disease states; administer maintenance fluid requirement (40–50 ml/kg per day) over the first 4–8 hour of treatment, followed by routine maintenance therapy. This allows for equilibration of fluid and electrolytes within the intracellular compartment and avoids potential complications such as oedema or effusion due to increased hydrostatic pressure, diuresis, and loss of administered electrolytes in the urine
   Shock, hypotension: up to 40–45 ml/kg per hour

6. *Glucose replacement therapy*
   Moderate hypoglycaemia: administer 5% dextrose solution intravenously or intraosseously, slowly to effect
   Profound hypoglycaemia with profound depression or seizures: administer 1–2 ml/kg of a 10% dextrose solution
   Maintain plasma glucose concentration at 80–200 mg/dl for euglycaemia

7. Colloid administered if severely hypoproteinaemic; total protein < 4.0 g/dl; albumin < 1.5 g/dl)
   Plasma: 6–10 mg/kg over 4–6 hours. Administer up to 3 times a day
   Dextran 70, hetastarch: 20–40 ml/kg per day. Can administer over 6 hours but maximum rate not to exceed 5–10 ml/kg per hour

---

Nutritional support

---

1. Encourage food and water intake once puppy or kitten is normothermic and adequately hydrated

---

Monitor effectiveness of therapy

---

1. Observe for improvement in the puppy's or kitten's general demeanour

2. Regularly assess the cardiopulmonary status (it is extremely easy to overhydrate the ill puppy and kitten, so attentive monitoring of breathing pattern is helpful for early recognition of overhydration)

3. Observe animal for signs of overhydration or too rapid fluid administration – serous nasal discharge, chemosis, restlessness, tachycardia, cough, altered breathing pattern, pulmonary crackles, ascites, polyuria, exophthalmos, diarrhoea and vomiting (Cornelius *et al.*, 1978)

4. Weigh the puppy or kitten 3–4 times a day to record weight gain or maintenance

5. Monitor urine output and the moistness of mucous membranes to assess hydration status

---

the catheter should be removed and a new catheter placed in another vein. When the catheter is not in use, the catheter should be flushed frequently with a small volume (less than 1 ml) of a solution containing 5 units of heparin per millilitre of 0.9% saline (heparinized saline) solution.

Fluid therapy should be discontinued when hydration is restored and the animal can maintain fluid balance by oral intake. As the animal recovers, fluid therapy should be tapered by decreasing the volume of fluid administered by 25–50% a day (DiBartola, 1992). During this time, fluid therapy may be changed from the intravenous or intraosseous route to the subcutaneous route when possible, based on the volume of fluid to be given daily. Do not give dextrose containing fluids subcutaneously.

Blood component therapy

Transfusion of blood components is often necessary in the adjunctive treatment of puppies and kittens. Blood components commonly used are whole blood, packed red blood cells and plasma (Authement *et al.*, 1987; Bucheler and Cotter, 1993). Indications for the use of fresh whole blood are haemorrhagic shock, anaemia, excessive traumatic haemorrhage, bleeding disorders (due to thrombocytopenia or clotting factor deficiencies) and non-immune haemolytic anaemia. Except for bleeding disorders, properly stored whole blood can usually be substituted for fresh whole blood. Routine treatment of most anaemias in the puppy and kitten can also be accomplished with packed red blood cells. Plasma is used primarily to correct clotting factor deficiencies and reversible hypoproteinaemias.

Whole blood collection

The safest and most accessible site for whole blood collection is the external jugular vein. The amount of blood that can be safely withdrawn via the external jugular vein from a

Table 4.5 Composition of solutions available for fluid therapy

Solution	Na^+ (mEq/l)	K^+ (mEq/l)	Ca^{2+} (mEq/l)	Mg^{2+} (mEq/l)	Cl^- (mEq/l)	Lactate (mEq/l)	pH	Osmolality (mosmol/l)	Caloric content (kcal/l)
Crystalloid solutions									
1. Replacement									
Lactated Ringer's	130	4	3		109	25	6.5	273	9
Ringer's	147	4	5		156		5.8	310	
2. Maintenance solutions									
One part 0.9% saline solution with two parts 5% dextrose solution; add 20 mEq KCl/l of final solution*	51	20			71			235	67
3. Dextrose solutions									
5% Dextrose in water							5.0	252	170
2.5% Dextrose in 0.45% saline	77				71		4.8	280	85
Colloid solutions									
1. Dextran 70 (6% w/v in 0.9% saline)	154				154		4.5–7.0	300–303	
2. Hetastarch	154				154				
3. Plasma (average for dog)	145	4.2	5	2.5	108	20	7.4	290	

* Guideline for preparation of a maintenance solution.

donor dog or cat is up to 22 ml/kg body weight every 2 weeks (Authement *et al.*, 1987). Donors may be minimally restrained or sedated and the venepuncture site surgically prepared. A haemostat is placed over the tubing of the plastic blood collecting bag and is removed only after the external jugular vein has been entered. Venepuncture should be clean with rapid blood flow to minimize activation of platelets and clotting factors and tissue thromboplastin contamination (Authement *et al.*, 1987). When the full blood volume is collected, the collecting tube is reclamped before removing the needle from the external jugular vein. Direct pressure should be applied over the collection site for 5–10 minutes after collection of blood for haemostasis.

Blood is best collected in a plastic bag containing citrate-phosphate-adenine (CPD-A) solution or acid-citrate-dextrose (ACD) solution (Authement *et al.*, 1987). The ratio of the volume of CPD-A or ACD anticoagulant to blood is 1 : 7 for storage of blood components (canine and feline blood in CPD-A has a storage life of 28 days versus 21 days for ACD at 4° C). If blood is given immediately after collection, a 1 : 10 dilution of anticoagulant to blood can be used. If heparin is used, 625 units is used per 50 ml of blood collected (Authement *et al.*, 1987). Procedurally, whole blood is collected in 450 ml CPD-A or ACD plastic blood-collecting bags to appropriate volume, with swirling of blood during collection to ensure adequate mixing with anticoagulant. To monitor the volume of blood being withdrawn, a triple-beam balance scale or digital electronic scale may be used. One ml of blood weighs approximately 1 g, so a unit containing 450 ml of blood should weigh 450 g plus the weight of the container with the anticoagulant. After collection, the collecting tube is tied off and the collected blood mixed thoroughly with anticoagulant in the collecting bag. The unit of collected blood is then used immediately or stored at appropriate temperature for later use.

If a small volume of whole blood is needed for immediate use, 7 ml of CPD-A or ACD anticoagulant may be drawn into a 50-ml plastic syringe and the rest filled with blood. Any open system, such as a plastic syringe or bag entered with a needle, should be used within 24 hours.

Packed red blood cells and plasma collection

Collection of red blood cells requires double or triple bags which consist of the main collection bag and one or two connected satellite bags. This prevents the system from being opened during the separation process (Schneider, 1995). After whole blood collection, packed red blood cells and plasma can be separated. Blood collected in plastic blood-collecting bags with CPD-A or ACD anticoagulant is taken directly to a local blood bank facility in an ice-filled cooler; the blood should not be allowed to come into contact with the ice (Authement *et al.*, 1987). At the blood bank facility, the blood-filled CPD-A or ACD bags will be centrifuged at 4° C in a centrifuge at a speed (rpm) of 5000 **g** for 10 minutes. Following centrifugation, extracted plasma is transferred into a satellite storage bag. The red blood cells remaining after extraction of the plasma are then labelled as packed red blood cells and can be stored for up to 21 days.

Fresh-frozen plasma is plasma that is frozen within 8 hours of the time of blood collection and is used primarily to supply clotting factors (treatment of haemophilia A, von Willebrand's disease, rodenticide toxicity and disseminated intravascular coagulation). It should be frozen (stored) at −70° C for optimal preservation of clotting factors for 1 year or in a conventional freezer for 3 months. Frozen plasma is plasma that is frozen after 8 hours from the time of collection or is fresh-frozen plasma that is older than 1 year of age. It is not used for supply of clotting factors, although it can be used in the treatment of haemophilia B (factor IX required) or rodenticide toxicity (factors II, VII, IX and X required) and has a shelf-life of up to 5 years if stored in a similar manner to fresh-frozen plasma.

Blood-typing

Blood-typing dogs is not essential prior to transfusion and recipient and donor animals with the same blood type may still be incompatible due to other plasma antigens. Typing will, however, help to minimize the incidence of reactions, and

Table 4.6 Blood types of dogs (modified from Hale, 1995)

Blood type (DEA)*	Population incidence (%)	Presence of naturally occurring antibody	Transfusion reaction with incompatible blood
1.1	42	No	No reaction with first transfusion. Acute haemolytic reaction with subsequent transfusion due to sensitization
1.2	20	No	No reaction with first transfusion. Acute haemolytic reaction with subsequent transfusion due to sensitization
3	6	Yes	Delayed reaction on first transfusion. Accelerated removal of red blood cells; no haemolysis
4	98	No	No reaction on first transfusion
5	23	Yes	Delayed reaction on first transfusion. Accelerated removal of red blood cells; no haemolysis
6	98–99	No	Unknown
7	45	Yes	Delayed reaction on first transfusion. Accelerated removal of red blood cells; no haemolysis
8	40	No	Unknown

* Dog erythrocyte antigen.

is particularly important in cats which, unlike dogs, have naturally occurring antibodies against other blood types which can cause life-threatening transfusion reactions in mismatched transfusions (Griot-Wenk and Giger, 1995; Tables 4.6 and 4.7). Animals kept as donors should probably be blood-typed. The release of new blood group cards (RapidVet-H, DMS Laboratories, Flemington, NJ, USA) has made blood-typing easy and requires only drops of blood. Blood-typing may also be important in animals kept for breeding, in order to prevent neonatal isoerythrolysis – again, particularly important in cats.

Alloantibodies can be transferred via colostrum up to 16 hours after birth and all type-B (and to a much lesser degree, type-A) kittens develop alloantibodies at a few weeks of age.

Table 4.7 Blood types of cats (modified from Griot-Wenk and Giger, 1995)

Blood type	Comment
A	Most common Have high anti-B titres Accounts for 95–99.7% of domestic short- and long-haired cats in the USA, 74% in Australia and 85–100% in the UK and Europe All Siamese cats and related breeds (Burmese, Tonkinese, Russian Blue) are type A
B	Uncommon but not rare Have high anti-A titres Frequency varies in selected breeds; 1–10% in Maine Coon and Norwegian Forest; 11–20% in Abyssinian, Birman, Persian, Somali, Sphinx and Scottish fold cats; 20–45% in exotic and British shorthair cats, Cornish and Devon rex
AB	Rare Have no anti-A or anti-B antibodies Found in domestic shorthair, Abyssinian, Birman, British shorthair, Norwegian Forest, Persian, Scottish fold and Somali breeds

Thus, cats do not need to be sensitized by a prior blood transfusion or pregnancy to develop alloantibodies and adverse reactions can occur with the first transfusion or in kittens from a primiparous queen (Griot-Wenk and Giger, 1995). Type-A kittens from a type-B queen and a type-A male are susceptible. In dogs, if a dog erythrocyte antigen (DEA) 1.1-negative bitch is bred to a DEA 1.1-positive male, she may produce DEA 1.1-positive puppies. If this occurs or the bitch has had a red cell transfusion and is sensitized to DEA 1.1, antibody to DEA 1.1 is transferred via the colostrum. The puppies, normal at birth, may show immune-mediated haemolytic anaemia 3–10 days after birth (Hale, 1995).

Cross-matching procedures

In addition to blood-typing in-house donor dogs and cats, cross-matching donor and recipient blood should be performed if possible. Incompatibilities revealed by cross-matching indicate earlier sensitization of the recipient (dogs) or naturally occurring isoantibodies (particularly important in cats). Puppies and kittens needing repeated transfusions should be given blood from donors with which they are cross-match-compatible.

Cross-matching is performed for major and minor compatibilities (Turnwald and Pichler, 1985). The major cross-match, performed with donor cells and recipient serum, determines whether the recipient has antibodies against donor cells. The minor cross-match, using recipient cells and donor serum, detects antibodies in donor serum against recipient cells and is of much less significance. Both tests are performed on fresh blood because anti-DEA antibodies fix complement. Blood transfusions should be of major compatibility.

Blood samples (5 ml) are collected from donor and recipient animals and allowed to clot. After centrifugation, the serum is withdrawn and placed in separate tubes. The clots are then gently broken down, and 0.3 ml of cells is aspirated from each sample and added to separate tubes, each containing 9.7 ml of normal saline solution. Cells should be washed at least once with the saline solution to remove plasma and prevent formation of small fibrin clots. After washing, supernatant is discarded and cells are resuspended to a dilution of 0.3 ml of cells to 9.7 ml of normal saline solution. The major cross-match is performed by adding 0.1 ml of recipient serum to 0.1 ml of donor red cell suspension. The minor cross-match is performed by adding 0.1 ml of donor serum to 0.1 ml of recipient red cell suspension. A control reaction is performed using recipient's serum and washed cells. Each test is done in triplicate and incubated for 15 minutes – one set at 37° C (98.6° F), one set at room temperature, and one set at 4° C (39.2° F). Incubation at various temperatures is necessary because incompatibility reactions can occur over a range of temperatures (Turnwald and Pichler, 1985).

Following incubation, each tube is centrifuged for 1 minute at 280 g and the supernatant is examined for haemolysis. The tubes are then gently tapped to check for agglutination. Compatible cross-matches do not show agglutination or haemolysis. If overt agglutination is not noted, a small amount of the suspended material is transferred to a clean glass slide and microscopically examined at low power. Any degree of agglutination or haemolysis in the major cross-match is considered an indication of incompatibility, and transfusion should not be performed. If slight agglutination or haemolysis is detected in the minor cross-match, transfusion can be performed on an emergency basis (Turnwald and Pichler, 1985).

Blood component administration

Stored blood components should be warmed to room temperature prior to administration to prevent inducing hypothermia in the recipient. To be warmed before administration, blood components can be passed through coils of transfusion tubing immersed in a water bath maintained at 37–38° C. Alternatively, a blood component container can be placed in a water bath or dry incubator maintained at that temperature or frozen plasma can be warmed slowly in a conventional microwave oven (Hurst *et al.*, 1987). Excessive heat should not be used to accelerate blood-component warming because fibrinogen precipitates at 50° C (122° F) and autoagglutination occurs when temperatures exceed 45° C (113° F).

If blood components have been opened or entered with a needle or warmed to 10° C (50° F) or more, the container should be given within 4 hours to reduce the possibility of bacterial growth (Cotter, 1988). Warmed blood components should not be returned to storage.

Microwave thawing of frozen plasma has been described (Hurst *et al.*, 1987) but has come under more recent scrutiny as to its effect on the plasma proteins. Warm-water baths for thawing plasma are preferred.

Appropriate filters and administration sets should be used when blood components are transfused. Filters are designed to retain blood clots and leukocyte/platelet aggregates, since pulmonary microembolism is a potential complication following transfusion of blood component. Most transfusions of blood components require the 170-size filter. Blood in a syringe also can be given through a standard blood infusion set or an infusion set with side-arm Luer connector for a syringe.

Blood components can be given intravenously to large puppies by the cephalic or external jugular veins through a 20-gauge indwelling catheter. Smaller puppies and large kittens can be infused by cephalic or external jugular veins using a 22-gauge indwelling catheter. Young puppies and kittens can be transfused by cephalic or external jugular veins using 23-gauge infusion sets. To reduce viscosity when using a small-bore needle, blood components can be mixed with normal saline solution before and during infusion. The use of fluid solutions other than normal saline solution is not recommended. Hypothermic, dehydrated puppies and kittens (younger than 3 months of age), in which venepuncture is often impossible, can be transfused by the intraosseous route. Absorption of the infused blood components is rapid – approximately 95% within 5 minutes (Clark and Woodley, 1959; Corley, 1963).

Before the infusion of blood components, baseline values on the recipient should be obtained, such as body weight and temperature, pulse and respiratory rate, mucous membrane colour, packed cell volume and total plasma protein concentration. An initial infusion rate of 0.25 ml/kg body weight is given over a 30-minute period, during which the recipient should be carefully watched for transfusion reactions (Turnwald and Pichler, 1985). With a slow initial infusion rate, a minimal amount of incompatible blood component is administered in the event that an incompatible recipient displays an immediate reaction. If no problems appear in the recipient after the initial 30-minute period, the rate of infusion can be increased. This is not an acceptable practice for type-B cats since even 1 ml of incompatible type-A blood can cause death. Cats of high-risk breeds for type-B blood should be blood-typed.

The required volume of blood should be infused over 3–4 hours. This guideline should be flexible because the infusion rate depends on the physical condition and hydration status of the recipient. With a hypovolaemic recipient, up to 22 ml/kg per hour is acceptable. Circulatory overload, a continuing problem in normovolaemic recipients, may be compounded in a recipient with cardiac or renal failure. Puppies or kittens in cardiac failure may not tolerate infusion rates exceeding 4 ml/kg per hour (Authement *et al.*, 1987).

The amount of whole blood necessary for infusion can be estimated. A simple guideline is that 2.2 ml/kg of whole blood raises the packed cell volume by 1% when the volume of the transfused blood is 40%. Packed red blood cells (packed cell volume 60–80%) are infused into the recipient in the same manner as whole blood. Packed red cells should be diluted prior to infusion. Normal saline solution is added at a dose of 0.5–1.0 ml/ml of packed red blood cells. The amount of normal saline solution to be added for infusion can vary with the recipient's circulatory function and hydration status.

If fresh plasma, fresh-frozen plasma or frozen plasma is being administered for active bleeding due to clotting factor deficiencies, a suggested dose is 6–10 ml/kg body weight two or three times a day for 3–5 days, or until bleeding is controlled (Authement *et al.*, 1987).

Complications of blood component therapy

Although complications of blood component transfusions are relatively rare in puppies and kittens, they do occur. Haemolytic reactions result from incompatible red blood cells given to a recipient that has developed antibodies from prior sensitization or transfusion. Type B cats generally have strong preformed anti-A antibodies and can react by haemolysis to the first transfusion. Most haemolytic reactions in puppies are delayed and are evident only as a shortened red blood cell survival after transfusion and the development of a positive direct

Coombs test. Haemolysis can also occur from overheating or freezing of blood components, concurrent administration of hypotonic solutions, mechanical damage of red blood cells from faulty equipment during collection, storage and administration, or infusion under pressure through a small-bore needle/catheter or a plugged filter.

Adverse effects of leukocytic, platelet and plasma protein incompatibility may include fever, neurological signs, vomiting and urticaria. Pretreatment with oral diphenhydramine hydrochloride at 4 mg/kg body weight 20–30 minutes prior to transfusion may reduce these reactions. If these reactions are evident during the transfusion, the infusion rate should be slowed and intramuscular diphenhydramine hydrochloride at 2 mg/kg body weight be administered if necessary (Turnwald and Pichler, 1985). Febrile reactions to infused blood components occur occasionally and are usually mild. Septic reactions are very rare if aseptic collection, proper storage and administration are used.

Antimicrobial therapy

Meaningful advances in the treatment of bacterial infections have been made in recent years, particularly in the development of new antibiotics. Many of these antibiotics have either an increased spectrum of activity or a diminished toxicity in comparison with previously available antibiotics (Dow and Papich, 1991). However, specific pharmacokinetic data for many of the new antibiotics have not been obtained in puppies and kittens, and therefore the use of these antibiotics remains somewhat empiric (Boothe and Tannert, 1992).

The β-lactam antibiotics are the first-choice drugs in the treatment of bacterial infections in puppies and kittens. This group includes the penicillins, cephalosporins, and the combination of β-lactam antibiotics and β-lactamase inhibitors (Tables 4.8 and 4.9). The β-lactam antibiotics act by inhibiting a series of bacterial enzymes necessary for cell wall synthesis (Goldberg, 1987; Kilgore, 1989). The spectrum of activity of β-lactam antibiotics is widely varied.

Drug distribution in puppies and kittens, especially those younger than 5 weeks, differs from that in adults because of differences in body composition – i.e. less total body fat, higher percentage of total body water, lower concentrations of albumin and poorly developed blood–brain barrier (Boothe and Tannert, 1992). Because of this, modifications to dosing amounts used for adult dogs and cats – as much as 30–50% reduction of the adult dose – or changes in dosing frequency may be necessary when antibiotics are administered to bacteraemic puppies and kittens.

These antibiotics should be administered intravenously or intraosseously, because systemic absorption following oral, subcutaneous or intramuscular administration may not be as reliable. Most drugs ingested by the lactating mother appear in her milk; the amount is generally 1–2% of the mother's dose.

Penicillins

Amoxycillin and ampicillin are clinically effective as broad-spectrum antibiotics, although they are sensitive to the β-lactamase enzymes. The new penicillins (ticarcillin, azlocillin, piperacillin, mezlocillin and carbenicillin) are ampicillin derivatives that have much greater activity against Gram-negative bacilli, especially *Pseudomonas aeruginosa*, than either ampicillin or amoxycillin alone (Lloyd and Martin, 1982;

Table 4.8 Dosage and route of administration for selected newer antibiotics

Antibiotics	Dose (mg/kg)*	Interval (hours)	Route
Amoxycillin clavulan	13.75	12	PO
Ampicillin–sulbactam	20	6–8	IV, IO
Imipenem/cilastatin	2–5	8	IV, IM, IO
Ticarcillin	40–75	6–8	IV, IM, IO
Ticarcillin/clavulanate	30–50	6–8	IV, IO

* These dosages are intended for adult dogs and cats and should be reduced by 30–50% for use in puppies and kittens.
PO = Oral; IV = intravenous; IO = intraosseous; IM = intramuscular administration.

Table 4.9 Dosage and route of administration for commonly administered cephalosporins

Antibiotics	Dose (mg/kg)*	Interval (hours)	Route
First-generation			
Cefazolin	10–30	6–8	IM, IV, IO
Second-generation			
Cefoxitin	10–20	6–8	IM, IV, IO
Cefotetan	10–20	6–8	IM, IV, IO
Third-generation			
Cefotaxime	25–50	6–8	IM, IV, IO
Ceftriaxone	25–50	12	IM, IV, IO
Ceftazidime	25–50	8–12	IM, IV, IO

* These dosages are intended for adult dogs and cats and should be reduced by 30–50% for use in puppies and kittens.
IM = intramuscular; IV = intravenous; IO = intraosseous administration; SC administration is not recommended due to unreliable absorption.

Prince and Neu, 1983; Tilmant, 1985). These antibiotics also inhibit *Escherichia coli* and some *Enterobacter*, *Salmonella* and *Serratia* spp. However, their antianaerobic activity is only moderate. Piperacillin and azlocillin are the penicillins most active against *P. aeruginosa in vitro*, although the other new penicillins appear to be clinically equivalent.

Both carbenicillin and ticarcillin act synergistically with aminoglycosides against *Pseudomonas* and some Enterobacteriaceae (Parry, 1987). The new penicillins inactivate the aminoglycosides in solution, so a new penicillin and an aminoglycoside should not be mixed in the same container. Neither carbenicillin nor ticarcillin is absorbed orally, but high serum concentrations occur after intravenous or intramuscular injection (Simmons and Keefe, 1983). Both antibiotics are excreted primarily by tubular resorption in humans, and 80% of the agent appears unchanged in the urine. Dosages should be reduced in animals with renal failure and in septicaemic puppies and kittens.

β-lactamase inhibitors

Ampicillin–sulbactam, ticarcillin/clavulanate and amoxicillin clavulanate combine β-lactam antibiotics with β-lactamase inhibitors (Table 4.8). Combination products improve the β-lactam antibiotics' effectiveness towards *E. coli*, *Klebsiella* spp., and some *Proteus* spp., but not towards *Pseudomonas* spp. (Simmons

and Keefe, 1983; Kilgore, 1989). Amoxycillin–clavulanic acid combination is especially useful for an amoxycillin-resistant *E. coli* urinary tract infection, and ampicillin–sulbactam combination is effective against many ampicillin-resistant isolates of *Pasteurella multocida* and *P. haemolytica*. Ticarcillin–clavulanic acid combination is also effective in Gram-negative bacilli and anaerobic infections.

Carbapenem

Imipenem cilastatin is a new carbapenem. Imipenem is combined with cilastatin to block the degradation of imipenem in the renal tubules. This combination has a broad spectrum of activity, including Gram-positive cocci, Gram-negative bacilli, Gram-negative aerobes and anaerobes. Imipenem cilastatin is useful as initial therapy for sepsis and intra-abdominal infections, which are caused by a wide variety of bacteria. The antibiotic is effective in treating animals who have osteomyelitis, complicated urinary tract infections or lower respiratory tract infections or are febrile and neutropenic. It penetrates the cerebrospinal fluid poorly.

Cephalosporins

The cephalosporins used most commonly in veterinary practices now are the first-, second-

and third-generation cephalosporins (Table 4.9). The first-generation cephalosporins are most active against Gram-positive bacteria, especially *Staphylococci* spp., and some Gram-negative bacteria such as *E. coli*, *Klebsiella pneumoniae* and *Proteus* spp. (Riviere, 1989). Second-generation cephalosporins are more active than first-generation cephalosporins against Gram-negative bacteria (*E. coli*, *Enterobacter*, *Proteus* and *Klebsiella* spp.) and can, in some situations, be substituted for potentially nephrotoxic aminoglycosides (Goldberg, 1987). Most anaerobic bacteria are susceptible to second-generation cephalosporins. As with first-generation cephalosporins, these antibiotics do not reach effective concentrations in cerebro-spinal fluid.

The third-generation cephalosporins are generally reserved primarily for serious infections caused by resistant strains of Gram-negative bacteria, especially bacteria of the Enterobacteriaceae family, e.g. *E. coli*, *Enterobacter*, *Serratia*, *Klebsiella* and *Citrobacter* spp. and most anaerobic bacteria (McElroy *et al.*, 1986; Riviere, 1989). Their activity is accompanied by diminished activity against Gram-positive infections. They are able to achieve therapeutic cerebrospinal concentrations. Therefore, third-generation cephalosporins are excellent first choices for the treatment of severely septicaemic puppies and kittens.

The major disadvantages of the cephalosporins include the lack of specific dosing regimens in puppies and kittens 2–16 weeks of age and, in most cases, the necessity of intravenous or intraosseous administration. The cephalosporins are a relatively non-toxic group of antibiotics. Adverse effects reported include coagulopathies and bleeding that is vitamin K_1-responsive, urticaria, anaphylaxis, immune-mediated reactions such as haemolytic anaemia, leukopenia, thrombocytopenia and positive Coombs antiglobulin tests, gastrointestinal side-effects (vomiting, diarrhoea, anorexia) and abnormal liver and renal function tests (Fekety, 1990).

Aminoglycosides

The risks of using aminoglycosides – neomycin, streptomycin, kanamycin, amikacin, gentamicin, tobramycin and netilmicin – in puppies and kittens 4–16 weeks of age may outweigh the benefit of these agents. The spectrum of activity of aminoglycosides includes many aerobic Gram-negative bacteria, especially *E. coli*, *Klebsiella pneumoniae*, *Pseudomonas aeruginosa*, *Proteus* spp. and *Serratia* spp. Since aminoglycosides frequently cause nephrotoxicity, the nephrotoxicity may be minimized by using the least nephrotoxic drug, i.e. amikacin rather than gentamicin, ensuring the puppy's or kitten's hydration status is normal, lengthening the dosing interval and using combination therapy with synergistic antibiotics when indicated for serious infections (Boothe and Tannert, 1992).

Potentiated sulphonamides

The Gram-positive and Gram-negative spectrum of the combination of sulphonamides with trimethoprim or ormetoprim is broad, including *E. coli*, some *Salmonella* spp., and other Gram-negative bacteria. Most potentiated sulphonamides have a wide margin of safety, but their dosage and dosing intervals should be modified in puppies and kittens 4–16 weeks of age because of a prolonged half-life, resulting from decreased metabolism by the liver and decreased renal excretion (Boothe and Tannert, 1992).

Modified tetracyclines

Tetracyclines are broad-spectrum bacteriostatic antibiotics that inhibit bacterial protein synthesis by blocking transfer RNA from binding to the ribosomal complex (Aronson, 1980). Minocycline and doxycycline are much more lipid-soluble than the parent tetracycline (Aronson, 1980; Shaw and Rubin, 1986). Gastrointestinal absorption of the tetracyclines is greatly reduced by the presence of dairy products and by divalent and trivalent cations (e.g. in magnesium-containing antacids). Minocycline and doxycycline are more active than tetracycline against anaerobic bacteria, some facultative anaerobes and intracellular parasites and bacteria. Minocycline is more active than other tetracyclines against *Nocardia* spp. and *Staphylococcus aureus*.

All tetracyclines, except doxycycline, should be used cautiously in animals with renal failure and in septicaemic puppies and kittens.

Doxycycline, in contrast, is excreted primarily in the intestine, so the dose does not have to be reduced for animals with renal failure. Doxycycline has a much longer elimination half-life than tetracycline, which allows the dosage interval to be extended beyond that for tetracycline administration to once or twice daily (Shaw and Rubin, 1986). Minocycline and doxycycline each undergoes some enterohepatic recirculation, and 10% of non-metabolized minocycline is excreted in urine. Tetracyclines administered to septicaemic puppies and kittens may alter enamel formation, causing discoloured teeth. The potential for causing discoloured teeth is a good reason for not routinely using tetracyclines in the treatment of ill puppies and kittens.

Quinolones

The quinolones (ofloxacin, ciprofloxacin, pefloxacin, enrofloxacin and norfloxacin) possess an extremely good spectrum of activity against Gram-negative bacteria, yet are associated with minimal toxicity. The mechanism of action of these antibiotics is by inhibition of DNA synthesis (Talley, 1991). Their spectrum of activity includes most Gram-negative bacteria, particularly *E. coli*, *Klebsiella* spp., *Enterobacter* spp., *Proteus mirabilis*, *Pseudomonas aeruginosa*, *Citrobacter* spp. and *Serratia marcescens*. They are ineffective against *Streptococcus* spp. and anaerobic bacteria (Talley, 1991).

The quinolones are generally rapidly and well-absorbed from the gastrointestinal tract. However, food does inhibit their absorption, and they should be dosed an hour before or 2 h after a meal. After absorption, they are well-distributed to almost all body tissues, including bone, prostate gland, bile and urine (Talley, 1991). Toxicity includes hypersensitivity reactions, seizures, erosion of articular cartilages in growing puppies and kittens and crystalluria which necessitates adequate hydration. Because of their limited spectrum of activity against *Streptococcus* spp. and anaerobes, enrofloxacin is probably not the first choice of antibiotic agents to be used in any septicaemic puppy and kitten. The risk of cartilage erosion should be emphasized and the quinolones should not be considered in a protocol requiring repeated administration.

Supportive care

In most instances, puppies and kittens suspected of having a severe illness that may often be fatal require immediate critical care management. A summary outline of an approach to the management of such puppies and kittens is presented in Table 4.10.

Table 4.10 Revision of external re-warming procedure

External re-warming procedure

1. Place animal in an incubator if available
2. Alternatively, use a re-warming device such as circulating hot-water blanket and cover animal with a light, insulating (space) blanket
3. Keep peripheral limbs warm. Peripheral warming is more efficient at elevating and maintaining core body temperature than covering the trunk only (Cabell *et al.*, 1997)
4. Take at least 20–30 minutes for gradual re-warming of the animal
5. Keep the animal sternal if possible; alternatively turn the animal every 30–60 minutes
6. Record rectal temperature every 30 minutes until normal

Parenteral fluid therapy

---

1. Use multiple electrolyte solution supplemented with 5% dextrose solution
2. Supplement the fluids with potassium chloride solution if plasma potassium concentration is less than 2.5 mEq/l
3. Administer warm fluids slowly by intravenous or intraosseous route

Table 4.10 (continued)

Glucose replacement therapy

---

1. Administer 5% dextrose solution intravenously or intraosseously, slowly to effect
2. Administer 1–2 ml/kg of a 10% dextrose solution to an animal that is profoundly depressed or having seizures
3. Maintain plasma glucose concentration at 80–200 mg/dl for euglycaemia

---

Antibiotic therapy

---

1. Collect bacterial culture samples (whole blood, urine, exudate, faeces) before initiation of antibiotic therapy
2. For blood culture, collect 1 ml of whole blood aseptically and inoculate blood directly into enriched tryptic or trypticase soy broth; dilute the whole blood 1:5–1:10 in enriched broth, and examine broth for bacterial growth 6–18 hours later
3. For urine culture, collect urine by cystocentesis and culture it by standard methods
4. For exudate and faecal cultures, collect and culture by standard methods
5. Begin empirical treatment with antibiotic agents immediately after collection of appropriate bacterial culture samples
6. Adjust the dose and dosing interval of antibiotic selected
7. Administer the antibiotic by the intravenous or intraosseous route

---

Oxygen and nutritional therapy

---

1. Administer oxygen by mask or intranasal catheter to counteract tissue hypoxaemia
2. Encourage food intake once patient is normothermic and adequately hydrated
3. Monitor the effectiveness of medical management
4. Observe the animal for improvement in general demeanour
5. Regularly assess the cardiopulmonary status (it is extremely easy to overhydrate the ill puppy and kitten, so attentive monitoring of breathing pattern helps in early recognition of overhydration)
6. Weigh the animal 3–4 times a day to record weight gain
7. Look for moistness of mucous membranes in assessing the animal's hydration status

---

References

Aronson, A.L. (1980) Pharmacotherapeutics of the new tetracyclines. *Journal of American Veterinary Medical Association*, **176**, 1061–1068.

Authement, J.M., Wolfsheimer, K.J. and Catchings, S. (1987) Canine blood component therapy: product preparation, storage, and administration. *Journal of American Animal Hospital Association*, **23**, 483–493.

Baines, F.M. (1981) Milk substitutes and the hand rearing of orphan puppies and kittens. *Journal of Small Animal Practice*, **22**, 555–578.

Bjorck, G. (1982) Care and feeding of the puppy in the postnatal and weaning period. In: Bjorck, G. (ed.) *Nutrition and Behavior in Dogs and Cats*, New York: Pergamon Press.

Boothe, D.M. and Tannert, K. (1992) Special considerations for drug and fluid therapy in the pediatric patient. *Compendium of Continuing Education for the Practicing Veterinarian*, **14**, 313–329.

Bucheler, J. and Cotter, S.M. (1993) Setting up a feline blood donor program. *Veterinary Medicine*, **88**, 838–845.

Cabell, L.W., Perkowski, S.Z., Gregor, T. and Smith, G.K. (1997) The effects of active peripheral skin warming on perioperative hypothermia in dogs. *Veterinary Surgery*, **26**, 79–85.

Corley, E.A. (1963) Intramedullary transfusion in small animals. *Journal of American Veterinary Medical Association*, **142**, 1005–1006.

Cornelius, L.M., Finco, D.R. and Culver, D.H. (1978) Physiologic effects of rapid infusion of Ringer's lactate solution into dogs. *American Journal of Veterinary Research*, **39**, 1185–1190.

Cotter, S.M. (1988) Blood banking I: Collection and storage. In: *American College Veterinary Internal Medicine Forum*, vol. 6. pp. 45–47.

Cullison, R.F., Menard, P.D. and Buck, W.B. (1983) Toxicosis in cats from the use of benzyl alcohol in lactated Ringer's solution. *Journal of American Veterinary Medical Association*, **182**, 61.

DiBartola, S.P. (1992) Introduction to fluid therapy. In: DiBartola, S.P. (ed.) *Fluid Therapy in Small Animal Practice*, pp. 321–340. Philadelphia: WB Saunders.

Dow, S.W. and Papich, M.G. (1991) Keeping current on developments in antimicrobial therapy. *Veterinary Medicine*, **86**, 600–604.

Fekety, F.R. (1990) Safety of parenteral third-generation cephalosporins. *American Journal Medicine*, **88 (suppl 4A)**, 38S–44S.

Goldberg, D.M. (1987) The cephalosporins. *Medical Clinics of North America*, **71**, 1113–1133.

Griot-Wenk, M.E. and Giger, U. (1995) Feline transfusion medicine. *Veterinary Clinics of North America [Small Animal Practice]*, **25**, 1305–1322.

Hale, A. (1995) Canine blood groups and their importance in veterinary transfusion medicine. *Veterinary Clinics of North American [Small Animal Practice]*, **25**, 1323–1332.

Hurst, T.S., Turrentine, M.A. and Johnson, G.S. (1987) Evaluation of microwave thawed canine plasma for transfusion. *Journal of American Veterinary Medical Association*, **190**, 863–865.

Kilgore, W.R. (1989) Clavulanate-potentiated antibiotics. In: Kirk, R.W. (ed.) *Current Veterinary Therapy X*, pp. 78–81. Philadelphia: WB Saunders.

Lewis, L.D., Morris, M.L.J. and Hand, M.S. (1987) *Small Animal Clinical Nutrition III*. Topeka, KS: Mark Morris Associates.

Lloyd, C.W. and Martin, W.J. (1982) A review of the new penicillins: azlocillin, mezlocillin and piperacillin. *American Journal of Intravenous Therapy and Clinical Nutrition*, **22**, 9.

McElroy, D., Ravis, W.R. and Clark, C.H. (1986) Pharmacokinetics of cefotaxime in the domestic cat. *American Journal of Intravenous Therapy and Clinical Nutrition*, **47**, 86–88.

Otto, C.M., Kaufman, G.M. and Crowe, D.T. (1989) Intraosseous infusion of fluids and therapeutics. *Compendium of Continuing Education for the Practicing Veterinarian*, **11**, 421–431.

Parry, M.F. (1987) The penicillins. *Medical Clinics of North America*, **71**, 1093–1112.

Prince, A.S. and Neu, H.C. (1983) New penicillins and their use in pediatrics. *Pediatric Clinics of North America*, **30**, 3–16.

Remillard, R.L., Pickett, J.P., Thatcher, C.D. and Davenport, D.J. (1993) Comparison of kittens fed queen's milk with those fed milker replacers. *American Journal of Veterinary Research*, **54**, 901–907.

Riviere, J.E. (1989) Cephalosporins. In: Kirk, R.W. (ed.) *Current Veterinary Therapy X*, pp. 74–77. Philadelphia: WB Saunders.

Schneider, A. (1995) Blood components: collection, processing, and storage. *Veterinary Clinics of North America [Small Animal Practice]*, **25**, 1245–1261.

Shaw, D.H. and Rubin, S.I. (1986) Pharmacologic activity of doxycycline. *Journal of American Veterinary Medical Association*, **189**, 808–810.

Sheffy, B.E. (1978) Nutrition and nutritional disorders. *Veterinary Clinics of North America [Small Animal Practice]*, **8**, 7–29.

Simmons, R.D. and Keefe, T.J. (1983) Penicillins: an expanding spectrum. *Modern Veterinary Practice*, **1**, 49–54.

Talley, J.H. (1991) Fluoroquinolones. *Postgraduate Medicine*, **89**, 101–113.

Tilmant, L. (1985) Pharmacokinetics of ticarcillin in the dog. *American Journal of Veterinary Research*, **46**, 479–481.

Turnwald, G.H. and Pichler, M.E. (1985) Blood transfusion in dogs and cats. Part II. Administration, adverse effects, and component therapy. *Compendium of Continuing Education for the Practicing Veterinarian*, **7**, 115–125.

5

General surgical principles

General considerations

It is difficult to separate anaesthetic and surgical considerations as most concerns regarding surgery on a puppy or kitten should be contemplated in the preoperative and anaesthetic planning. Probably the biggest concern specific to surgery on the puppies and kittens is duration of surgery. By taking measures to reduce the duration of surgery, morbidity can be reduced, particularly that associated with hypothermia (Hosgood, 1995). The efficiency of the surgical process should be maximized at all times (Table 5.1).

Skin preparation should be performed quickly, again to minimize the duration of anaesthesia. Avoid using alcohol since it evaporates very quickly from the skin and has a cooling effect, exacerbating hypothermia. Avoid getting other parts of the animal wet. Warm chlorhexidine solution is the preparation of choice since it has prolonged residual activity, is effective against Gram-positive and Gram-negative organisms, is effective in the presence of organic matter and does not irritate the skin. It can be removed between scrubs with normal saline solution but a final residual film is left on the skin.

Table 5.1 Concepts to improve efficiency during surgery in puppies and kittens

Concept	Comment
Clip the surgical site immediately prior to anaesthetic induction	Useful in the cooperative or premedicated animal Do not clip the day before surgery; since microlacerations of the skin may increase the risk of surgical site contamination
Intravenous catheter placement	Always place a venous catheter. This preserves the integrity of the vein and provides ready access should a complication develop Have catheter placed, if possible, before the animal is anaesthetized to reduce duration of anaesthesia, regardless of whether an injectable induction protocol is used
Surgical planning	Be familiar with procedure Know the anatomy Select the best approach to facilitate exposure and uninhibited progress Have the appropriate equipment sterilized and readily accessible Be prepared for problems and have contingency plans formalized
Suture material	Have appropriate suture material selected and readily available Have appropriate staplers (and staples) available if they can be used
Haemorrhage	Have access to radiosurgery or electrosurgery if at all possible Have blood collected prior to surgery if blood loss is anticipated Have personnel available to collect blood from donors if needed

Perioperative antimicrobial therapy

The perioperative period is that period around surgery, loosely defined as the time immediately prior to anaesthesia induction to several hours postoperative. The considerations for use of perioperative antimicrobials in puppies and kittens are similar to those in adult animals and are usually based on the classification of the surgical procedure, the duration of surgery and the health of the animal (Table 5.2). Antimicrobials should not be used as a replacement for poor aseptic technique. For invasive surgical procedures with the potential for development of infection after surgery, perioperative administration of antimicrobials should be considered. Perioperative antimicrobial administration requires that an antimicrobial is administered immediately prior to surgery to allow effective blood levels to be present at the time of contamination. If the surgery lasts more than 90 min, antimicrobials are administered every half-life of the drug for the duration of the surgery, and for one or two more doses after the surgery (no more than 24 hours postoperative). Antimicrobials administered beyond 6 hours postoperative show limited benefit in preventing surgical infection. Administration of antimicrobials after this time would be considered antimicrobial treatment, only indicated if infection (as opposed to contamination) is present.

Consideration of the type of bacterial contamination that may occur or the infective agent present should be made such that a narrow-spectrum antimicrobial can be selected. Typically, contamination from the skin and

Table 5.2 Indications for use of perioperative antimicrobials in puppies and kittens

Condition	Comment
Clean surgical procedure	An elective procedure in which the respiratory, gastrointestinal and urogenital tracts are not entered. No drains are placed, no trauma, no inflammation or break in aseptic technique, e.g. tail amputation, excision of skin tumour, castration. Minimal risk for infection of the surgery site. Perioperative antimicrobials are not indicated
Clean-contaminated procedure	A procedure in which the respiratory, gastrointestinal and urogenital tracts are entered in a controlled manner without unusual contamination of surrounding tissues. An otherwise clean procedure is converted to a clean-contaminated procedure if a drain is placed, e.g. cystotomy, enterotomy, routine ovariohysterectomy. Minimal risk for infection of the surgery site. Perioperative antimicrobials are not indicated unless the health of the animal is compromised
Contaminated procedure	A procedure involving acute traumatic wounds (< 6 hours old) or surgery in the presence of acute, non-purulent inflammation. Surgery is also classified as contaminated if there is gross spillage from the gastrointestinal tract, a major break in aseptic technique, penetration of the respiratory and urogenital tracts in the presence of infection. Considered high risk for infection of the surgery site, e.g. ovariohysterectomy for pyometra, intestinal anastomosis with spillage. Perioperative antimicrobials are indicated, even in the uncompromised animal
Dirty procedure	A procedure involving delayed treatment of traumatic wounds (> 6 hours old), surgery that encounters the presence of gastrointestinal contents, foreign bodies or purulent inflammation. Considered very high risk for infection of the surgery site and infection often already present. Perioperative antimicrobials and antimicrobial treatment postoperative are indicated
Surgery duration > 90 minutes	Procedures longer than 90 minutes are associated with increased risk of surgical contamination and consequently increased infection of the surgery site. Perioperative antimicrobials are indicated and should be administered every half-life of the drug during the surgery
Health	A normal, healthy animal undergoing an elective procedure using aseptic technique does not require perioperative antimicrobials. A sick animal undergoing a necessary procedure is less able to mount a host defence and is a candidate for receiving perioperative antimicrobials. A sick animal should not undergo an elective procedure

respiratory tracts results in the presence of Gram-positive organisms, contamination from the gastrointestinal tract results in the presence of Gram-negative and anaerobic organisms, and contamination from the urogenital tract can result in the presence of both Gram-positive and Gram-negative organisms. A narrow-spectrum agent should be selected because use of a broad-spectrum antimicrobial can cause the selection of resistant bacteria and kill normal resident microflora.

Because of the differences in drug absorption, distribution, metabolism and excretion between puppies and kittens and adult animals, the use of antimicrobials requires careful consideration and doses may have to be adjusted accordingly. Intramuscular absorption of drugs may be unreliable because of the small muscle mass and poor muscle blood supply in the puppy and kitten. Oral drug absorption is more reliable

but still inconsistent, and in fact, may result in higher blood concentrations in puppies and kittens than in adult animals. Intravenous or intraosseous administration gives the most reliable blood levels, although the dosages must be adjusted to compensate for delayed distribution, metabolism and excretion (Chapter 4).

Instrumentation and tissue handling

Great care is required when handling the delicate tissue of puppies and kittens. During pre-surgical clipping of the hair, skin should not be lacerated. Using appropriate-sized clipper blades will facilitate precise clipping. The use of paediatric surgical instruments facilitates proper tissue handling and they should be purchased if paediatric surgery is a large portion of your practice (Table 5.3; Fig. 5.1).

Table 5.3 Selected paediatric surgical instruments for addition to a general surgery pack

Instrument	Use/comment
$3\frac{1}{2}$-inch Backhaus towel clamps	Less traumatic and bulky than standard-sized towel clamps
5-inch Hartmann mosquito forceps (straight and curved)	
5-inch Micro mosquito forcep (curved, delicate)	
5-inch Metzenbaum scissors (straight, delicate)	Easier to use than standard-sized Metzenbaum scissors
5-inch Micro Adson tissue forceps (delicate)	Very fine-tipped atraumatic thumb forceps which grasp tissue more firmly than plain tissue forceps
5-inch Plain tissue forceps (delicate)	Fine-tipped atraumatic thumb forceps
6-inch DeBakey tissue forceps	Although long, they are very easy to use and cause minimal trauma associated with grasping tissue
$3\frac{3}{8}$-inch Bishop–Harmon thumb forceps (1 × 2 teeth, 0.5 mm)	Fine rat-toothed forceps useful for delicate tissue
$6\frac{1}{4}$-inch Mixter gallduct forceps or $7\frac{1}{2}$-inch Kantowitz thoracic forceps	Excellent for blunt dissection around delicate structures (e.g. patent ductus venosus, portosystemic shunt)
$5\frac{3}{4}$-inch Babcock forceps (paediatric)	Essential for any gastrointestinal surgery or urogenital surgery. Considered atraumatic in their use for grasping viscera
Bard–Parker tonsil scalpel handle, no. 7	Long-handled. Allows finer control than standard-sized scalpel handle
Derf needle holder	Smaller than standard-sized needle holders. Useful for suturing with 3-0 to 5-0 suture
Iris scissors	Very small, usually sharp-pointed scissors useful for controlled cutting of delicate tissue, e.g. vessels after ligation, ureters, urethra
Castroviejo needle holder ($5\frac{1}{2}$-inch)	Ophthalmic-type needle holder essential for use with suture material 5-0 and smaller
$3\frac{1}{2}$-inch spread paediatric Gosset abdominal retractor	Similar to a Balfour abdominal retractor but smaller size for animals less than 6 kg
$1\frac{3}{4}$-inch Barraquer eye speculum (10 or 15 mm blades)	Can be used as an abdominal retractor in very small animals less than 4 kg
Finochetto–DeBakey infant rib spreader	Essential for thoracic surgery

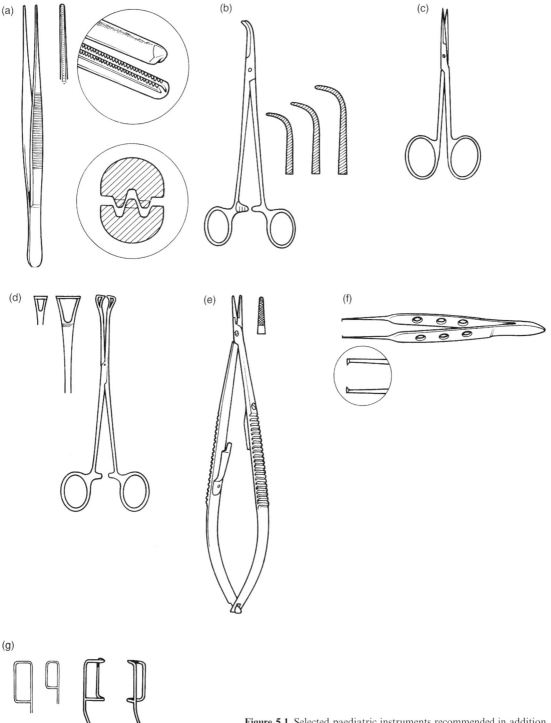

Figure 5.1 Selected paediatric instruments recommended in addition to a general surgical pack. (a) DeBakey's tissue forceps; (b) Mixter gallduct forceps; (c) Iris scissors; (d) Babcock paediatric tissue forceps; (e) Castroviejo needle holder; (f) Bishop–Harman thumb forceps; (g) Barhaquer eye speculum

The use of magnification will facilitate paediatric surgery. Head loupes offer the most practical and versatile magnification equipment. These can be mounted to the frame of eye glasses or on a headband and are usually hinged such that they can be lifted up out of the line of sight. Some companies can fit prescription lenses to the eye glasses. Most models come with a halogen or fibreoptic light that can be clipped to the loupe (Fig. 5.2) or to the headband if using the glasses-mounted loupe (Surgitel, General Scientific Corportation, Ann Arbor, MI 48103, USA; Orascoptic Dimension-3, Orascoptic Acuity, Orascoptic Research Inc., Madison, WI, USA). Generally, magnification between 2.0× and 3.5× is adequate. Magnification of 2.75× provides a field-of-view between 58 and 136 mm and a working distance between 250 and 553 mm. Magnification of 3.5× provides a field-of-view between 50 and 110 mm and a working distance between 252 and 512 mm.

Meticulous haemostasis is essential during surgery since a small volume of blood loss can represent a relatively large percentage of blood volume loss. Radiosurgery or electrosurgery may facilitate haemostasis but should be used appropriately. It is important to have the unit set correctly to the wave required, whether cutting, coagulation, cutting–coagulation or fulguration. Excessive use, high settings or use of a charr-covered electrode causes disseminated tissue damage and will delay wound healing. Use of a fine-tipped bipolar handpiece allows precise placement of the radiowave or current and avoids excessive tissue damage (Fucci and Elkins, 1991). Bleeding vessels that cannot be coagulated should be ligated using a fine, soft absorbable suture material, such as 4-0 or 5-0 polyglactin 910, poliglecaprone 25 or chromic cat gut. Haemostatic clips may be useful on small, fragile vessels to avoid tearing during hand ligation (see surgical staples).

Suture selection

Before selecting a suture material, the strength of the tissue, the rate of healing of the tissue and the physical condition of the animal should be considered (Smeak and Wendelburg, 1989). In the otherwise healthy animal, a rapid gain in wound strength is observed by 7 days postoperative. Healing of neonatal tissue is faster than adult tissue, with a more complex collagen structure and less inflammatory response. Most absorbable suture material provides adequate tensile strength during this period. Soft, non-irritating suture material, such as polyglactin 910 or poliglecaprone 25, is preferred. Poliglecaprone 25 is a new monofilament, absorbable suture that is more pliable than polydioxanone but still stiffer than polyglactin 910. In addition, it may be the preferred suture since its rate of absorption is moderate (completely absorbed by 91–119 days) compared with polyglactin 910 (60–90 days) and polydioxanone (180 days). Polydioxanone and poliglecaprone 25 have less tissue drag and better knot security than polyglactin 910 but the prolonged rate of absorption of polydioxanone compared to polyglactin 910 and poliglecaprone 25 make it less useful (Table 5.4). Use of polydioxanone may be desirable in debilitated animals where healing is delayed and it is preferable to use non-absorbable suture material such as polypropylene or nylon.

The development of suture sinuses is associated with the use of non-absorbable suture, whether monofilament or multifilament, far more often than with absorbable suture and the duration of a suture's presence in puppies and kittens should be factored into decision-making. Multifilament or coated non-absorbable suture materials such as polyester, silk or caprolactam should not be used in deep tissue and are only suitable for use in skin. Suture material of the smallest possible diameter should be used: 4-0 to 5-0 suture material is suitable for most tissues of very young animals less than 3 months, increasing to 3-0 to 4-0 suture material for older, larger animals 3–6 months of age. Suture patterns should be selected for their effectiveness and ease of placement. Continuous suture patterns in the linea alba

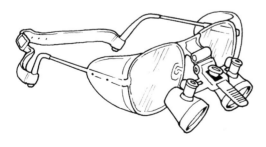

Figure 5.2 Head loupe for magnification during surgery.

Table 5.4 Properties of suture material and their indications for use in the puppies and kittens

Suture description	Suture type
A. Absorbable multifilament without prolonged absorption	Catgut (plain or chromic) Polyglactin 910 Polyglycolic acid
B. Absorbable monofilament without prolonged absorption	Poliglecaprone 25
C. Absorbable monofilament with prolonged absorption	Polydioxanone Polygluconate
D. Non-absorbable monofilament	Polypropylene Nylon Polybutester Stainless steel
E. Non-absorbable, coated, multifilament	Caprolactam Silk Polyester
F. Skin staples	

Patient status	Linea alba	Soft tissue	Skin
Healthy	A, B Catgut contraindicated due to unpredictable absorption	A, B Poliglecaprone 25 may be preferred due to monofilament nature, less tissue drag and less bacterial adherence	D, E, F Polyester contraindicated as poor knot security
Concurrent disease that delays wound healing	C	C	D, E, F Polyester contraindicated as poor knot security
Severely debilitated	C, D	C, D	D, E, F Polyester contraindicated as poor knot security

and skin are safe and help decrease operative time.

The skin of puppies and kittens is thin and delicate. Skin tension should be alleviated with a subcutaneous or subcuticular closure and, if apposition of the skin edges is achieved, skin sutures may not be required. This is desirable to avoid the dam or queen inadvertently chewing the sutures. If skin sutures are required, they should be loosely placed using very fine non-absorbable suture material such as 4-0 or 5-0 nylon. Tight sutures with small bites less than 2–3 mm from the skin edge may cause skin necrosis, especially if swelling occurs.

Surgical needles

Proper selection of surgical needles is critical since the needle can induce the most trauma associated with suturing. Use of swaged needles is essential. Selection of the smallest needle possible will minimize tissue trauma. Select a needle appropriate to the size of the suture; some small-gauge suture materials come on many different needles. Use of a cutting needle in dense tissue will minimize trauma associated with passing the needle through the tissue. If selecting a cutting needle, use of a reverse cutting needle, with the cutting edge on the convex

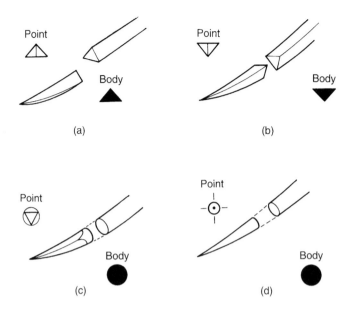

Figure 5.3 Conformation of cutting needles: (a) cutting needle; (b) reverse cutting needle; (c) tapered cutting needle; (d) tapered needle

or outer edge of the needle, will reduce the likelihood of tearing through the tissue (Fig. 5.3). These needles are stronger than the conventional cutting needle with the cutting edge on the concave or inside edge of the needle. Tapered cutting needles also minimize tissue trauma since they have a cutting point, either reverse or conventional, but a tapered body. These are useful in tissue that may have a dense and delicate component such as the gastrointestinal tract. Reverse cutting needles are applicable for use in the dermis, fascia, oral surgery and some intestinal surgery.

Surgical staples

Surgical stapling devices are available for use in gastrointestinal, parenchymatous organ and thoracic surgery (Table 5.1; Figs 5.4 and 5.5; Pavletic, 1990). The thoracoabdominal stapler is probably the most versatile stapling instrument. Fascial staples for closure of the linea alba are available but not suitable for most puppies and kittens, as the tissue thickness must be greater than 2 mm, generally – for dogs greater than 20 kg-body weight. Surgical stapling instruments are available as reusable instruments with disposable cartridges or as completely disposable units. Stapling instruments are extremely useful in puppies and kittens since they result in minimal tissue trauma, often result in a more secure method of closure than suturing and significantly shorten surgery time. These factors reduce morbidity and consequently, should not be considered cost-prohibitive. Skin staples substantially reduce the time required for skin closure and tend to discourage the animal or mother from licking the wound (Fig. 5.6). They require a special instrument to remove them.

Tissue adhesives

Tissue adhesives are cyanoacrylate polymers that are catalysed by minute amounts of water

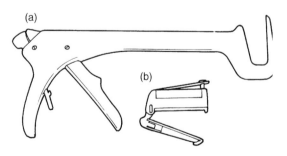

Figure 5.4 (a) Thoracoabdominal stapler and (b) cartridge.

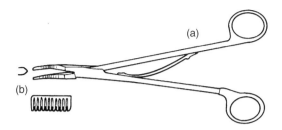

Figure 5.5 (a) Haemostatic staple applicator and (b) staples.

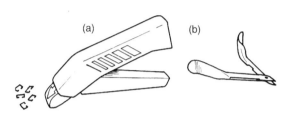

Figure 5.6 (a) Skin stapler and (b) remover.

on the wound surface. Shorter-chain derivatives (methyl and ethyl-cyanoacrylate) have proven histiotoxicity. These compounds are often the components of household 'super glues'. Longer-chain derivatives (butyl- and isobutyl-cyanoacrylate) are much less histiotoxic and are preferred (Hampel, 1991).

The cyanoacrylate polymer is self-sterilizing with a setting time between 2 and 60 seconds. The healing tissue cannot penetrate the cyanoacrylate and must advance around the polymer. Hence, meticulous use is required. The cut surfaces should be dry and free from blood; the cyanoacrylate should be spot-welded along the top of the cut edges and not placed directly on the cut surface. The amount of adhesive used should be minimized. Although the adhesive is relatively inert, granulomas, wound infection and delayed healing have been reported. Cyanoacrylate have been used in oral surgery, intestinal anastomoses, controlling haemorrhage from parenchymatous organs, microvascular anastomoses, fracture repair, prosthetic implant maintenance and skin graft placement.

Fibrin-based glues may provide additional mechanical strength in wounds in the lag phase of healing, that is, 0 to 3–5 days. These glues, as opposed to cyanoacrylate glues, are designed to be used as an adjunct to sutured (or stapled) closures, for example, to reduce the incidence of early leakage from intestinal anastomoses. Experimental and clinical evidence is still equivocal to date and this, along with their expense, may limit their application.

Wound protection and bandaging

Protection of the surgical incision from self-mutilation is imperative to avoid wound breakdown. In puppies and kittens that are not weaned, protection of the surgical incision from licking by the bitch or queen is extremely important. Keeping the incision covered with a bandage or separating the young from the mother, except for feeding, is necessary. In weaned puppies and kittens, protection of the incision through the use of an Elizabethan collar, either commercial or fashioned from cardboard or plastic, is preferred to bandaging to avoid bandaging complications. Inadvertent compression of the neck, thorax or abdomen can easily occur with circumferential bandages. Always use a three-layered bandage: a primary or contact layer, a secondary or padded layer and a tertiary or protective layer. Omitting the secondary padded layer may result in a tight bandage.

Tight bandages or bandages that do not extend far enough beyond the incision cause swelling proximal and distal to the bandage. If a limb requires bandaging, the entire limb should be incorporated in the bandage. Application of a surgical skin spray to the surgical incision will protect the uncovered surgical wound from moisture and contamination. In contrast to surgical incisions, open wounds obviously require bandage protection.

Suture removal

Suture removal in healthy puppies and kittens can be performed 7 days postoperative. In debilitated animals or when radiosurgery or electrosurgery had been used on the surgical wound margins, suture removal should be delayed to 10–14 days postoperative.

Table 5.5 Surgical stapling devices and indications for use

Stapling device	Size	Indications
Thoracoabdominal (TA)*	Staple lines of 90, 55 and 30 mm TA 30V3 (white, vascular) 3 mm wide, 1 mm compression TA 3.5 (blue) 3.5 mm wide, 1.5 mm compression TA 4.8 (green) 4.8 mm wide, 2.0 mm compression	Places two rows (or three rows for vascular staple); requires manual incision distal to staple line Most versatile stapler Complete and partial lung lobectomy Partial hepatectomy and splenectomy Intestinal anastomosis Partial gastrectomy
Gastrointestinal anastomosis (GIA*)	Staple lines of 50 and 90 mm	Places four rows of staples and automatically cuts between the rows Gastrointestinal anastomosis Excision of fluid-filled mass (pyometra, urachal cyst) Cholecystoduodenostomies Partial lung lobectomies
End-to-end anastomosis (EEA*)	Outer diameter cartridges of 31, 28 and 25 mm producing anastomoses with an internal diameter of 21, 18 and 15 mm, respectively	Places two rows of staples and automatically cuts on the outside of the staples Small and large intestinal anastomosis Oesophageal anastomosis Gastroduodenostomies
Ligate-and-divide staplers	Two sizes; compress to 7.3 mm wide and 5.33 mm wide with range of tissue compression from 1–2 mm thick to <1 mm thick	Places two staple ligations and automatically cuts between the two staples Procedures that require many ligatures (e.g. splenectomy)
Vascular staple units (Surgiclips*)	Available in three sizes: Small (yellow) – approximately 2 mm high before compression and 3 mm wide Medium (blue) – approximately 4 mm high before compression and 5 mm wide Medium-large (green) – approximately 6 mm high before compression and 8 mm wide Large (orange) – approximately 8 mm high before compression and 10 mm wide	Fire a single vascular staple
Skin staples (Precise Vista skin stapler† Autosuture‡)	Available in 12-, 25- and 35-staple cartridges Two sizes available: Regular with a 9.9 mm span prior to closure, 4.8 mm wide and 3.4 mm high when closed; Wide with a 11.98 mm span prior to closure, 6.5 mm wide and 3.6 mm high when closed	Disposable, quick, convenient and effective for closure of skin Partially used cartridges can be resterilized with ethylene oxide

*US Surgical Corporation Norwalk, CT
†3M, St Paul, MN
‡Pilling-Weck, Research Triangle Park, NC

References

Fucci, V. and Elkins, A.D. (1991) Electrosurgery: principles and guidelines in veterinary medicine. *Compendium of Continuing Education for the Practising Veterinarian*, **13**, 407–415.

Hampel, N. (1991) Effects of isobutyl-2-cyanoacrylate on skin healing. *Compendium of Continuing Education for the Practicing Veterinarian*, **13**, 80–83.

Hosgood, G. (1995) Anesthesia and surgical considerations. In: Hoskins, J.D. (ed.) *Veterinary Pediatrics: Dogs and Cats from Birth to Six Months*, pp. 561–575. Philadelphia: WB Saunders.

Pavletic, M.M. (1990) Surgical stapling devices in small animal surgery. *Compendium of Continuing Education for the Practicing Veterinarian*, **12**, 1724–1740.

Smeak, D.D. and Wendelburg, K.L. (1989) Choosing suture materials for use in contaminated or infected wounds. *Compendium of Continuing Education for the Practicing Veterinarian*, **11**, 467–475.

6

Abdominal cavity and gastrointestinal disorders

Abdominal cavity

Umbilical hernia

Umbilical hernias are almost always congenital. The umbilical ring should close shortly after birth following rupture of its contents, leaving the umbilical cicatrix. An umbilical hernia develops if the umbilical ring is malformed or too large to allow contraction at birth, or develops if contraction of the umbilical ring does not occur.

Umbilical hernias can occur in any breed or mixed-bred dog or cat but have been reported most often in the Airedale, Bull Terrier, Basenji, Cocker Spaniel, Collie, Pekinese, Pointer and Weimaraner dog breeds and the Cornish Rex, Persian and Himalayan cat breeds. Umbilical hernia has been reported in conjunction with peritoneopericardial hernias, incomplete caudal sternal fusion and cranioventral abdominal wall defects (Hayes, 1974, Robinson, 1977; Evans and Biery, 1980; Bellah *et al.*, 1989; Wallace *et al.*, 1992). Congenital heart defects (Bellah *et al.*, 1989) and portosystemic shunts may be associated with supraumbilical defects (Lunney, 1992). In addition, other congenital defects or developmental abnormalities such as crypt-

orchidism may be present and a thorough physical examination of a puppy or kitten with an umbilical hernia is warranted to detect other concurrent anomalies.

Clinical signs

An umbilical hernia is a true hernia composed of a hernial ring and a hernial sac (peritoneum) surrounding the contents. False hernias lack the peritoneal sac. An umbilical hernia presents as a mass in the ventral abdomen where the umbilical cicatrix should be located. Palpation of the hernia will indicate the size of the hernial ring, and the nature and reducibility of the contents. Typically the mass is non-painful and not associated with inflammation or overlying skin changes. Small umbilical hernias are often an incidental finding on physical examination and contain herniated falciform or omental fat which is not reducible due to constriction of the ring around the base of the herniated fat. Occasionally, larger defects may be observed and herniated intestine or other abdominal viscera may be palpated. If strangulation of abdominal viscera occurs, these animals may present with abdominal pain, vomiting and depression. Palpation of the hernia in these animals causes pain and reveals the overlying skin and contents of the hernia to be firm and warm.

Animals with concurrent peritoneopericardial hernias may present with clinical signs of respiratory distress.

Diagnosis

Diagnosis is usually based on physical examination alone, although a swelling in the location of the umbilicus does not rule out an abscess or neoplasia. If there is any doubt to the contents of the swelling, fine-needle aspiration (26-gauge needle) and cytological examination of the aspirate may be indicated. If there is associated respiratory distress or signs suggestive of intestinal obstruction, radiographic studies may be required to evaluate the diaphragm and abdominal cavity.

Treatment and surgical technique

In very young puppies less than several days of age small hernias that can be reduced at the time of presentation may resolve spontaneously. Very small hernias that contain fat and appear to be non-reducible rarely cause clinical signs. Small hernias can easily be repaired at the time of ovariohysterectomy if a midline coeliotomy is performed. If the umbilical hernia is large and appears to contain abdominal viscera, repair should be as soon as possible.

An elliptical incision (with the length four times the width) is made around the hernia, judging the amount of redundant skin that requires excision. Alternatively, a ventral midline skin incision is made over the hernia and redundant skin is excised at the time of closure. Care is required to avoid incising into the contents of the hernia. Regardless of the size of the hernia, the author prefers to open the hernial sac and inspect the contents. For small hernias, the falciform fat and hernial sac are excised and the margin of the hernial ring is debrided. The external rectus fascia is closed in a simple interrupted or a simple continuous suture pattern using absorbable suture material with a prolonged absorption (Fig. 6.1). Sutures should avoid penetrating the rectus muscle and internal rectus sheath and should be of an adequate-sized bite from the cut edge of the rectus fascia (at least 3 mm for very small dogs and cats). For large hernias, the hernial sac is opened,

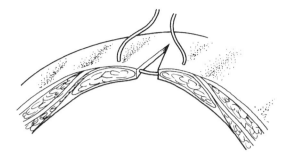

Figure 6.1 Closure of the external rectus fascia for repair of umbilical hernias or abdominal wall closure.

the contents inspected and returned to the abdominal cavity and the hernial ring is debrided. In animals where strangulation or visceral damage is suspected, the ventral midline skin incision may be extended and the hernial ring is enlarged to facilitate exploration of the abdomen. In addition, the region of the cranial ventral abdomen and diaphragm may require examination to rule out concurrent defects. The external rectus fascia is then sutured as described above. Rarely is prosthetic mesh required to close defects. A plane of anaesthesia that allows good abdomen muscle relaxation is recommended to facilitate abdominal closure of large defects. Subcutaneous and skin closure is routine.

Postoperative considerations and prognosis

Activity should be restricted for 7–10 days after which the suture line should be examined and sutures removed. The prognosis is excellent for most cases. The heritability of umbilical hernias is unclear but likely. Umbilical hernias have been observed in littermates, and as a concurrent congenital anomaly in animals after selective inbreeding. Neutering of affected animals is recommended until there is conclusive evidence to the contrary.

Inguinal and scrotal hernias

Inguinal hernias form when tissue or organs protrude through the inguinal canal. Indirect hernias, where tissue protrudes through the normal evagination of the vaginal process in females, or the vaginal tunic in a male, are most common. A direct hernia occurs when the peritoneal evagination occurs separate from and lies along the vaginal process or the vaginal tunic as a separate protrusion of tissue (Dean *et al.*, 1990). An indirect inguinal hernia in a male animal may progress to a scrotal hernia where the herniated tissue lies in the space between the parietal and visceral tunics adjacent to the testicle (Fig. 6.2).

Inguinal hernias are most frequently reported in middle-aged intact female dogs but are also seen as a congenital defect in young puppies and kittens (Fox, 1963; Strande, 1989; Waters *et al.*, 1993). Congenital inguinal hernia may be more common in male puppies, although the defect in older female dogs may represent a congenital defect that was not detected earlier. Bilateral hernias have been reported in approximately 25% of affected dogs (Waters *et al.*, 1993). Because of this, and the association of inguinal hernias with other problems such as cryptorchidism (Strande, 1989; Waters *et al.*, 1993) and umbilical hernia, a thorough physical examination is always warranted.

Inguinal hernias have been reported in several breeds and mixed breeds of dogs including the Basset Hound, Basenji, Cairn Terrier, Pekinese and West Highland White Terrier (Fox, 1963; Hayes, 1974). The author has also observed inguinal hernias in mixed-breed cats. Scrotal hernias are rare.

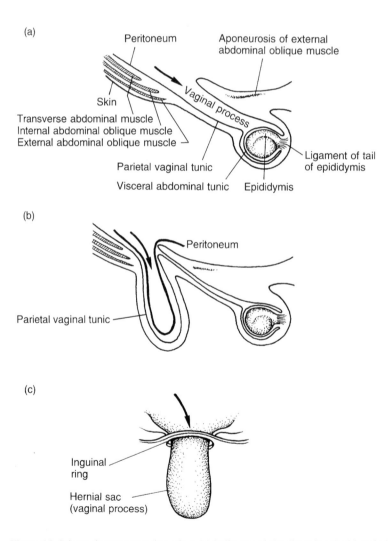

Figure 6.2 Schematic representation of an (a) indirect and (b) direct inguinal hernia in a male dog. Arrow indicates inguinal herniation. (c) Indirect hernia in a female dog.

Clinical signs

Clinical signs vary depending on the size of the defect but generally the animals present with a soft, non-painful mass in the inguinal region. Elevation of the hind limbs may facilitate reduction of the hernia and palpation of the defect in the abdominal wall. Animals with scrotal hernias present with a varying degree of scrotal swelling. Since the inguinal canal is smaller in the male dog, strangulation of hernial contents is more common in the male than the female. Strangulated hernias may be painful and discoloration of the herniated tissue may be visible through the skin.

Diagnosis

Diagnosis is usually based on clinical signs. Inguinal hernia needs to be differentiated from subcutaneous fatty tissue accumulation, abscess, haematoma and inguinal lymphadenopathy (especially prominent in a puppy with dermatitis). If bowel or urinary bladder herniation is suspected, radiographic and ultrasonographic examination may facilitate the diagnosis. Intraoperative examination may be required to differentiate an inguinal hernia from a femoral hernia, where the hernia is ventral to the inguinal ligament.

For scrotal hernias, careful palpation is required to differentiate the swelling from orchitis or severe scrotal inflammation. In the case of a hernia a cord-like structure should be palpable alongside the spermatic cord, extending from the external inguinal ring to the scrotum.

Treatment and surgical technique

A ventral midline incision can be used for all inguinal hernias (Dean *et al.*, 1990; Peddie, 1980). This facilitates exposure of both inguinal rings and abdominal exploration, should that be required. The incision extends from the cranial edge of the pubis as far cranially as required to expose the hernial sac. The incision is continued through the subcutaneous tissue down to the external rectus fascia. The skin is undermined using blunt dissection until the inguinal ring and hernial sac are exposed. In a large male puppy with a scrotal hernia, to avoid excessive undermining of the penis and prepuce, incisions can be made over the inguinal rings.

The hernial sac is dissected from the subcutaneous tissue, the hernial sac is opened and the contents examined. Any adhesions between the hernial sac and the contents are broken down and the contents are then reduced. Extension of the hernial ring can be performed to facilitate reduction of contents. Aspiration of urine from a herniated urinary bladder will facilitate reduction of the urinary bladder. The redundant hernial sac is then trimmed at the margin of the hernial ring or for large hernias, the redundant hernial sac is excised, and the remainder of the sac is subsequently closed. The edges of the hernial ring may require debridement if excising the hernial sac does not result in a freshly cut edge. The hernial ring is then closed using simple interrupted sutures through the rectus fascia (Fig. 6.3). Care must be taken to avoid the external pudendal vessels and genitofemoral nerve which exit from the caudomedial aspect of the inguinal ring. In males, if castration is not intended, care is required to avoid complete inguinal ring closure and compromise of the spermatic cord which traverses the inguinal ring. In suspected cryptorchid animals, inspect the inguinal ring thoroughly as a poorly developed testicle can lodge within the inguinal ring and go undetected.

If castration is intended, it can be performed once the hernial sac is opened. Bilateral castration should always be performed. Scrotal ablation may be required if the scrotum is redundant.

The subcutaneous tissue is closed to eliminate dead space over the inguinal area in the region of the dissection. Although elimination of any dead space with sutures is preferred, if closure is difficult, a closed-suction drain can be placed (see section 7.45, nasopharyngeal polyps). The skin is closed routinely.

Postoperative considerations and prognosis

Activity should be restricted for 7–10 days, after which the suture line should be examined and sutures removed. The prognosis is excellent for most cases. If a drain has been placed, meticulous drain management is required to avoid contamination and introduction of infection into the surgical wound. The drain should be covered by a bandage and the collection system changed as frequently as required to avoid clotting and obstruction of the drain. The volume and

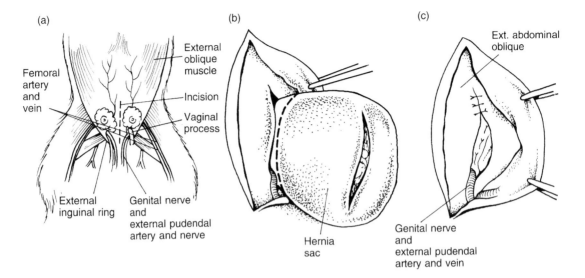

(a)

Femoral
artery
and
vein

External
oblique
muscle

Incision

Vaginal
process

External
inguinal ring

Genital nerve
and
external pudendal
artery and nerve

(b)

Hernia
sac

Genital nerve
and
external pudendal
artery and vein

(c)

Ext. abdominal
oblique

Figure 6.3 (a) Closure of an inguinal hernia through a midline incision. (b) After exposure of the hernial sac, it is opened and the contents examined and reduced. The redundant hernial sac is excised and may be closed. (c) The hernial ring is closed using simple interrupted sutures through the rectus fascia, taking care not to compromise the external pudendal vessels and genitofemoral nerve, which exit from the caudomedial aspect of the inguinal ring.

nature of the drainage should be monitored. Drains should be removed as soon as possible to avoid complications, usually after 2–3 days. The heritability of inguinal hernias is unclear but the condition has been observed in littermates and has been produced by selective inbreeding (Fox, 1963). Neutering of affected animals is recommended until there is conclusive evidence to the contrary.

Oral cavity

Dentistry

Paediatric dentistry is probably best restricted to disorders of dentition, occlusion and possibly traumatically induced problems. In addition, the early inception of a preventive home care programme is extremely important to the long-term dental care of the animal.

Dogs and cats are edentulous when they are born. The incisors begin erupting when they are 2 weeks of age, and all deciduous dentition is present by 8 weeks of age (Table 6.1). The permanent dentition begins erupting at 3 months of age and is complete by 7 months (Table 6.2).

Normal dental anatomy is depicted in Figure 6.4. The number of tooth roots varies between teeth (Tables 6.3 and 6.4). This becomes important during teeth extraction.

Table 6.1 Deciduous dentition of cats and dogs

Dental formula	Time of eruption (weeks)	
Dog	Incisors	2–4
2(I3/3, C1/1, P3/3) = 28	Canines	3–5
	Premolars	4–12
Cat	Incisors	2–4
2(I3/3, C1/1, P3/2) = 26	Canines	3–4
	Premolars	3–8

I = Incisors, C = Canines, P = Premolars

Table 6.2 Permanent dentition of cats and dogs

Dental formula	Time of eruption (months)	
Dog	Incisors	3–5
2(I3/3, C1/1, P4/4,	Canines	4–7
M2/3) = 42	Premolars	4–6
	Molars	4–7
Cat	Incisors	3–5
2(I3/3, C1/1, P3/2,	Canines	4–5
M1/1) = 30	Premolars	4–6
	Molars	4–5

I = Incisors, C = Canines, P = Premolars, M = Molars

Table 6.3 Number of tooth roots for teeth in the dog

Upper teeth	Incisors	Canine	P1	P2	P3	P4	M1	M2	
Roots	1	1	1	2	2	3	3	3	

Lower teeth	Incisors	Canine	P1	P2	P3	P4	M1	M2	M3
Roots	1	1	1	2	2	2	1	2	3

P = Premolar, M = Molar

Table 6.4 Number of tooth roots for teeth in the cat

Upper teeth	Incisors	Canine	P2*	P3	P4	M1
Roots	1	1	1 or 2 (fused)	2	3	1, 2 or 3

Lower teeth	Incisors	Canine	P3†	P4	M1
Roots	1	1	2	2	2

* The premolars are numbered assuming that P1 is missing in the cat.
† The lower premolars are numbered assuming P1 and P2 are missing in the cat.
P = Premolar, M = Molar

Table 6.5 Selected dental terminology

Term	Definition
Apical	Direction towards the root tip or away from the incisal or occlusal surface
Buccal	Facing towards the cheek or lip
Coronal	Direction of the tip of the crown
Crown	The part of the tooth above the gingival surface
Cusp	Point or tip of tooth
Furcation	Space between the roots of the same tooth
Gingival sulcus	Space created around the tooth by the free gingiva; that part of the gingiva not attached to the tooth. It should be 2–3 mm deep
Interalveolar septa	Bony partition between adjacent teeth
Labial	The surface of the tooth facing the lip
Lingual	The surface of the tooth facing the tongue; sometimes referred to as palatal for teeth in the maxilla
Mesial	Facing towards the rostral end of the arch or towards the midline (incisor teeth)
Occlusal surface	Flat grinding surface of the molars
Periodontal ligament	A thin layer of connective tissue surrounding the tooth root
Proximal surface	The surface of the teeth in contact with each other; distal are away from the front of the face; mesial are towards the front of the face

Disorders of dentition (Table 6.6)

Table 6.6 Disorders of dentition

Disorders of dentition	Characteristics
Enamel hypoplasia	Caused by interruption of the ameloblasts during the second to fifth months of age
	The enamel is irregular, pitted, thinner than normal or even absent in some places. It may appear heavily stained
	Pyrexia, severe parasitism and nutritional deficiencies can be causes
	Daily brushing of the teeth, regular dental prophylaxis, weekly application of 0.4% stannous fluoride gel to strengthen the enamel, and avoidance of hard chew toys or bones is advised
Split crown	Occurs occasionally during crown development
	No treatment is required
	Cosmetic restoration over the deficits can be performed
	Plaque may accumulate in the fissure and stringent home care is advised
Enamel staining	Tetracycline staining occurs if an animal is placed on tetracycline or derivative during the enamel-forming stage (2–5 months of age)
	If the bitch or queen is given tetracycline during pregnancy, the deciduous teeth may be stained
	The teeth are structurally sound
	Bleaching can be performed for cosmetic reasons

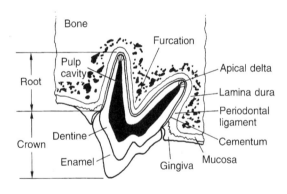

Figure 6.4 Normal dental anatomy.

Anatomical disorders

Normal occlusion in dogs is described as scissor occlusion; the upper incisors slightly overlap the lower incisors. The lower canine teeth should occlude in the interdental space between the upper third incisor (lateral) and the upper canine tooth. No tooth surfaces should touch. In the cat, scissor occlusion is also normal. Abnormalities are not uncommon and interfere with the normal self-cleaning mechanisms of the teeth and can result in excessive accumulation of food and dental calculus on the teeth (Table 6.7). Corrections may be possible, but where impossible, client education and strict preventive care are imperative.

Basic prophylaxis and home care

Probably the biggest factor in the effectiveness of home care and basic prophylaxis is owner–animal interaction. Hence, training of both the client and the animal should begin as early as possible since it may take several months before the animal will tolerate long periods of restraint. A prophylaxis programme should be initiated before the eruption of permanent teeth. Ideally, daily inspection and cleansing are advised; however, at worst, cleansing should be at least three times a week. This allows evaluation for proper eruption and shedding of teeth and for evaluation of other oral lesions.

Home care is best performed with the animal in a passive posture (lying or sitting at command). Training should begin with the owner lifting the lips to examine the incisors and canines and pulling the lips caudally to inspect

Table 6.7 Occlusal abnormalities

Abnormality	Characteristics
Anterior cross-bite	Most common malocclusion (undershot jaw)
	Lower incisors are rostral to the upper incisors and the occlusion is reverse scissor
	Exaggerated anterior cross-bite is found in all brachycephalic breeds; the mandible is of normal length but the maxilla is brachygnathous (too short)
Mandibular brachygnathism	Overshot jaw
	Far less common
	Mandible is shorter than normal and the lower canine teeth may even be caudal to the upper canine teeth
Posterior cross-bite	Occurs occasionally in Boxers, Collies and other dolichocephalic (long-nosed) breeds
	Mandible is wider than the maxilla in the region of the premolars and heavy amounts of calculus may accumulate on the buccal surfaces of the lower premolar and molar teeth
Wry mouth	Result of the growth centres of one or more quadrants of the mouth being asynchronous. Varying degrees of disparity occur and, depending on the quadrant affected, one side of the face may be shorter, the nose twisted to one side, or the mandible twisted (Hawkins, 1991). This is a common malocclusion in flat-nosed cats, often resulting in one lower canine tooth protruding outside the upper lip when the mouth is closed. Tissue trauma may occur to the upper lip or internally in the contact area. Orthodontic repositioning, coronal amputation and vital pulpotomy are treatment alternatives
Oligodontia	Too few teeth – usually insignificant to tooth function but important for the show dog
	Incisors or premolars are usually missing
	Radiographic evaluation of the permanent teeth crowns can be performed at 12–16 weeks
	Complete absence of teeth (anodontia) is very rare in dogs and cats
Polyodontia	Supernumerary teeth
	Usually involves the premolars or incisors
	Supernumerary tooth distinguished from a retained deciduous tooth by examining the anatomy of the crown and by radiography
	Up to 9% of dogs have supernumerary teeth
Dental interlock	Deciduous teeth erupt abnormally such that the upper deciduous canine teeth are rostral to the lower deciduous canine teeth and prevent forward growth of the mandible. Extraction of the upper deciduous canine teeth results in correction of the growth if genetic potential has not been surpassed
Lingually displaced mandibular canine teeth	Base narrow lower canine teeth
	Cause soft- or hard-tissue damage or even oronasal fistula
	May be in conjunction with retained deciduous teeth, in which case the permanent canine teeth are lingually or mesially displaced
	Early extraction of retained deciduous teeth may allow correction
	Treatments include a variety of orthodontic corrections or crown height reduction of the canine teeth as alternatives to extraction of permanent teeth (Oakes, 1993). Occasionally the upper third incisor must be extracted to provide space for the lower canine tooth
Rostrally displaced maxillary canine teeth	Genetic condition common in Shetland Sheepdogs
	Also seen in Scottish Terriers and other medium- and small-breed dogs
	Upper canine tooth is displaced rostrally and hits the upper third incisor tooth
	Periodontal disease and upper-lip ulceration will develop if left untreated
	Treatment involves extraction, amputation or shortening of the crown or orthodontic correction
	Neutering the animal is advised since it is a genetic condition
	Rostrally displaced upper canine teeth can occur in the cat

Table 6.7 (continued)

Abnormality	Characteristics
Crowded and rotated teeth	Common in dogs with small jaws
	Both mandibular second incisors are displaced buccally or lingually
	If crowding results in significant compromise of periodontal tissue, extraction of one or more crowded incisors is indicated
	Premolar and molar crowding is common in brachycephalic dogs; typically, the premolar teeth are normal but rotated relative to the long axis of the jaw
	Affected teeth are predisposed to periodontal disease (Harvey and Emily, 1993)
Retained deciduous teeth	Common condition in toy-breed dogs; less frequent in large-breed dogs and cats
	Retained incisors and canine teeth are common, causing the permanent tooth to erupt in an abnormal position
	Retained deciduous incisor causes the permanent tooth to erupt more lingually
	Retained deciduous maxillary incisors cause a level or anterior cross-bite
	Retained deciduous canines cause the permanent teeth also to erupt more lingually, which may cause soft-tissue trauma of the gingival tissue or palate
	Retained maxillary canine teeth cause the permanent teeth to erupt more rostrally, which may interfere with the mandibular canines causing tooth damage and attrition
	Retained deciduous teeth should be removed as soon as possible after identification; careful extraction is required to prevent damage to the permanent tooth or fracture of the deciduous tooth root, which are longer than the crown of the tooth. Any fractured root segments should be removed
Impacted or undescended upper deciduous canine teeth	Seen in Miniature Poodles and Shetland Sheepdogs
	May or may not be in conjunction with retained deciduous teeth
	An undescended or impacted tooth predisposes the animal to an inapparent oronasal fistula with or without nasal discharge, and odontoma/ameloblastoma tumour development around the tooth from primordial cells
	Impacted teeth should be extracted or corrected using orthodontic bands
	Partially impacted teeth have all or part of the coronal aspect of the tooth covered by soft-tissue with the root of the tooth in the bone (Harvey and Emily, 1993). If the soft tissue covering the tooth becomes cystic or in the line of occlusion, trauma can occur during mastication. Operculectomy is performed to remove the soft tissue over the crown of the tooth. Further eruption of the tooth may be stimulated by this procedure

the premolars and molars. Gradually, the animal should be accustomed to having its mouth opened, its teeth rubbed with a cloth, then progressing to sponge-tipped applicator and soft brush.

The objective of prophylaxis for the puppy or kitten is the prevention of plaque build-up and development of periodontal disease. The most effective way to achieve this is by daily brushing or cleansing. Use of cotton-gauze or a soft toothbrush is adequate; a brush is preferred as it can get into the gingival sulcus, a common site of plaque build-up. A huge variety of oral hygiene products are on the market (Table 6.8), available as powders, pastes, gels and liquids. A flavoured paste can be used. Alternatively, particularly in animals predisposed to

enamel abnormalities or caries, an unflavoured stannous fluoride gel is recommended (Aller, 1989).

Advice on diet and appropriate chew toys is important. Semi-moist diets are associated with enhanced plaque formation. Rawhide and hard biscuits can help; however, very hard toys should be avoided as they may cause tooth fracture or damage. Once the puppy or kitten reaches 6 months of age, veterinary evaluation of the teeth every 6 months is advised.

Cleft palate

Cleft palates and oronasal fistulas are abnormal communications between the oral and nasal

Table 6.8 Common oral hygiene products

Product ingredient	Comment
Sodium bicarbonate (baking soda)	May be bitter unless flavoured. Use with caution in animals on sodium-restricted diets
Hydrogen peroxide	Reduces plaque directly. It is antibacterial but limits lactoperoxidase system. Do not use plain hydrogen peroxide – it is cytotoxic to the mucosa and ingestion may cause foaming at the mouth and vomiting
Lactoperoxidase	Augments salivary lactoperoxidase system which produces antibacterial substances (Fig. 6.5)
Chlorhexidine	Antibacterial. It binds to oral mucosa and provides residual antibacterial activity. 0.12% marketed as rinse. Prolonged use may stain teeth. It is indicated for animals with, or predisposed to, periodontitis
Stannous fluoride	Indicated for enamel problems. Avoid excessive use as fluorosis can potentiate hyperkalaemia and bone and tooth development

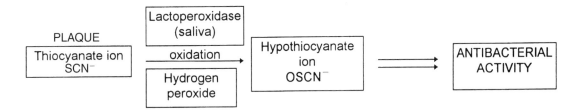

Figure 6.5 Lactoperoxidase activity in mouth.

cavities. Cleft palates are usually congenital while oronasal fistulas are acquired (Harvey, 1987).

Cleft palates may be clefts of the primary palate (harelip) or the secondary palate (hard and soft palate) (Harvey, 1987). Cleft palates are rare in cats. Primary cleft palates are anterior to the incisive foramen and involve the lip (Fig. 6.6). Isolated cleft of the primary palate is rare but more common in males; brachycephalic breeds have the highest risk. The left side appears to be affected more often than the right side.

Secondary cleft palates are posterior to the incisive foramen and involve the hard and soft palates (Harvey, 1987) (Fig. 6.7). Clefts of the secondary palate, alone or in combination with cleft primary palate, occur more frequently than primary lesions alone.

Acquired oronasal fistulas may be secondary to trauma, surgical resection of maxillary lesions and, most commonly in dogs, secondary to severe periodontal disease with maxillary bone resorption. Failure of repair of congenital cleft

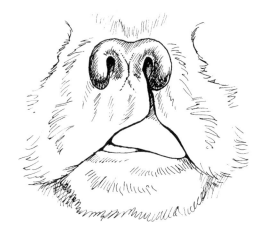

Figure 6.6 Primary cleft palate.

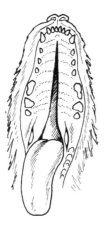

Figure 6.7 Secondary cleft palate with extension into the soft palate.

palates may also result in secondary oronasal fistulas. Acquired oronasal fistulas secondary to head trauma and maxillary fracture are not uncommon in the cat.

Clinical signs

The predominant clinical sign of cleft palates or oronasal fistulas is nasal discharge. It can be either purulent or haemorrhagic, and unilateral or bilateral. Nasal regurgitation of fluid or food may be evident in animals with congenital cleft palates. Difficulty suckling is particularly apparent in animals with primary cleft palates.

Diagnosis

Diagnosis is by visual examination of the oral cavity. This should be performed routinely at birth to screen for obvious problems. Thorough examination may require sedation or anaesthesia, especially for lesions secondary to periodontal disease if the fistula is small.

Treatment and surgical technique

Surgical correction of all types of clefts and oronasal fistulas is the treatment of choice. Surgical correction of cleft palates is possible once the animal has attained a suitable size for anaesthesia and surgery, usually by 6–8 weeks after birth.

Preoperative radiographs of the maxilla in animals with oronasal fistulas secondary to neoplasia, infection or trauma are recommended to examine the extent of bone destruction. Preoperative radiographs of the thorax are also indicated to rule out the presence of aspiration pneumonia.

Repair of cleft palate or oronasal fistula is based on creating a mucoperiosteal and/or gingival/buccal mucosal flap to cover the defect (Table 6.9).

Absorbable and non-absorbable sutures (except stainless steel) can be used in an appositional suture pattern (simple interrupted). If possible, a two-layer closure is advised to minimize tension on the epithelial suture line. Non-absorbable sutures have to be removed, often requiring sedation or anaesthesia of the animal; however, this provides an opportunity to examine the suture line.

The use of electrosurgery in the oral cavity is unclear. Excessive use should be avoided to prevent tissue damage, avoid delayed wound healing, and avoid the likelihood of wound dehiscence.

In healthy wounds, perioperative antibiotics are unnecessary. If there is moderate to severe periodontal disease, perioperative antibiotics should be used.

The goals of primary cleft palate corrective procedures is first to close the floor of the nasal orifice so it is confluent with the mucosal side of the lip closure, followed by closure of the nasal and cutaneous lip clefts (Kirby *et al.*, 1988). This is a difficult procedure and requires a certain level of surgical experience.

The two most frequently used procedures for treatment of secondary cleft palates involve creation of sliding bipedicle flaps and over-

Table 6.9 Important considerations during surgery for repair of cleft palate or oronasal fistula

Surgical considerations
Create a flap larger than the defect
Ensure that apposed edges are cleanly incised since a flap sutured to an intact epithelial surface will not heal
Attempt to have the suture lines lie over connective tissue rather than the defect itself
Minimize tension on suture lines by adequately mobilizing the flaps and using large bites of tissue when placing sutures
Preserve the major palatine artery when elevating mucoperiosteal flaps near its point of penetration of the palatine bone (approximately 1 cm medial to the carnassial tooth)

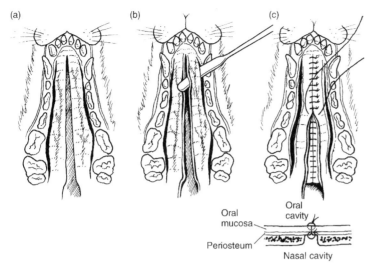

Figure 6.8 Secondary cleft palate repair using sliding, bipedicle mucoperiosteal flaps. (a) Bilateral incisions are made in the mucoperiosteum along the dental arcade. (b) The mucoperiosteal layer is elevated on both sides of the defect and the edges of the defect are incised, pulled towards the midline and (c) sutured in two layers (nasal and oral mucosa).

lapping flaps (Ellison *et al.*, 1986; Harvey, 1987; Kirby, 1990). Sliding bipedicle flaps are created on either side of the cleft, along the length of the defect, by making bilateral releasing incisions in the mucoperiosteum along the dental arcade (Harvey, 1987; Fig. 6.8). The mucoperiosteal layer is elevated on both sides of the defect and the edges of the defect are incised and sutured in two layers (nasal and oral mucosa). This procedure does place the suture line over the defect.

For overlapping flaps, a mucoperiosteal pedicle at the margin of the defect is created, reflected and overlapped by the opposite incised edge of the defect (Harvey, 1987; Fig. 6.9). This procedure avoids having the suture line over the defect and is usually associated with less tension on the suture line than the bipedicle procedure.

Combinations or modifications of these two procedures are feasible. Defects that extend into the soft palate can be closed by incising the margins of the defect, undermining the oral and nasal mucosa and apposing the nasal mucosa and oral mucosa in separate layers. Releasing incisions as described above for the hard palate may facilitate closure.

Acquired oronasal fistulas secondary to trauma and tooth extraction require careful debridement and excision of devitalized and infected tissue.

For simple tooth extraction, the gingiva is elevated and the tooth removed. For complicated tooth extraction, creation of a gingival flap and removal of alveolar bone may be necessary. For maxillary teeth, closure of the now created oronasal fistula may be performed with a gingival/buccal mucosal flap (Fig. 6.10), a mucoperiosteal flap elevated from the hard palate or a combination of both in a double reposition flap procedure.

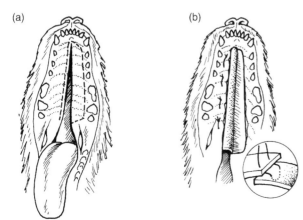

Figure 6.9 Secondary cleft palate repair using a mucoperiosteal flap. (a) An incision (broken line) in the mucoperiosteum is made on one side of the defect to create the flap. The flap and incised opposite margin of the defect are elevated. (b) The flap is reflected and placed underneath the incised opposite margin and sutured in place.

(a)

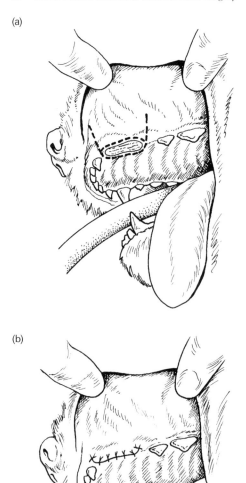

(b)

Figure 6.10 Acquired oronasal fistula repair using a buccal gingival flap. (a) The incision around the fistula or the fresh incision from tooth extraction extends into the buccal gingiva. The buccal flap is elevated and advanced over the defect. (b) The flap is sutured to the muco-periosteum of the hard palate in a two-layer closure.

The gingival/buccal mucosal flap is an advancement flap created in the buccal mucosa at the edge of the fistula (Harvey, 1987; Kirby, 1990). The flap is elevated and advanced until it will cover the defect without tension. The flap is positioned over the defect and sutured (in two layers if possible) to the edges of the defect. This procedure is suitable for oronasal fistulas positioned close to the gingival margin. The exposed submucosal tissue facing the nasal cavity is covered with nasal epithelium by 30 days.

Mucoperiosteal flaps elevated from the hard palate may be hinged, advanced or rotated over the defect, depending on the location of the fistula and the availability of nearby tissue (Harvey, 1987; Kirby, 1990). Mucoperiosteal flaps are often used for oronasal fistulas located towards the centre of the hard palate, or in combination with gingival/buccal mucosal flaps. A secondary defect is often created and the exposed bone of the hard palate is covered by epithelium in 3–4 weeks.

The double reposition flap is used to repair large oronasal fistulas that require several flaps to cover the defect, or for repair of failed closures of oronasal fistulas near the gingival margin (Ellison *et al.*, 1986). A hinged muco-periosteal flap, based at the medial edge of the defect, is elevated and reflected over the defect. This flap and the exposed palatine bone are then covered by a gingival/buccal mucosa advancement flap.

Advantages of the double reposition flap include providing a strong closure and a more bacterial-resistant epithelial surface in both the nasal and oral cavities (Ellison *et al.*, 1986).

Recently, the successful use of a microvascular free flap using the myoperitoneum (transversus abdominus muscle) and its right cranial abdominal artery and vein (a branch of the phrenicoabdominal artery and vein) to close a large defect in the hard palate of a dog was reported (Degner *et al.*, 1996). The right cranial abdominal artery and vein were anastomosed to the infraorbital artery and vein. This procedure, while requiring technical expertise, does offer an alternative for very large defects where creation of mucoperiosteal flaps may be prohibited by the size of the defect.

Postoperative considerations and prognosis

Postoperative considerations include oreventing dehiscence, enteral feeding and monitoring of the surgical site. Prevention of self-mutilation is extremely important. An Elizabethan collar should be placed on the animal immediately after recovery.

The necessity for enteral feeding to bypass the oral cavity is controversial. Proponents feel it prevents irritation of the suture line and impaction of food around the suture line. Definitive evidence of any beneficial effect of food bypassing the oral cavity on healing is, however, lacking. Pharyngostomy, oesophagostomy or gastrostomy (percutaneous endoscopic gastrostomy) tube-feeding is suitable. The duration of enteral feeding is arbitrary but should probably cover at least the first 7 days.

Inspection of the surgical site daily is important to monitor healing (Kirby, 1990). If required, non-absorbable sutures can be removed in 14 days. Open palatine defects usually take 3–4 weeks to become completely covered with epithelium. Unless the area is obviously infected (e.g. necrotic stomatitis) postoperative antibiotics are unnecessary.

Dehiscence or failure of repair is the most common complication of oronasal fistula repair and is often the result of technical difficulties and poor tissue integrity (Kirby, 1990). Congenital defects often require staged procedures and it may be difficult to get a final complete closure in very large defects. The prognosis for defects of the soft palate is less favourable. However, if the defect can be closed, the long-term prognosis thus becomes very good.

Papillomatosis

Oral papillomas caused by papillomavirus commonly occur in dogs younger than 1 year of age, and may spread through a kennel in 2–4 weeks. The cauliflower-like growths begin as smooth, cream-coloured elevations, which later become rough and grey. Histologically, a thick squamous epithelium covers branching cords of dermal papillae. The oral mucosa and commissures of the lips are most commonly affected. The number and size of lesions are variable. Although usually not necessary, a biopsy may be required with early atypical lesions or hyperpigmented contracted lesions that form during regression. Therapy is usually unnecessary because the lesions regress spontaneously in 6–12 weeks. Surgical excision may be a means of stimulating regression and eliminating confluent pedunculated masses, which may impair the prehension and mastication of food. Lifetime immunity generally follows recovery.

Stomatitis

Stomatitis or inflammation of the oral cavity may be due to any infectious, physical or chemical agent or traumatic insult that significantly alters the replication, maturation or exfoliation of the healthy oral mucosa (Table 6.10).

Table 6.10 Characteristics and causes of stomatitis

Type and causative agents	Characteristics	Comment
Viral stomatitis		Because oral lesions from most viral infections are only part of the disease, their treatment is usually supportive
Feline rhinotracheitis virus (FRV) and feline calicivirus (FCV)	Buccal, lingual and nasal ulcers commonly accompany these viral respiratory infections, although ulcers are generally more severe in FCV than in FRV infections	Most common cause of stomatitis in young cats
Feline leukaemia virus (FeLV) and feline immunodeficiency virus (FIV)	May be associated with oral lesions such as a persistent glossitis, periodontitis, palatitis and gingivitis, presumably because of virus-induced immunosuppression	
Canine distemper virus	May cause stomatitis in affected puppies	Severe clinical signs referable to other organ systems usually more prominent than oral lesions
Feline parvovirus (feline panleukopenia virus)	May cause stomatitis in kittens	Severe clinical signs referable to other organ systems usually more prominent than oral lesions

Table 6.10 (continued)

Type and causative agents	Characteristics	Comment
Physical agent-induced stomatitis	Traumatic insult to the oral mucosa followed by secondary bacterial infection and scar tissue (which may obscure foreign body) Oral burns from electrical cords are not uncommon in young dogs and cats that chew through the insulation of the cords. Pulmonary oedema, seizures and cardiac arrhythmias frequently accompany these electrical shock injuries	Removal of the foreign object(s) usually effects a cure
Chemical agent-induced stomatitis	Oral lesions from ingestion of caustic or corrosive substances are uncommon Continual exposure to environmental chemicals, especially pesticides, fertilizers and irritant plants may cause severe oral lesions	Immediate, liberal flushing of the mouth with copious amounts of water is indicated Chemical neutralization with most chemical antidotes is ineffective if administration is delayed Supportive care includes cleansing and occasional debridement of the oral lesions, treatment of secondary bacterial infection and frequent feeding of a nutritionally complete, soft, palatable diet to ensure adequate caloric intake
Immune-mediated stomatitis Pemphigus complex, bullous pemphigoid and lupus erythematosus	Autoantibodies to intercellular epidermal antigens cause acantholysis and intraepidermal vesicobullous ulceration of the skin and oral cavity Bullous pemphigoid: autoantibodies against antigens at the basement membrane zone cause subepidermal vesicobullous ulceration of the skin and oral cavity Systemic lupus erythematosus: oral ulceration may occur in conjunction with its other multisystemic manifestations Pemphigus foliaceus: rarely affects the oral cavity Unusual in either the dog or cat for oral lesions to occur without skin involvement, especially at other mucocutaneous junctions (eyelids, nostrils, anus, vagina and prepuce)	May first appear in the dog or cat at 4–6 months of age Treatment includes supportive and immunosuppressive therapy
Other causes Mineral and vitamin deficiencies	Rare Vitamin B-complex vitamins and possibly zinc deficiencies may contribute to development of oral lesions in growing malnourished dogs or cats	
Heavy-metal poisoning	Thallium	
Coagulation abnormalities	May be caused by rodenticide poisoning, thrombocytopenia, clotting factor deficiencies and disseminated intravascular coagulation	Petechiae of the oral mucosa or gingival bleeding are observed. Dogs affected with cyclic haematopoiesis often develop a recurrent stomatitis that coincides with absolute neutropaenia
Proliferative eosinophilic granuloma (oral)	Reported in Siberian Huskies and many breeds of young cats (kittens as young as 8 weeks of age)	

General therapy

The definitive cause of a stomatitis cannot always be determined by history, physical examination, cytological evaluation, bacterial and fungal culture or tissue biopsy. In many cases, bacterial cultures reveal the normal mixed flora of the oral cavity; therefore, antimicrobial sensitivities are often unreliable. In these cases, symptomatic therapy is often efficacious.

A gauze sponge can be used for mechanical cleaning of the mucosal surface. Daily flushing of the mouth with chlorhexidine (diluted to 0.1–0.2% solution in water) followed by rinsing the mouth with copious amounts of water will help cleanse the affected areas. Soft, palatable food may need to be provided for several days during the initial healing phase. Ampicillin, amoxycillin or cephalosporins may be administered daily in an oral liquid form for both a local antimicrobial effect and subsequent systemic effect after absorption. Antimicrobial therapy may be indicated for up to 3 weeks.

Oesophagus

The oesophagus is generally implicated in disease in the regurgitating puppy or kitten. Several conditions can cause these signs and must be differentiated, particularly to rule in or out any disease that requires surgical treatment, since delayed surgery will substantially increase the morbidity and mortality of most problems.

Megaoesophagus

Primary megaoesophagus is characterized by motor disturbances of the oesophagus that result in abnormal or unsuccessful transport of ingesta between the pharynx and stomach. Although a complete understanding of the pathophysiology of primary megaoesophagus is still lacking, it is believed by most investigators that primary megaoesophagus results from a dysfunction of the primary motor system of the oesophagus with or without secondary dysfunction of the gastro-oesophageal sphincter.

Both congenital and acquired forms of megaoesophagus occur in young dogs and cats. The incidence of congenital megaoesophagus is highest in Great Danes, followed by German Shepherd Dogs and Irish Setters. In the cat, Siamese and Siamese-related breeds have the highest incidence.

Acquired megaoesophagus may occur spontaneously in any young dog or cat. In most instances, the underlying cause is undetermined; however, megaoesophagus may occur in several systemic diseases that affect the nervous system or skeletal muscles (Table 6.11).

Clinical signs

Clinical signs associated with congenital megaoesophagus usually begin at weaning (Table 6.12). Regurgitation is most characteristic. The time interval between eating and regurgitation can be related to the degree of dilation or to the general activity of the animal. Usually both liquids and solids are poorly tolerated.

Diagnosis

Diagnosis of megaoesophagus is usually obvious. Survey thoracic radiographs consistently

Table 6.11 Diseases that may be associated with megaeosophagus

Disease type	Condition
Autoimmune/inflammatory	Systemic lupus erythematosus, ganglioradiculitis, polyneuritis
Infectious	Toxoplasmosis, canine distemper
Endocrine	Hypothyroidism, hypoadrenocorticism
Muscular	Inherited myopathies, polymyositis
Toxic	Tick paralysis, botulism, lead poisoning, anticholinesterase compounds
Neurologic	Dysautonomia, myasthenia gravis

Table 6.12 Clinical signs of megaoesophagus

Clinical sign
Effortless regurgitation of oesophageal contents; may occur immediately after feeding or up to 12 h or more later
Weight loss
Polyphagia
Weakness
Dehydration
Impaired skeletal mineralization; result of poor nutritional status
Ballooning of the cervical region of the oesophagus that is synchronized with respiration
Recurrent laryngotracheal aspiration; often leads to recurrent pneumonia
Oral foetor; result of stagnation of fermenting ingesta retained in the dilated oesophagus

reveal a dilated oesophagus. The oesophageal lumen typically contains sufficient air and ingesta to allow visual observation on the lateral projection of a pair of soft-tissue stripes that arise in the mid-thorax region and converge towards the gastro-oesophageal junction. Cranially, the dorsal wall of the oesophagus may merge with the longus colli muscle to outline a sharp margin. Ventrally, the ventral wall of the oesophagus will create a silhouette with the dorsal wall of the air-filled trachea, creating a wide soft-tissue band called the tracheal stripe. When the cervical oesophageal segment is dilated, a sabre-shaped radiolucent shadow is seen dorsal to the trachea and tapering towards the thoracic inlet. A partially fluid-filled oesophagus will present as a homogeneous grey shadow. With marked oesophageal dilatation, ventral displacement of the trachea and heart occurs. In the dorsoventral or ventrodorsal projection, the caudal thoracic oesophagus is seen as V-shaped pair of lines to either side of midline with the convergence at the gastro-oesophageal junction. Evidence of aspiration pneumonia is frequently present and consistent with the signs of dysphagia and regurgitation.

When the oesophagus is not observed visually on survey radiographs, a contrast oesophagogram is required. A contrast study better defines the degree of oesophageal dilatation, lack of function and extent of involvement. The con-

trast study will help rule out congenital vascular ring anomalies or other causes of localized obstruction that might contribute to megaoesophagus and outlines the funnel shape of the caudal region of the oesophagus to rule out invasive processes that may cause irregular or asymmetric narrowing. If no contrast medium enters the stomach, as noted on initial contrast radiographs, the animal's forequarters should be elevated for several minutes to allow for gravitational flow of the contrast medium into the stomach, and follow-up radiographs should be done.

Treatment

For primary megaoesophagus, proper dietary management in terms of frequent, elevated feedings with foods of appropriate consistency for the particular animal (some handle bulky foods well; others tolerate gruels better) generally result in spontaneous improvement in a number of animals identified at an early age. With the elevated feedings, minimal stress and distension of the oesophagus occur until such time as normal oesophageal motor function develops. If stasis of oesophageal contents is allowed however, gradual overdistension and atony result, contributing to persistent megaoesophagus.

Prognosis

The earlier the dysfunction is recognized and dietary management instituted, the better the prognosis. Puppies and kittens diagnosed at the time of weaning and managed appropriately have a better prognosis than those recognized later, around 4–6 months of age. Once severe megaoesophagus occurs, complete recovery is unlikely. Aspiration pneumonia and malnourishment limit the longevity of these animals.

If the underlying cause of acquired megaoesophagus can be identified and successfully treated, the signs of megaoesophagus may subside. However, the development of megaoesophagus secondary to systemic disease is correlated with an extremely poor response to therapy. Death results from aspiration pneumonia, gastro-oesophageal intussusception, cachexia and other related organ dysfunctions.

Oesophageal foreign bodies, perforation, fistulas, diverticuli and stricture

Oesophageal foreign body is a common problem in puppies and sometimes kittens, and can be life-threatening. The most common sites of lodgement are in the thoracic oesophagus at the diaphragmatic hiatus, followed by lodgement at the base of the heart (Parker *et al.*, 1989; Spielman *et al.*, 1992). Lodgement also occurs at the thoracic inlet and at the level of the cricopharyngeal sphincter (Spielman *et al.*, 1992). The most commonly ingested foreign bodies in dogs are bones. Oesophageal perforation associated with foreign bodies can occur as a direct result of ingestion of a sharp pointed object or secondary to ischaemic necrosis due to pressure on the oesophageal wall. For this reason oesophageal foreign bodies should be removed as soon as possible.

Other causes of oesophageal perforation include ingestion of caustic substances, penetrating external trauma such as bite wounds, incisional dehiscence, traumatic endoscopy, iatrogenic tears during intraluminal stricture dilatation and oesophageal neoplasia. Prolonged clinical signs of oesophageal disease and evidence of increased numbers of immature neutrophils on a haematological evaluation may indicate oesophageal perforation and further diagnostic tests should be performed (Spielman *et al.*, 1992).

Oesophageal fistulas can be congenital or, more commonly, acquired and may communicate with the trachea, bronchus or lung parenchyma. Congenital fistulas are probably due to failure of separation of the gastrointestinal and respiratory tracts during embryogenesis (Basher *et al.*, 1991). Acquired oesophageal fistulas are most commonly associated with foreign-body ingestion and are most frequently located between the oesophagus and the right caudal lung lobe in dogs, and between the oesophagus and the accessory lobe and the left caudal lung lobe in cats (Fingeroth, 1993). An untreated oesophageal perforation may develop into an oesophageal fistula (Flanders, 1989; Parker *et al.*, 1989) and a cervical oesophageal perforation may form a cutaneous fistula.

Oesophageal diverticuli are congenital defects which result from inherent weakness in the oesophageal wall or incomplete separation of the respiratory and gastrointestinal tracts during embryogenesis (Fingeroth, 1993). Pulsion or traction diverticuli occur but are rare in small animals. A pulsion diverticulum is an outpouching of mucosa and submucosa between muscular layers and results from intraluminal forces. A traction diverticulum is an outpouching of all layers of the oesophagus and usually results from extraluminal forces. A normal developmental redundancy of the oesophagus may be seen in brachycephalic breeds and Shar-Peis and should not be confused with a congenital diverticulum (Stickle and Love, 1989; Twedt, 1995).

Oesophageal strictures may develop secondary to ingestion of caustic chemicals, trauma, lodgement of foreign bodies, resection and anastomosis or gastric reflux oesophagitis.

Clinical signs

Common clinical signs associated with any oesophageal disease include dysphagia, regurgitation, ptyalism and repeated attempts to swallow. Depending on the disease and its duration, the animal may otherwise appear normal. If perforation or fistula formation is present the animal may appear lethargic and be febrile. Subcutaneous emphysema may be observed with perforation. A cervical swelling and associated cellulitis may be noted in cervical perforation or fistulation. Coughing is a common finding if aspiration pneumonia, oesophageal perforation or a broncho-oesophageal fistula is present.

Diagnosis

The breed and medical history may be important in the differentiation of certain surgical and non-surgical problems. If oesophageal disease is indicated from the history and physical examination, thoracic radiography is essential. Since most foreign bodies in dogs are bones, plain radiography may be satisfactory to make that diagnosis. Other radiographic findings associated with oesophageal disease include pneumomediastinum, aspiration pneumonia, gaseous dilation of the oesophagus and a mediastinal mass (Stickle and Love, 1989).

Oesophagography and oesophagoscopy are the most helpful diagnostic tools in diagnosing oesophageal disease. Obstruction due to strictures must be differentiated from persistent right aortic arch (PRAA) (see Chapter 8). The location of the stricture must be at the base of the heart to implicate PRAA. Remember PRAA is not a common disease. Breed profile and prior medical history (ingestion of caustic materials, prior surgery with possible intraoperative oesophageal reflux) may also help in the differential diagnosis of strictures.

Oesophageal perforation can be diagnosed with oesophagography or oesophagoscopy but false-negatives can occur with both techniques (Parker *et al.*, 1989). Oesophagoscopy should be performed prior to any contrast study as the contrast agent will coat the oesophageal mucosa and may obscure detection of any perforation.

A positive-contrast oesophogram is indicated if thoracic radiographs are non-diagnostic and oesophagoscopy cannot be performed. Barium paste and liquid barium are the most commonly used contrast agents. However, if perforation is suspected, a water soluble organic iodine contrast medium should be used instead of barium until a perforation can be ruled out. The normal canine oesophagus has linear mucosal striations throughout its length, while the distal feline oesophagus usually has circular mucosal folds that form a herring-bone pattern with positive contrast (Stickle and Love, 1989).

Treatment and surgical technique

Due to the morbidity of oesophageal surgery, non-surgical removal of a foreign body with a fibreoptic endoscope or rigid proctoscope may be attempted prior to surgery if the equipment is available (Tams, 1990). If removal with an endoscope is unsuccessful, it may be possible to push a foreign body from the distal thoracic oesophagus into the stomach in order to allow removal by gastrotomy, thus avoiding a thoracotomy. In some cases, the foreign body may be pulled through the cardia from the distal oesophagus via a gastrotomy incision. These techniques for removal are discouraged, particularly if the foreign body has been present greater than 36–48 hours, due to the increased risk of perforation through devitalized tissue.

Oesophagoscopy has the advantage of allowing visualization of oesophageal mucosa to enable evaluation of any damage. A foreign body may be grasped with forceps and removed with the endoscope or proctoscope. If a mass is present, endoscopy can be used to obtain a biopsy without the need for surgery. Complica-

tions of oesophagoscopy include perforation of a compromised oesophagus, and an inability to evaluate the structures completely surrounding the oesophagus for evidence of perforation that is not visible from the mucosal surface.

Foreign bodies can be treated by oesophagotomy or, if severe oesophageal damage has occurred, by resection and anastomosis. Oesophageal diverticulum can be treated by resection of the diverticulum or, in the case of a pulsion diverticulum, by resection of the mucosa and closure of the muscle defect.

Oesophageal fistula connected with the respiratory tract may require lung lobectomy. Cutaneous fistula (usually in the cervical region) requires repair of the oesophageal defect and debridement of the fistulous tract which is left to heal by second intention. The tract does not require excision if the oesophageal defect can be closed.

Oesophageal stricture is best treated non-surgically using repeated balloon dilatation under general anaesthesia. Balloon dilatation has less risk of perforation than bougienage, which has been used historically, since it allows controlled, circumferential, radial dilatation with even pressure on all aspects of the cicatrix. It has, however, also been associated with tears and perforation in a small number of animals (Willard *et al.*, 1994).

The catheter can be passed through an endoscope so visualization of the dilatation procedure is possible. The balloon length should be longer than the cicatrix to maximize benefit from the dilatation and prevent tearing at the region of the end of the balloon (Willard *et al.*, 1994). Multiple treatments may be required but a standard protocol for repeated treatments is not known. An endoscope large enough to have a 2.8-mm biopsy channel is required for passage of the balloon catheter. This may preclude its use in very small puppies or kittens. Use of cuffed endotracheal tubes may be an alternative for small animals that cannot undergo endoscopy but there is a disadvantage of non-visualization of the procedure (Hardie *et al.*, 1987). Adjunctive therapy with H_2-blockers (see Table 6.15), prednisolone (to reduce oesophagitis and scar reformation) and metoclopramide (to reduce oesophageal reflux) has been used (Hardie *et al.*, 1987; Smith and Clark, 1992). Failure to respond to dilatation may require resection and anastomosis of the affected segment, but recurrence of the stricture after surgery is also possible (Willard *et al.*, 1994).

Oesophagotomy and oesophageal resection and anastomosis

General principles

The oesophagus is predisposed to postoperative dehiscence due to several inherent characteristics, including a segmental blood supply and lack of a serosal covering to facilitate formation of a seal. Constant movement of the oesophagus and irritation of the luminal surface by ingesta and saliva also play a role in the development of postoperative complications. Excessive tension on an anastomotic suture line after resection can also result in failure and tension should be avoided (Flanders, 1989; Oakes *et al.*, 1993). Gentle, atraumatic tissue handling is imperative (Flanders, 1989). Perioperative antibiotics are indicated since the surgery is classified as clean-contaminated and may be contaminated if perforation is present.

The cervical oesophagus is approached through a ventral midline incision extending from the level of the caudal mandible to the manubrium with the animal in dorsal recumbency. The skin incision is extended through the subcutaneous tissues, and the sternohyoideus muscles are separated along the midline and retracted, exposing the trachea. The trachea is retracted to the right side to expose the oesophagus. The carotid sheath and left recurrent laryngeal nerve are protected.

The thoracic oesophagus is best approached through a lateral intercostal thoracotomy. A right lateral approach is indicated for much of the oesophagus since it is displaced to the right of midline by the trachea cranially and the aorta caudally. The location of the expected lesion determines the intercostal space chosen.

Oesophagotomy

Stay sutures are placed in the oesophagus for atraumatic immobilization and the affected segment is isolated from the rest of the cervical region or thorax using moistened laparotomy sponges. A stomach tube or oesophageal stethoscope may help to facilitate identification of the oesophagus as well as to provide support while incising the oesophagus. The oesophageal incision is made longitudinally in a healthy portion

of the oesophagus. If a foreign body is present, the oesophagus is incised just distal to it, and the foreign body is grasped with an instrument and removed with gentle traction and manipulation. The tissues are inspected for damage and viability. It is important to explore the surrounding mediastinum and thorax for damage or additional foreign bodies. If non-viable oesophageal tissue is suspected, various patching techniques or resection and anastomosis should be considered. The wound is lavaged thoroughly prior to closure.

Closure of the oesophagus is best performed using a two-layer, simple interrupted suture pattern. This pattern results in the greatest immediate wound strength and best tissue apposition and healing when compared with single-layer techniques (Oakes *et al.*, 1993). The first layer should incorporate the mucosa and submucosa with the knots tied in the lumen of the oesophagus. The second layer should incorporate the muscularis and adventitia and the knots should be tied externally (Fig. 6.11). Sutures should be placed carefully and be approximately 2 mm apart. The holding layer of the oesophagus has been shown to be the submucosa, therefore the first layer is the most important (Dallman, 1988). An absorbable, monofilament, minimally reactive suture material (3-0 or 4-0) such as polydioxanone or poliglecaprone 25 with a swedged-on taper or reverse-cutting needle is recommended for oesophageal surgery (Flanders, 1989).

Oesophageal resection and anastomosis

Resection of the oesophagus should be considered only if necessary due to the complications associated with oesophageal healing and

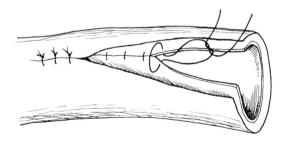

Figure 6.11 Oesophagotomy closure using two layers of simple interrupted sutures, in the mucosa and submucosa, and in the muscular layers. Knots are placed within the lumen during the mucosal/submucosal closure.

excessive tension. Tension has been reported to be present when only 2 cm of the oesophagus is removed. If a larger segment of oesophagus needs to be removed, an oesophageal reconstruction technique may be attempted. Small perforations can be debrided and closed primarily in two layers (Flanders, 1989; Parker *et al.*, 1989). If resection is necessary, the oesophageal segment is isolated as described above and held with stay sutures. The oesophageal lumen is occluded with atraumatic intestinal clamps such as a Doyen or Pean forceps and the oesophageal segment is resected along the outside edge of the clamps.

The oesophageal lumen is closed in a two-layer, interrupted pattern as described for oesophagotomy closure. The first layer should incorporate the mucosa and submucosa and the knots should be tied intraluminally as described for oesophagotomy. The first suture should be placed on the far side between the dorsal and ventral stay sutures, and subsequent sutures should be placed on either side in alternating fashion until closure is complete. The final sutures placed in the inner layer may be preplaced in order to facilitate tying of the knots in the lumen. The second layer is placed in the muscularis and adventitia and is also placed in an interrupted pattern with the knots external.

To minimize tension at the anastomotic site, several procedures have been attempted. Oesophageal immobilization via dissection from surrounding structures provides minimal advancement and may risk damage to the segmental blood supply. A circular myotomy of the outer muscular layer of the oesophagus while preserving the inner muscular layer may provide tension relief in some cases. This can be performed at a site proximal and distal to the anastomosis (Attum *et al.*, 1979; Flanders, 1989). Following closure of the intrathoracic oesophagus, a section of omentum may be pulled through an incision in the diaphragm or a subcutaneous tunnel and placed over the oesophageal incision in order to provide a seal and enhance blood supply to the area (Flanders, 1989; Hosgood, 1990).

Postoperative considerations and complications

Postoperative care after oesophageal surgery or dilatation should be aimed at decreasing mechanical trauma to the affected oesophageal site while providing nutritional support to the animal. Feeding tubes have been advocated to reduce mechanical trauma caused by food and peristaltic activity and are certainly indicated in debilitated animals, animals with other problems that may cause inappetence (aspiration pneumonia) or those with substantial oesophageal inflammation. Gastrostomy tubes are superior to pharyngostomy, oesophagostomy or nasogastric tubes since the physical presence of a tube across the oesophageal incision can delay healing or predispose to stricture (Flanders, 1989; Parker *et al.*, 1989). Animals not requiring a feeding tube can be fed soft food (which can be in the form of a slurry for animals with stricture), beginning 24 hours after surgery (Flanders, 1989).

Oesophageal stricture has been reported after oesophageal surgery and may be due to tissue damage by a foreign body, excessive surgical trauma or reflux oesophagitis. Oesophageal inflammation may cause decreased effectiveness of oesophageal peristaltic activity and decreased lower oesophageal sphincter tone resulting in continued gastro-oesophageal reflux and oesophagitis (Spielman *et al.*, 1992). H_2-receptor blocking agents or omeprazole should be used to control oesophagitis by increasing the pH of gastric fluid refluxed into the oesophagus. Metoclopramide may be indicated to reduce oesophageal reflux as it will improve gastro-oesophageal tone and promote gastric emptying. Cisapride may also be indicated (see Table 6.15). Postoperative antibiotics should be continued if there was contamination or evidence of infection at surgery.

The prognosis for animals with oesophageal stricture that undergo balloon dilatation is good for return to eating soft food or normal food without regurgitation (Hardie *et al.*, 1987; Smith and Clark, 1992; Willard *et al.*, 1994). For animals with oesophageal foreign bodies with perforation that require surgery, a 57% mortality has been reported (Parker *et al.*, 1989).

Stomach and intestines

Gastritis and enterocolitis

Gastritis and enterocolitis frequently occur in dogs and cats from weaning and throughout adulthood. Gastritis can be associated with a

Table 6.13 Causes of gastritis and enterocolitis in puppies and kittens

Cause	Comment
Dietary indiscretion	Ingestion of rancid or contaminated foodstuffs that leads to a food intoxication
	Ingestion of foreign material such as bones, pins, needles, plastic objects, food wrappings, rocks and small toys mechanically irritates the gastric mucosa and thereby causes gastritis and enterocolitis. The incidence of ingesting foreign objects is much higher in puppies and kittens than adult animals, probably because of their developmental chewing habits and curious natures
	Intolerance of lactose ingested as milk and miscellaneous food intolerances, such as fatty or spicy food
	Trichobezoars (hairballs) are frequently seen in the vomitus or diarrhoeic stools of some long-haired cats and dogs
	The ingestion of grass and plants by seemingly healthy animals is not uncommon, possibly owing to their natural instinctual behaviours. Many young dogs and cats with gastric or intestinal disorders, for some unknown reason, frequently ingest and then vomit grass or plant material
Drugs	Antimicrobial agents, non-steroidal anti-inflammatory drugs and anthelmintics can induce gastritis and enterocolitis
Chemicals	Inadvertent ingestion of heavy metals, cleaning agents, fertilizers and herbicides may cause signs of gastritis and enterocolitis
Mycotic infections	Not an important cause of gastritis or enterocolitis in dogs and cats younger than 6 months of age. The primary fungi infecting the intestinal tract are *Histoplasma capsulatum*, *Aspergillus* spp. and *Pythium* spp.
Others	Renal failure, liver disease, neurological disease, shock, sepsis, hypoadrenocorticism, stress and possibly altered behaviour may play a role in the cause of gastritis and enterocolitis in the puppy or kitten

	Gastritis	*Enterocolitis*
Bacterial infections	Incidence is extremely low because the acidic gastric lumen does not favour the growth and colonization of bacteria. Gastric chlamydial infection may occur in young cats	Many agents can be associated with varying degrees of enterocolitis: *Salmonella* spp., *Escherichia coli*, *Campylobacter jejuni*, *Yersinia enterocolitica*, *Bacillus piliformis* and *Clostridium perfringens* are most common as they normally reside in the intestine
Viral infections	Canine distemper, canine adenovirus-1 (CAV-1), coronaviruses and parvovirus may cause gastric lesions and vomiting as a part of a more extensive disease condition	Canine distemper, parvovirus-2 (CPV-2), coronavirus and rotavirus are important causes of enterocolitis in young dogs
		Other viruses identified in unformed stools of dogs are a minute parvovirus (canine parvovirus-1; CPV-1), adenovirus, caliciviruses, paramyxovirus-like virus, astrovirus, picornavirus, and human echovirus and coxsackievirus
		Feline parvovirus-1 (feline panleukopenia virus) and coronaviruses are the most common causes of viral enterocolitis in young cats
		Other viruses identified in cats include rotavirus, astrovirus, calicivirus, reovirus type III and non-culturable enteric Picornaviridae-like virus

Table 6.13 (continued)

	Gastritis	Enterocolitis
		In cats with refractory diarrhoea, feline leukaemia virus (FeLV), feline immunodeficiency virus (FIV) and feline infectious peritonitis (FIP) virus should be considered
Endoparasites	Seldom produce gastric lesions or signs. *Physaloptera* spp., *Ollulanus tricuspis* (cats), ascarids and occasionally tapeworms may be associated with gastric irritation and vomiting	Generally do not produce intestinal lesions but contribute to generalized unthriftiness, diarrhoea, weight loss or failure to gain adequate body weight
		The younger the animal, the more likely it is to show clinical signs
		Endoparasitism often complicates other existing intestinal disorders such as virus- or bacterial-induced enterocolitis

multitude of factors but more commonly results from dietary indiscretions, infectious diseases and possibly endoparasites (Table 6.13).

Clinical signs

Gastritis

Vomiting is typically the primary clinical sign of gastritis. Vomiting as an event first appears in puppies and kittens with a full stomach at 3 and 10 days of age, respectively. Observation of the amount, colour and consistency of vomitus is useful for obtaining insight into the origin of a gastric disorder and the degree of mucosal damage. If the vomitus consists of food, the degree of digestion indicates the length of time food has remained in the stomach. Vomitus can contain varying amounts of mucus and fluid from gastric and swallowed salivary secretions. Yellow or green stained vomitus indicates intestinal reflux of bile into the stomach. Vomitus containing faeces usually indicates intestinal stasis or possibly intestinal obstruction. Fresh blood from gastric bleeding may be present as small red flecks or as large blood clots. Blood that has been retained in the stomach soon becomes partially digested and has a brown 'coffee grounds' appearance. The presence of blood in vomitus usually signifies a more serious gastric disorder. Other clinical signs associated with gastric disorders may include nausea, belching, inappetence, polydipsia and pica. Melaena, or black tarry stools, is seen with upper

gastrointestinal bleeding and may imply gastric mucosal damage.

Enterocolitis

Diarrhoea is the primary clinical sign of enterocolitis and often occurs secondary to many non-intestinal diseases. The onset is typically abrupt and follows a short course that ranges from transient and self-limiting to fulminating and explosive. By using the history, physical examination and stool characteristics (i.e. frequency, volume, consistency, colour, odour and composition), diarrhoea can be localized to the small intestine, large intestine, or both.

Diagnosis

Gastritis

Gastritis is generally diagnosed and treated on the basis of the animal's history, signs and physical findings. Symptomatic treatment of most cases of gastritis and vomiting is begun without extensive diagnostic procedures. Most animals show improvement within 12–24 hours following little or no therapy and usually are treated on an outpatient basis. Those animals with persistent vomiting, evidence of dehydration, abdominal pain, organomegly or palpable abdominal mass, or failure to respond to previous symptomatic treatment require further medical and laboratory evaluation. The general principles in the treatment of gastric disorders include removing the inciting cause; providing proper conditions to promote mucosal repair; correcting fluid, electrolyte and acid–base abnormalities; and alleviating secondary complications of gastritis, e.g. abdominal pain and diarrhoea.

Enterocolitis

The diagnosis of acute enterocolitis is based an the animal's history, signs and physical findings, often without detailed diagnostic procedures. A review of the animal's vaccination status, diet, current medications and possible exposure to chemicals or infectious diseases is warranted. Endoparasites, ingestion of questionable food or foreign material and/or infectious diseases should always be considered the primary cause of enterocolitis in the young dog or cat until proven otherwise. Animals that experience severe illness or fail to respond to symptomatic therapy usually require a more detailed medical and laboratory evaluation. Diagnostic efforts should then be aimed at detecting an underlying non-intestinal disease as the contributing cause of the diarrhoea. Diagnostic evaluations considered for short-term diarrhoea are faecal identification of endoparasites, virological tests, faecal

cultures for bacteria and survey abdominal radiographs for detection of intestinal foreign material or an obstruction.

Treatment

Dietary restriction is the initial management for gastritis and entercolitis (Table 6.14) as well as parenteral fluid therapy, if indicated. Most animals show improvement within 24–48 hours following little or no therapy and are usually treated on an outpatient basis.

Medicants

Antiemetic drugs may be given to control refractory vomiting in dogs and cats older than 3 months of age (Table 6.15) and when the presence of a pyloric dysfunction or a gastric foreign object has been ruled out. These drugs inhibit vomiting but do little for primary treatment of gastritis. Antiemetic drugs act centrally by suppressing the chemoreceptor trigger zone, the emetic centre or the vestibular apparatus. The phenothiazine tranquillizers (chlorpromazine) have a broad-spectrum pharmacological

Table 6.14 Guidelines for initial management of gastritis in a puppy or kitten

Treatment	Comment
Withhold food for 24–48 hours and water for 12–24 hours	If no vomiting occurs during this period of management, over the next 2–5 days the animal is gradually returned to full feed and water
	Most young dogs and cats with vomiting will respond to dietary and water intake restriction
Reintroduce water and food gradually	Water is offered initially in small, frequent amounts or provided in ice cubes, enough to keep the mouth moist and to supply a modest fluid replacement
	Feed small amounts frequently (3–6 times daily) of a highly digestible, low-fibre diet – cooked rice or cooked cereals supplemented in a 50:50 ratio with low-fat cottage cheese, boiled chicken, lean boiled ground beef or commercial baby foods
	Commercial diets formulated for gastrointestinal disease may also be prescribed. Initially feed one-third the amount needed to meet normal maintenance caloric needs and gradually increase the amount over the next few days to meet the animal's maintenance caloric needs
Parenteral fluid therapy	Initiated when electrolyte or acid–base imbalances or dehydration occurs
	Volume administered should supply daily maintenance needs (approximately 40–60 ml/kg per day), correct existing dehydration and replace fluid losses caused by continued vomiting or diarrhoea
	Vomiting in gastritis and diarrhoea in enterocolitis generally result in volume depletion and losses of sodium, chloride and potassium with a metabolic acidosis
	Isotonic, balanced electrolyte solution (lactated Ringer's solution) with potassium supplementation is recommended

Table 6.15 Therapeutic agents available for management of gastrointestinal disorders (modified from Hoskins and Dimski, 1995)

Agent	Dosage	Comments
Antidiarrhoea		
Chlordiazepoxide and clidinium	Dog: 1–2 tablets b.i.d.–t.i.d. PO	Causes central nervous system depression and anticholinergic effects. Contraindicated in infectious enteritis and gastrointestinal obstruction; not recommended for dogs < 10 kg
Dicyclomine	0.15 mg/kg t.i.d. PO (paediatric dose)	Anticholinergic effects. Dose unclear for dogs and cats
Diphenoxylate	Dog: 0.06–0.1 mg/kg t.i.d.–q.i.d. PO	Narcotic analgesic effects
Loperamide	Dog: 0.08 mg/kg t.i.d.–q.i.d. PO	Narcotic analgesic effects. Tablet or liquid form
Paregoric	Dog: 0.05–0.06 mg/kg t.i.d. PO	Narcotic analgesic effects. Useful for dogs < 10 kg
Propantheline	0.25 mg/kg t.i.d. PO	Anticholinergic effects. Contraindicated in infectious enteritis and gastrointestinal obstruction
Antiemetic		
Chlorpromazine	Dog and cat: 0.5 mg/kg t.i.d. IM Dog: 1.0 mg/kg t.i.d. PO or rectal Dog: 0.05 mg/kg IV	
Dimenhydrinate	4 mg/kg t.i.d. PO	Antihistamine antiemetic. Good for motion sickness if given before event
Diphenhydramine	2–4 mg/kg t.i.d. PO	Antihistamine antiemetic. Good for motion sickness if given before event
Metoclopramide	0.2–0.4 mg/kg t.i.d. PO, SC 1–2 mg/kg per 24 hours IV as slow infusion	For gastric motility disorders and reflux oesophagitis
Prochlorperazine	0.1 mg/kg q.i.d. IM	
Propantheline	0.25 mg/kg t.i.d. PO	Questionable efficacy. Parasympatholytic effects
Triethylperazine	Dog: 0.25 mg/kg t.i.d. IM Dog: 0.5 mg/kg t.i.d. rectal Cat: 0.125 mg/kg t.i.d. IM	Very effective
Trimethobenzamine	Dog: 3 mg/kg t.i.d. IM	Antihistamine antiemetic. Appropriateness for cats unknown
Gastric protectants		
Sucralfate	Dog: 100–1000 mg PO Cat: 100–200 mg PO	Requires acidic pH for activation. Administer 30–40 minutes before H_2-receptor blockers. Use low dose for animals < 4 months. Not absorbed systemically. May cause constipation with daily use
H_2-receptor blocker Cimetidine	5 mg/kg b.i.d.-t.i.d. IM, IV, PO	For gastric ulceration. Do not use on animals < 2 months. Impedes hepatic biotransformation enzymes
H_2-receptor blocker Ranitidine	2–4 mg/kg b.i.d. IV, SC, PO	For gastric ulceration. Do not use on animals < 2 months. Does not impede hepatic biotransformation enzymes
H_2-receptor blocker Famotidine	0.5–1.0 mg/kg s.i.d. PO	For gastric ulceration. Do not use on animals < 2 months
Omeprazole	Dog: 1–2 mg/kg s.i.d.	For gastric ulcers and reflux oesophagitis. Longer acting than H_2-receptor blockers. Prolonged administration not recommended
Misoprostol	Dog: 2–5 μg/kg t.i.d.	For NSAID-induced gastric ulceration. Synthetic analogue of prostaglandin E. May cause diarrhoea. Contraindicated in pregnant animals

Table 6.15 (continued)

Agent	Dosage	Comments
Laxatives		
Bisacodyl	5 mg s.i.d. PO	5-mg tablet and 5-mg suppository. 6–12 hours required for effect. Animals should be well-hydrated
Bran	1–2 tablespoons mixed in 400 g of canned food. Given s.i.d.–b.i.d.	Powder; 12–24 hours required for effect
Dioctyl sodium sulphosuccinate	Dog: 50–200 mg s.i.d. PO Cat: 50 mg s.i.d. PO	Available as 50- and 100-mg capsules, 1% liquid, or 4 mg/ml syrup. 12–72 hours required for effect. Animals should be well-hydrated. Do not use with mineral oil
Dioctyl calcium sulphosuccinate	Dog: 100–150 mg s.i.d. PO Cat: 50–100 mg s.i.d. PO	Available as 50- and 240-mg capsules. Considerations as for dioctyl sodium sulphosuccinate
Lactulose	Dog: 1 ml/4.5 kg t.i.d. PO; adjust dose to induce 2–3 bowel movements per day Cat: 0.25–1 ml; adjust dose to induce 2–3 bowel movements per day Retention enema for hepatoencephalopathy: 5–20 ml lactulose diluted 1:3 in water t.i.d.–q.i.d.	Overdose causes diarrhoea, flatulence, intestinal cramping, dehydration and acidosis
Mineral oil	5–25 ml b.i.d. PO or perrectum	Liquid. Caution with oral administration (aspiration pneumonia). Administer between feeding. 6–12 hours required for effect
Psyllium	1–3 teaspoons mixed with food s.i.d.–b.i.d.	Powder. 12–24 hours required for effect
White petrolatum	1–5 ml s.i.d. PO; then 2–3 times/week	Paste. Administer between feeding. 12–24 hours required for effect
Prokinetic agents Cisapride	Dog: 0.1–0.5 mg/kg t.i.d. to b.i.d. PO Cat: 2.5–5.0 mg per cat t.i.d. to b.i.d. PO	Administer 30 minutes before feeding It may cause elevated heart rate

effect in blocking the emetic centre and the chemoreceptor trigger zone, and some anticholinergic action. These drugs are effective in blocking viscerally stimulated vomiting caused by gastritis and can be used in animals with protracted vomiting. The phenothiazines should not be used in a dehydrated or a hypotensive animal or if a hepatopathy is suspected.

Anticholinergic drugs reduce gastric motility and smooth-muscle spasms. In addition to blocking the parasympathetic stimulation of smooth muscles, these drugs block the cephalic and gastric phases of gastric acid secretion, but they do not block histamine- or gastrin-stimulated acid secretion. They have the adverse effect of slowing gastric emptying, which results in gastric distension and further gastric acid secretion. Overuse of the anticholinergic drugs can cause gastric atony and a pharmacological gastric outflow obstruction, resulting in further vomiting. Anticholinergic drugs used in the therapy of gastric disorders include atropine and propantheline. These drugs are often combined with an antiemetic for veterinary use.

Cisapride a serotonin-4 receptor agonist, increases gastrointestinal motility, increases the lower esophageal sphincter tone and increases esophageal peristalsis. It can be used for gastroesophageal reflux, gastroduodenal reflux and gastric motility disorders. It has met with limited success in the treatment of constipation and feline megacolon. Cisapride may be indicated in conjunction with antiemetic therapy for the treatment of protracted vomiting, once gastric outflow obstruction has been ruled out as a cause of the vomiting.

Oral protectants, such as kaolin and pectin, and antimicrobial agents are usually not indicated in the treatment of gastritis in the young dog or cat. Protectants may bind certain bacteria or toxins, but they do not coat or protect the irritated gastric mucosa. Any potential benefit is frequently outweighed by difficulty in owner administration and vomiting that occurs because of gastric distension. However, sucralfate in tablet form or given as a slurry (crush sucralfate 1 g and mix with 10 ml water; give 5 ml of slurry 4–6 times daily) may be protective when the gastric mucosa is irritated or ulcerated.

Protectants, however, are often used for the treatment of diarrhoea, although they are probably not as beneficial in animals as once thought. There is some evidence that pectin plus salicylates can absorb and inactivate enterotoxins, such as those produced by *Escherichia coli*. One effect of salicylates is inhibition of prostaglandins, which may decrease enterotoxin-induced intestinal hypersecretion. Of the salicylates, bismuth subsalicylate appears to be more effective as an oral antidiarrhoeal compound. The dose is about 0.25 ml/kg body weight divided into four to six equal daily doses. Bismuth subsalicylate should be administered with caution in cats because of their increased sensitivity to aspirin and should not be administered to cats younger than 4 months of age. Its taste is unpleasant, but some of the resistance to administration may be overcome by keeping the product in the refrigerator and administering it cold.

Antimicrobial agents are not required unless a bacterial infection is suspected.

Secretory blockers (H_2-receptor antagonists), e.g. cimetidine, ranitidine, and famotidine, are effective in reducing gastric acid production by blocking the H_2-receptors of the parietal cells (Table 6.15). Use of these drugs has been recommended in the symptomatic treatment of gastric and duodenal ulcers and in syndromes resulting in gastric acid hypersecretion. They may be useful as adjunctive therapy in some types of gastritis. However, they probably should not be administered to dogs or cats younger than 2 months of age.

The use of narcotic analgesics as antimotility drugs is warranted in the treatment of some diarrhoeas (Table 6.15). The rationale behind their use is their direct action on the smooth muscle of the small intestine and colon, causing increasing tone and segmentation. This produces increased resistance to luminal transit of ingesta. These drugs effectively relieve abdominal pain and tenesmus and reduce the frequency of stools. Anticholinergic and related antispasmodic drugs have an uncertain role in the management of diarrhoea. Anticholinergic drugs block the effect of acetylcholine, the major neurotransmitter of the gastrointestinal smooth muscle, resulting in both decreased peristalsis and decreased segmentation. With their use, motility of the small intestine and colon can be stopped, which allows the occurrence of bacterial overgrowth, thus compounding the hypomotility and possibly the diarrhoea problem. Therefore, the narcotic analgesics, such as paregoric, diphenoxylate hydrochloride and loperamide hydrochloride, are the preferred motility modifiers to be used in the symptomatic treatment of diarrhoea. If the diarrhoea is caused by an infectious agent such as *Salmonella,* the narcotic analgesics may be detrimental because they may trap organisms and their toxins within the intestine, and the infection may persist longer.

Because of the frequent occurrence of endoparasites as the primary or secondary cause of enterocolitis in the young dog or cat, routine administration of an appropriate antiparasitic drug is recommended. The use of antimicrobial agents in the treatment of diarrhoea is controversial. If antimicrobial agents only succeed in inhibiting the normal intestinal flora, they are detrimental. In diarrhoea, antimicrobial therapy is only warranted when there is evidence of inflammation in the gastrointestinal tract (numerous inflammatory cells in the faeces), damaged intestinal mucosa (blood in the stool), a systemic inflammatory reaction (fever and leukocytosis) and abnormal faecal culture results.

Gastrointestinal surgery (Table 6.16)

Table 6.16 General principles of gastrointestinal surgery

Consideration	Comment
Contamination	Perioperative antibiotics primarily directed against Gram-negative bacteria (and anaerobes for large-bowel surgery) are indicated
	The operated segment of the gastrointestinal tract should be isolated from the abdominal cavity with moistened laparotomy sponges
	If contamination of the peritoneal cavity occurs, vigorous, copious lavage with warm normal saline should be performed. Lavage with antibiotics or antiseptics is not indicated. Postoperative antibiotic medication may be required depending on the degree of contamination, the status of the animal and the effectiveness of lavage
	Have clean instruments set aside to close abdominal incision after closure of the gastrointestinal tract and lavage of the peritoneal cavity. These are your clean instruments. All others used in the gastrointestinal procedure are contaminated. Reglove before abdominal closure
Wound closure	The gastrointestinal tract is highly vascular and healing is generally rapid. The submucosa is the holding layer for wound strength for the entire gastrointestinal tract
	Colonic healing is the slowest and is at the greatest risk for dehiscence, although morbidity and mortality of small and large intestinal surgery in the dog and cat do not appear significantly different (Wylie and Hosgood, 1994)
	Gastrointestinal dehiscence is more common in debilitated animals, animals on immunosuppressive therapy (corticosteroids) or after surgery for foreign bodies or trauma where there is bowel compromise
	Monofilament absorbable suture (3-0 to 4-0) is indicated for closure. Polydioxanone is preferred. Single-layer, appositional closure (simple interrupted) suture patterns are indicate for the small and large intestine. Inverting closure is indicated for the stomach only
	Gastrointestinal (GI) or thoracoabdominal (TA) staplers may be used for gastric closure and reduce surgery time and the risk of spillage. End-to-end anastomosis (EEA) staplers can be used for intestinal surgery but the small size of some puppies and kittens may prohibit their use
	Omental or serosal patching can be used to support incisions. The omentum is placed over the incision and sutured loosely if necessary. A serosal patch requires an adjacent segment of intestine to be sutured to the affected bowel such that it lies over the incision without compromising luminal flow
Postoperative considerations	Unless there was gross spillage, postoperative antimicrobial medication is not indicated
	Fluid requirements of the animal are maintained parenterally until the animal will drink water voluntarily without vomiting
	Small amounts of water can be given within 12 hours of surgery and, if no vomiting occurs, a bland, easily digestible diet can be offered within 24 hours

Gastric foreign bodies

Gastric foreign bodies are not uncommon in young puppies and kittens. Small objects may pass and animals should be closely observed for 48 hours. Failure to pass an object, consistent presence of an object on serial radiographs or development of clinical signs are indications for removal.

Clinical signs

Clinical signs primarily consist of persistent vomiting, which may be intermittent. Physical examination is often unremarkable, although if vomiting has been persistent for several days, dehydration may be present. The mucous membranes may be dry and tacky and the animal may appear somewhat depressed. A gastric foreign body, depending on the size of the animal, may be palpated on physical examination.

Laboratory findings may be consistent with dehydration (elevated packed cell volume and total solids). Metabolic acidosis is the most common blood chemistry abnormality.

Diagnosis

Diagnosis is based on history of observation of ingestion and radiographic findings. Radiopaque material may be observed on plain radiographs. For radiolucent material, contrast studies using water-soluble iodinated medium should be performed.

Treatment and surgical technique

Emetics should be used with extreme caution and are only indicated when the foreign body is small, rounded and smooth and has been present for less than 24 hours. Apomorphine can be used in the dog (1–5 mg SC) and xylazine for the cat (1 mg/kg SC).

Endoscopic removal under general anaesthesia can be used for small, smooth foreign bodies that are deemed easy to pass through the oesophagus. Retrieval is performed using a special basket that passes through the endoscope.

Large foreign bodies or those with rough edges that might injure the oesophagus require gastrotomy. Gastrotomy is performed through a cranial ventral midline coeliotomy and the general principles of gastrointestinal surgery apply (Table 6.16). If the stomach is full of fluid, passing a stomach tube at surgery will facilitate removal of fluid and reduce the risk of contamination during gastrotomy. Stay sutures (4-0) are placed to maintain traction while a stab incision is made in an avascular area of the fundus, along the greater curvature. Make sure the incision is far enough away from the epiploic vessels to allow for an inverting closure. The incision is continued until it is large enough to allow easy removal of the foreign body. Gavage of the stomach is not recommended due to the risk of peritoneal contamination. The stomach is closed in a two-layer closure with a simple continuous closure of the mucosal and submucosal layers followed by a continuous inverting closure (Connell or Lembert patterns) of the muscularis and serosal layers. The peritoneal cavity is lavaged with warm normal saline and closed in a routine three-layer closure.

Postoperative considerations and prognosis

The general principles of postoperative management for gastrointestinal surgery apply (Table 6.16). The prognosis for complete recovery is excellent.

Congenital pyloric stenosis

Congenital pyloric stenosis is an uncommon condition where there is thickening or hypertrophy of the pyloric circular smooth-muscle layer that results in delayed gastric emptying of solid foods. It is primarily reported in young male dogs and brachycephalic breeds. The exact pathogenesis or inheritance is unknown. Excessive levels of gastrin have been proposed due to the trophic effects of gastrin on the gastric smooth muscle. Congenital pyloric stenosis is rare in cats but has been reported in the Siamese. Concurrent megaoesophagus was reported in 8 of 15 cats and no cats had evidence of gross muscle hypertrophy. These findings suggested this may be a different disease than that of the dog with an underlying autonomic disorder (Pearson *et al.*, 1974).

Clinical signs

Clinical signs of vomiting become obvious when the animals are weaned since outflow of solid foods is affected. The animals may appear stunted in comparison to the littermates. Aspiration pneumonia may be present.

Diagnosis

Diagnosis is based on history, clinical signs and evidence of delayed gastric emptying on radiographic studies (gastric distension, delayed emptying of contrast material). Ultrasonographic examination of the pyloric area may demonstrate thickening. Diagnosis is confirmed by exploratory coeliotomy and possible histopathologic examination of biopsy samples.

Treatment and surgical techniques

Treatment requires pyloroplasty. Generally, a Fredet–Ramstedt pyloromyotomy or a Heineke–Mikulicz pyloroplasty is recommended (Fig. 6.12). This condition is the only true indication for these procedures; they are

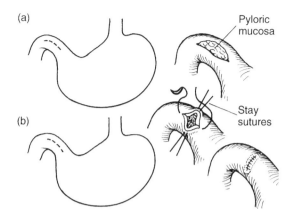

Figure 6.12 Pyloroplasty techniques. (a) Fredet–Ramstedt pyloromyotomy requires a longitudinal incision through the seromuscular and submucosal layers of the pylorus to expose the bulging mucosa. The incision is left open. (b) Heineke–Mikulicz requires a full-thickness longitudinal incision through the pyloric wall, which is then sutured transversely.

generally not effective for the adult-onset disease of chronic hypertrophic pyloric gastropathy. A cranial ventral midline coeliotomy is performed and the general principles of gastrointestinal surgery apply (Table 6.16). If the stomach is full of fluid, passing a stomach tube at surgery will facilitate removal of fluid and reduce the risk of contamination during myotomy. Stay sutures (4-0) are placed in the proximal duodenum and pyloric antrum to maintain traction.

For the Fredet–Ramstedt pyloromyotomy, a longitudinal incision is performed through the serosa, muscularis and submucosa to permit unrestricted bulging of the mucosa, relieving constriction of the pylorus. The mucosa must be completely exposed to allow this procedure to be effective. Tissue from the submucosal to serosal layers can be taken for histological examination. The incision is left open.

For the Heineke–Mikulicz pyloroplasty, a similar incision is made but it penetrates the mucosa and enters the pyloric lumen. A full-thickness tissue sample can be taken for histological examination. The incision is closed transversely using monofilament absorbable suture material (3-0 or 4-0) in a simple interrupted pattern with the sutures penetrating all tissue layers.

Postoperative considerations and prognosis

The general principles of postoperative manage-ment after gastrointestinal surgery apply (Table 6.16). The prognosis for complete recovery is fair, with over 50% of animals responding to surgery.

Intestinal obstruction

Intestinal obstruction is not uncommon in puppies and kittens and is generally due to foreign bodies or intussusception and occasionally, strangulation.

Common intestinal foreign bodies include rocks, coins, rubber and plastic objects, nuts, jewellery and cloth. Partial or complete obstruction may occur. These sorts of objects often have difficulty passing aborally through the gastro-intestinal tract and lodge in the jejunum. Linear objects including fabric (tights), dental floss, string, Christmas tree decorations, plastic bags, binding from golf balls and fishing line pose a more difficult problem as they tend to become lodged in a section of the gastro-intestinal tract, usually the pylorus, or under-neath the tongue, and cause extensive damage as the remainder of the linear object passes down the gastrointestinal tract. The small intes-tine tends to move cranially over the fixed linear object, resulting in pleating of the intestine and complete or partial obstruction. This creates tension on the mesenteric border of the intest-inal tract and can cause perforation at multiple sites and subsequent peritonitis.

Intussusception is a common cause of intest-inal obstruction in young dogs and occurs most commonly at the ileocolic junction. Intus-susception is characterized by the inversion of one segment of intestine (intussusceptum) into another (intussuscipiens). Intussusception may be associated with intestinal parasitism and diarrhoea, foreign bodies and abdominal sur-gery. Other causes of abnormal intestinal moti-lity such as enteritis, acute inflammation or orally administered anthelminthics may contri-bute to the development of intussusception. Intussusception generally causes a partial obstruction, with clinical signs being more severe the more cranial the location of the lesion.

Clinical signs

Clinical signs vary with the location of the obstruction and generally are more severe with proximal and complete obstruction. Vomiting and abdominal pain are common with high obstructions. A palpable abdominal mass may be detected with both foreign bodies and intussusception. With low obstructions, abdominal pain, bloody mucoid diarrhoea, anorexia, intestinal prolapse through the rectum and tenesmus may occur. A prolapsed intussusception must be differentiated from a prolapsed rectum. If the mass is a prolapsed intussusception, a probe can be inserted for a considerable distance.

Diagnosis

Diagnosis is based on clinical signs and survey radiographic findings (Table 6.17). Most diagnoses can be made from plain radiographs and contrast radiography using barium is discouraged. Oral barium usually gives equivocal results because of ileus and is contraindicated if there is any chance of intestinal perforation. If contrast medium is used, water-soluble iodine contrast medium is recommended. Ultrasonography is a more useful alternative to contrast radiography in confirming a diagnosis.

Treatment and surgical techniques

Treatment includes preoperative supportive therapy, intravenous fluids and electrolytes, and surgical removal of the foreign body or correction of the intussusception.

Foreign bodies are removed through a longitudinal enterotomy performed on the antimesenteric border of the intestine, just distal to the foreign body. Principles of intestinal surgery apply (Table 6.16). The bowel is occluded prior to enterotomy to prevent spillage. The enterotomy is closed with simple interrupted sutures which penetrate all layers of the intestine. The mucosa should be inverted manually as the sutures are tied. Excessive everted mucosa can be debrided prior to closure if necessary.

If the integrity of the intestine is questionable, resection and anastomosis is required. The affected bowel segment is located and isolated using saline-soaked abdominal sponges. The luminal contents are milked away from the site of incision and atraumatic intestinal clamps (Doyens/Peans) or an assistant's fingers are applied to prevent ingesta from moving back to the incision site. Crushing clamps can be used on the segment to be removed. The mesenteric vessels going to the segment are double-ligated using 3-0 or 4-0 absorbable suture, usually one or more radial vessels, followed by double ligation of the arcade vessels at the mesenteric border at either end of the segment. The vessels (between the two ligatures) and the

Table 6.17 Characteristic plain radiographic features of intestinal obstruction

Feature	Comment
Poor detail	Decreased definition of serosal surfaces is found with lack of intra-abdominal fat or presence of intra-abdominal fluid associated with peritonitis. Note that young animals have inherent poor detail due to lack of fat and, sometimes, a small amount of normal peritoneal fluid
Free intra-abdominal gas	Free gas is a sign of intestinal perforation and appears as small bubbles, often accumulating in the perirenal region, or collecting between the stomach and diaphragm. This makes the diaphragm outline very obvious, appearing as a white line demarcated by the radiolucent pulmonary field on one side and accumulated free gas on the other
Bowel loop dilatation	Dilatation of bowel loops with fluid or air is characteristic of obstruction, tending to be dilated proximal to the obstruction. Normal-size bowel loops may also be apparent distal to the obstruction
Abnormal positioning of bowel	Displacement of the bowel may occur secondary to an intra-abdominal mass. Stacked loops may occur with linear foreign bodies such that the bowel appears to be in layers parallel to each other
Radiopaque lumen contents	This may represent a radiopaque foreign body or small particles of ingesta and debris that have accumulated proximal to a chronic obstruction
Irregular gas shadows	Sharply demarcated gas shadows, particularly crescent-shaped shadows, often indicate gas trapped around obstructions, either foreign bodies or other bowel loops as in intussusception

mesentery are cut using scissors, followed by resection of the isolated bowel segment. The bowel is incised using a scalpel blade, with the incision angled at 30° from the mesenteric border to avoid producing an avascular antimesenteric area of bowel.

Prior to anastomosis, excessive mucosa can be trimmed with Metzenbaum scissors. The intestinal ends are examined for luminal disparity. The simplest technique for correction of size disparity is to spatulate the smaller lumen using an antimesenteric incision (Fig. 6.13). When disparity exists, avoid techniques that make the larger lumen smaller for risk of stricture and impaction causing future obstruction. The intestine is closed with a single layer of simple interrupted 4-0 sutures that pass full-thickness through the intestine. The first suture is placed at the mesenteric border, the second at the anti-

mesenteric border and the subsequent two halves of the anastomosis are then completed. The sutures must achieve apposition but should not crush through the mucosa. Sutures are approximately 3 mm apart and 1–2 mm from the incision edge. Sutures too close to the edge will pull out. Tight sutures or sutures too close together will cause ischaemia and dehiscence. Omentum is placed over the anastomosis.

Reduction of the intussusception may be possible for acute conditions. This must be attempted with caution. The intussuscipiens (ensheathing layer) is held in one hand and the apex of the intussusceptum (invaginating layer) is gently squeezed cranially (as you would squeeze a tube of toothpaste) as gentle traction is applied to the intestine cranial to the intussusception. If reduction is possible, the bowel must be examined closely for viability and evidence of tears. Intussusceptions that cannot be reduced and chronic intussusceptions that should not be attempted to be reduced are resected *in situ*.

For intussusceptions that have prolapsed through the anal orifice, gentle traction performed via a coeliotomy with gentle lubrication of the prolapsed segment via an assistant can be performed. If reduction cannot be achieved or there is excessive trauma to the prolapsed segment, resection must be performed at the anal junction from an external approach (see section on rectal prolapse). Enteroplication and colopexy are then performed.

Recurrence of the intussusception or intussusception at a different site are common postoperative complications and enteroplication is indicated. Animals undergoing intestinal plication appear to have a reduced incidence of recurrence (Oakes *et al.*, 1994). Adjoining loops of intestine are placed side-by-side in a series of gentle loops. Adjacent loops of intestine are sutured to each other with absorbable or nonabsorbable monofilament suture placed midway between the mesenteric and antimesenteric borders (Fig. 6.14). Generally, only the small intestine can be plicated. The descending colon can be stabilized by performing a colopexy. The colon is sutured to the left sublumbar body wall with the colon in slight cranial traction. Scarification of the body wall using a sponge or scalpel may promote adhesion formation. For plication and colopexy, the sutures are placed in a simple interrupted or simple

(a)

(b)

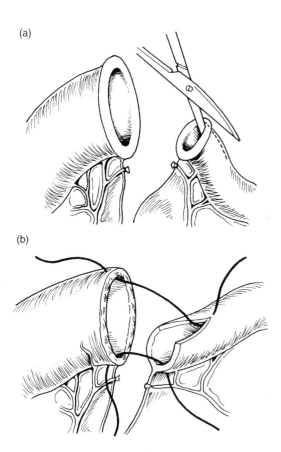

Figure 6.13 (a) Size disparity in intestinal anastomosis is corrected by performing an antimesenteric incision on the smaller segment to create a spatulated opening. (b) The remainder of the anatomosis is routine.

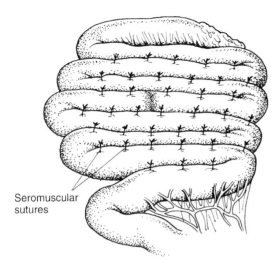

Figure 6.14 Plication of the entire jejunum and ileum is indicated to prevent recurrent intussusception. The bowel is folded in gentle loops with sutures passing through the seromuscular layer of each segment.

continuous pattern and should penetrate the seromuscular layer (Oakes *et al.*, 1994). A double row of sutures may be required for colopexy.

Postoperative considerations and prognosis

The general principles of postoperative management after gastrointestinal surgery apply (Table 6.16). The inciting cause of an intussusception must be treated if it is identified (e.g. intestinal parasites). The prognosis for complete recovery is good.

Faecal impaction

Faecal impactions resulting from a mixture of faeces and non-digestible hair or bones are the most common cause of infrequent defecation in dogs and cats younger than 6 months of age. Other causes of faecal impaction may include ingested foreign objects, narrowed pelvic canal following traumatically induced fractured pelvis, collapsed pelvic canal associated with pathological fractures due to nutritional imbalances, and congenital defects and inflammatory disease of the anus. Of these, foreign objects and fractured pelvis are the more likely causes of faecal impaction.

Clinical signs

Animals with faecal impaction usually present with a history of failure to defecate for days. The owner may have observed the animal making frequent, unsuccessful attempts to defecate and, in some cases, straining to pass small amounts of liquid faeces, often containing blood or mucus. Some animals present with the misleading complaint of diarrhoea. The disruption and irritation of the intestinal mucosa promote secretion and accumulation of fluid that cannot penetrate the densely packed faecal materials and thus produce diarrhoea. If defecation has not been observed, the animal may present because it is depressed, listless, inappetent or anorexic, and vomiting intermittently. Animals presenting with faecal impaction are generally dehydrated. Cats may assume a crouching, hunched attitude indicative of abdominal pain, and obvious abdominal distension is observed occasionally.

Diagnosis

Abdominal palpation typically reveals a hard faecal mass or masses that may fill the entire length of the large intestine. Rectal examination combined with abdominal palpation is useful in determining the amount of faeces retained, the compressibility of the material present, and possible identification of the underlying cause of the faecal impaction such as a foreign object or objects or a narrowed pelvic canal. Survey abdominal radiographs confirm the presence of faecal impaction and any opaque foreign objects.

Treatment

Treatment of faecal impaction requires gentle removal of impacted faecal material and, if possible, identification and remedy of the underlying cause. The animal with mild to moderate faecal impaction can generally be treated with oral laxatives and frequent small-volume enemas. The animal with more severe faecal impaction is often dehydrated and requires fluid replacement therapy for dehydration and electrolyte imbalances before correction of the faecal impaction is attempted. Breakdown and removal of the impacted faecal masses should be accomplished as slowly and gently as possible. It is less traumatic for the young animal if the faecal mass is softened and removed over 2 or 3 days rather than attempting removal of all the faecal impaction at one time. In dogs and cats older than 4 months of age with mild to moderate faecal impaction and after fluid replacement therapy has been accomplished, oral administration of a colon electrolyte/propylene glycol lavage preparation such as Colyte (Reed and Carnrick) or NuLytely (Braintree Laboratories), about 20–30 ml/kg body weight every 12 hours, can be used for complete removal of residual faeces.

Laxatives are mild in their effects and usually cause elimination of formed faeces. Their effects depend on dosage; major drugs and dosages are presented in Table 6.15. The dioctyl sodium sulphosuccinate and dioctyl calcium sulphosuccinate laxatives act as detergents to alter surface tension of liquids and promote emulsification and softening of the faeces by facilitating the mixture of water and fat. The animal must be well-hydrated before compounds containing these substances are administered, since they decrease jejunal absorption and promote colonic secretion. They should not be administered in conjunction with mineral oil, because they aid in the absorption of the mineral oil.

Mineral oil (liquid petrolatum) and white petrolatum are non-digestible and poorly absorbed laxatives. They soften faeces by coating them to prevent colonic absorption of faecal water and promote easy evacuation. A small amount of oil absorption does occur, but the primary danger of giving mineral oil is laryngotracheal aspiration due to its lack of taste. Bulk-forming laxatives such as psyllium and bran increase the frequency of evacuation of the upper large intestine via stimulation produced by added bulk or volume. They soften faeces by the retention of water. Metamucil, which contains natural psyllium and generic bran, is best given with moistened food to ensure a high degree of water intake.

Another useful laxative is bisacodyl; this compound exerts its action on colonic mucosa and intramural nerve plexuses. Stimulation is reportedly segmental and axonal, producing contraction of the entire colon independent of its resting tone. It should be used only in well-hydrated animals older than 4 months of age and is contraindicated when obstruction is present. Lactulose, a synthetic disaccharide of galactose and fructose, may be used for its laxative effects in the young dog and cat. Following oral administration, lactulose is metabolized to organic acids by intestinal bacteria and promotes an osmotic catharsis of faeces. The dose is individualized on the basis of stool consistency and is titrated until a semiformed stool is obtained with 2–3 soft bowel movements per day. Overdosage may induce intestinal cramping, profuse diarrhoea, flatulence, dehydration and acidosis. Cats, in general, dislike the taste of lactulose.

Enemas act by softening faeces in the distal large intestine, stimulating colonic motility and the urge to defecate. The enema fluid used should be at room temperature or tepid. Tap water, normal saline solution and sodium biphosphate solution add bulk; petrolatum oils soften, lubricate and promote the evacuation of hardened faecal material; and soapsuds solutions promote defecation by their irritant action. Normal saline solution and tap water (about 5 ml/kg body weight) are generally preferred for enemas in animals younger than 6 months of age. If ineffective, a soapy water solution can be used after ensuring that the animal is well-hydrated. About 5 ml/kg body weight of a mild soap solution is slowly instilled through a lubricated enema tube. In general, better results with normal saline solution, tap water or soapy water enemas are obtained if the enema is repeated several times using small volumes. Small volumes are retained for longer periods, allowing time to soften and break down faecal impactions. Mineral oil (5–20 ml) can be instilled directly into the rectum if faeces are extremely hard. The use of cisapride for the treatment of constipation and feline megacolon has met with limited success (Table 6.15). Cisapride is only indicated after the colon is evacuated and the cause of the impaction, if identified, has been recovered.

Prevention

After the successful relief of faecal impaction, attention is directed to the prevention of recurrence. If possible, non-digestible materials should be eliminated from the diet, regular grooming instituted, and the opportunity for regular defecation provided. In all instances, the goal should be to have the animal pass soft, formed faeces and to defecate regularly. Commercial veterinary laxatives containing petrolatum as their active ingredient are useful for preventing hair impaction in cats.

Rectal prolapse

Rectal prolapse is a common condition in puppies and kittens and may vary in degree from prolapse of the mucosa (incomplete prolapse) at the anal orifice to prolapse of several centimetres of full-thickness rectum (complete prolapse). Prolapse of an intussusception through the anal orifice can also occur and must be differentiated from a rectal prolapse (see above). Rectal prolapse is generally the result of excessive straining to defecate and small mucosal prolapses are often associated with diarrhoea. They are also seen in animals with sacral neurological dysfunction which may be of traumatic (tail avulsion) or congenital (Manx Cats, English Bull Dogs) origin. The underlying cause of rectal prolapse must be addressed.

Clinical signs

Prolapse of the rectal mucosa appears as a red, swollen doughnut of tissue protruding from the anal orifice. If all layers of the rectum are prolapsed, the prolapsed tissue appears more as a cylinder of tissue with the mucosal surface exposed.

Diagnosis

Diagnosis is based on clinical signs and physical examination to differentiate a rectal prolapse from a prolapsed intussusception.

Treatment and surgical technique

The inciting cause of rectal prolapse must be addressed. Conservative treatment of acute rectal prolapse requires application of a lubricant and gentle pressure to the prolapse as it is manually reduced into the pelvic canal. An anocutaneous pursestring suture is placed loosely to allow the passage of soft stool and should remain in place for 4–5 days.

Severely oedematous prolapses or traumatized necrotic tissue must be amputated. This is performed from an external approach at the level of the anus. Four stay sutures are placed in the external layer of the rectum at 0, 90, 180 and 270°. The external layer of the rectum is incised approximately 180° at the base of the prolapse, distal to the stay sutures, exposing the internal layer of rectum (Fig. 6.15). The internal layer is subsequently incised 180° and the two cut edges are apposed using simple interrupted sutures of 3-0 or 4-0 absorbable monofilament suture. After this section is closed, the remaining 180° of rectum is excised and closed similarly. Any rectum remaining prolapsed after resection is gently pushed into the pelvic canal. An anocutaneous pursestring suture is placed as described above. Colopexy is indicated in animals with extensive prolapses but is not indicated in animals with small mucosal prolapse and should be avoided to obviate the need for a coeliotomy.

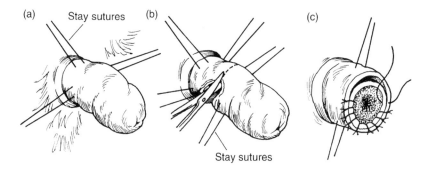

(a) Stay sutures   (b)   (c)

Stay sutures

Figure 6.15 Excision of rectal prolapse. (a) The prolapsed rectum is cleansed and several stay sutures placed full-thickness through the prolapse. (b) The external layer of the rectum is incised at the base of the prolapse, distal to the stay sutures, exposing the internal layer of rectum. (c) The internal layer is incised and the two cut edges are apposed using simple interrupted sutures of 3-0 or 4-0 absorbable monofilament suture. Any rectum remaining prolapsed after resection is gently pushed into the pelvic canal and a temporary anocutaneous pursestring suture is placed.

Postoperative considerations and prognosis

Oral stool softeners are administered for 5–7 days. The pursestring suture can be removed in 4–5 days. Avoid any rectal manipulation (e.g. body temperature measurement, administration of enemas). The prognosis is fair to good for complete recovery, depending on the amount of rectum resected. Recurrence is common if the inciting cause cannot be addressed. Recurrence after conservative therapy may require amputation and colopexy. Recurrence after amputation may also require colopexy. Faecal incontinence (reservoir incontinence) may occur in animals in which considerable amounts of rectum are resected. The prognosis for animals with neurological disease is poor since recurrence is common and the cause cannot be treated.

Anus and perineum

Atresia ani

Atresia ani is the congenital absence of an anal orifice. It is seen relatively infrequently in very young puppies and kittens and may be of several types, according to the anomaly present (Table 6.18).

Occasionally, these defects may be associated with fistula formation resulting in rectovaginal fistula, rectovestibular fistula, anovaginal cleft or rectal urethral fistula.

Clinical signs

A history of absence of defecation is most common, although occasionally it may go unnoticed. Abdominal distension or an obvious defect in the perineum may be apparent. Faeces may be voided through an inappropriate orifice, most commonly the vulva, if a fistula

Table 6.18 Categorization of atresia ani

Type	Anomaly
Type 1	The anus is strictured
Type 2	The anus is imperforate
Type 3	The rectum is discontinuous with an imperforate anus
Type 4	The cranial rectum is discontinuous with a normal terminal rectum and anus

is present. The animal may be unthrifty and exhibit tenesmus.

Diagnosis

Diagnosis is by clinical signs and radiography. Imperforate anus appears as a dimple in the skin at the usual site of the anus. Examination for external anal sphincter presence and function is important. Pinching the bulb of the penis or the vulva should result in contraction of the sphincter in the apparent region of the anus. Radiography is indicated to determine the presence of segmental defects or the location of the fistula. Plain radiography is best performed with the perineum elevated so that gas moves into the terminal rectum. Contrast material can be infused retrograde through a fistula if present. Evaluation of the urinary tract using excretory urography and cystourethrography is probably indicated to rule out other anomalies of any communication between the two body systems. An anovaginal cleft results in the mucosa of the anus or rectum and the vagina being continuous along the perineal raphe. The anus is often incomplete ventrally, with its dorsal border forming the dorsal part of the cleft. If the anus is atresic, a rectal fistula may form the dorsal part of the cleft. In the male, an anogenital cleft appears as an incomplete separation between the rectum/anus and the urethra. Hypospadia is often concurrently present.

Treatment and surgical techniques

Type I atresia is treated by bougienage or resection of the strictured tissue and rectal pull-through. Bougienage is best performed using balloon catheters (see section on oesophageal stricture) and may require multiple treatments. It is rarely successful. Excision of the stricture requires pulling the cut edge of the rectal mucosa distally so that a mucosa-to-skin closure is performed. Excision of the stricture may result in loss of external anal sphincter tissue and incontinence is likely. In addition, normal colon and rectal function is not always observed. Whether this is a congenital dysfunction or secondary to severe distension is unclear.

Type II atresia is treated by surgically perforating the tissue over the anal dimple and performing a mucosa-to-skin closure. A cruciate incision is made in the skin over the anal dimple, avoiding the anal sacs and their openings. The triangular flaps created by the skin incisions can be excised at this point or preferably prior to anastomosis with the rectum, when the size of the anal orifice can be better determined. The sphincter muscle is identified and the distal rectum is mobilized. The rectum is brought through the sphincter muscle and sutured to the subcutaneous tissue with simple continuous sutures of 4-0 to 5-0 monofilament absorbable suture. The rectum is then incised in the vertical plane and a mucosa-to-skin closure using simple interrupted sutures of 4-0 to 5-0 monofilament absorbable suture is performed. The rectum and colon should subsequently be evacuated of faeces prior to the animal recovering from anaesthesia to facilitate return to normal function.

Type III atresia is treated as for type II, except that dissection to isolate the distal rectum can be difficult and may have to be quite deep if there is substantial segment aplasia. This may require an abdominal approach to mobilize the terminal rectum in combination with rectal pull-through for creation of the anal orifice.

Rectovaginal or rectocutaneous fistulas are often present with type II atresia. The fistula is dissected through an incision between the anus and the vulva and ligated at its communication with the rectum and vagina. The length of fistula between these two locations can be excised.

Type IV atresia requires an abdominal approach with mobilization of the cranial rectum and anastomosis with the caudal rectum. Pubic symphysiotomy may be required.

Postoperative considerations and prognosis

Stool softeners are recommended to facilitate defecation but enemas or any anal/rectal stimulation should be avoided. Rectal temperature measurement should be avoided. The prognosis is generally poor and the presence of other congenital anomalies worsens the prognosis. Most animals are usually incontinent even with surgical reconstruction. True type II atresia with normal external anal sphincter function carries the best prognosis for normal function if associated problems such as megacolon have not been prolonged.

Table 6.19 Patterns of portosystemic shunts

Shunt type	Comments
Portocaval	Single, extrahepatic
	Most common in small breeds
	Left gastric to abdominal cava commonly reported and is the most common form described in cats
	Portoazygous shunts also reported in dogs and cats
	Splenic to abdominal cava also reported in cats
Patent ductus venosus	Single, intrahepatic
	Most common in large breeds
Portal atresia	Rare in dogs and cats
	Intrahepatic portal veins are absent or hypoplastic; extrahepatic portal vein is malformed
Acquired portosystemic shunts	Multiple portopostcaval anastomoses open in response to sustained portal hypertension of prehepatic or intrahepatic origin
	They do not develop in association with posthepatic portal hypertension (e.g. congestive heart failure or caval syndrome of heartworm disease)
Microscopic portosystemic shunting	May occur congenitally in certain breeds of dogs and cats; reported in Cairn Terriers (Phillips *et al.*, 1993; Schermerhorn *et al.*, 1993)
	Causes mixing of systemic and portal blood
	Similar but milder clinical signs as animals with macroscopic shunts
	May occur concurrently with macroscopic shunting
Intrahepatic arteriovenous fistula with acquired portosystemic shunts	Rare
	Isolated hepatic arteriovenous fistulas reported as an incidental finding in dogs

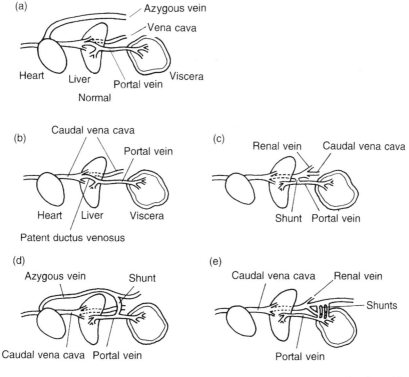

Figure 6.16 Types of portosystemic shunts. (a) Normal; (b) ductus venosus (intrahepatic); (c) single extrahepatic portocaval shunt; (d) portoazygous shunt; (e) multiple extrahepatic portocaval shunts.

The hepatic system

Portosystemic shunts

Portosystemic shunts are vascular anomalies that divert blood from the portal circulation into the systemic circulation, bypassing the liver. Portosystemic shunts may be congenital or acquired, single or multiple, and intrahepatic or extrahepatic (Table 6.19; Fig. 6.16). Portosystemic shunts, as a result of diverting blood from the liver, cause failure of liver growth with reduced hepatic function such as protein and urea production and ammonia clearance. Hepatoencephalopathy can develop from gut-derived encephalotoxins that alter cerebral metabolism.

Clinical signs

Clinical signs of congenital portosystemic shunts are typically observed in a pure-bred dog less than 1 year of age of either gender. Small breeds, such as the Yorkshire Terrier, Miniature Schnauzer, Maltese Terrier and Shih Tzu are commonly affected with single, extra-hepatic shunts while large-breed dogs such as Labradors are commonly affected with single intrahepatic shunts.

In general, animals may be underweight with stunted growth. A poor hair coat may be observed. Signs may be precipitated by ingestion of meals containing protein or by administration of drugs that are metabolized by the liver, such as anaesthetics (Table 6.20).

Occasionally, older dogs that have escaped detection at an earlier age due to lack of obvious signs of encephalopathy are presented for polydipsia or polyuria or urate urolithiasis, or occasionally delayed-onset hepatoencephalopathy (Johnson *et al.*, 1989).

Diagnosis

Diagnosis is based on clinical signs, results of blood work, radiography, ultrasonography, scintigraphy or exploratory coeliotomy (Tables 6.21 and 6.22).

Table 6.20 Clinical signs of portosystemic shunt

Clinical sign	Comment
Neurological signs	Abnormal behaviour, dementia, seizures, apparent blindness and circling are observed in most animals with portosystemic shunts at some time
Urological signs	Result from ammonium biurate crystal and calculus formation and decreased urea production
	Renal and cystic calculi may develop
	Haematuria, polyuria, pollakiuria and stranguria may be observed
	Polydipsia may be observed and is thought to be primary in some dogs (Grauer and Pitts, 1987)
Gastrointestinal signs	Result from abnormal bile metabolism
	Vomiting, diarrhoea, anorexia, pytalism (especially in cats)
Ascites and coagulopathies	More often present in animals with multiple acquired portosystemic shunts

Table 6.21 Haematologic, serum chemistry and urinalysis alterations in animals with congenital portosystemic shunts

	Comment
Haematology	
Hypoproteinaemia	
Leukocytosis	
Microcytosis	Observed in more than 60% of dogs and 30% of cats with congenital portosystemic shunts
Poikilocytosis	Observed in some cats
Serum chemistry	
Low blood urea nitrogen (BUN)	
Hypoproteinaemia/ hypoalbuminaemia	
Hyperammonaemia	May be normal
Hypoglycaemia	May be normal
Low creatinine	May be normal
Hypocholesterolaemia	
Normal liver enzymes	Usually normal unless there is a superimposed hepatic insult
	Elevated serum alkaline phosphatase is not an uncommon result of increased biliary canalicular activity and may be indicative of subcellular hepatocyte organelle injury
Conjugated bile acids	Elevated resting and postprandial bile acid concentration. This is indicative of any hepatobiliary dysfunction
Urinalysis	
Low specific gravity	
Ammonium biurate crystals	Persistent presence in freshly voided urine sample

Table 6.22 Comparison of clinical features of congenital portosystemic shunts to those of primary hepatobiliary disease and acquired portosystemic shunt in dogs and cats (modified from Bunch, 1995)

Clinical feature	Congenital	Acquired
Age at presentation	< 1 year	≥ 4 years
Stunted appearance	+	−
Thin body condition, poor hair coat	+/−	−
Other congenital defects	+	−
Signs of hepatoencephalopathy	+	+
Intermittent vomiting and diarrhoea	++	
Polyuria/polydipsia	+/− (Uncommon)	+
Urate urolithiasis	+	−
Ascites, gastrointestinal bleeding, jaundice	+	−
Microcytosis (dogs)	++/−	
Poikilocytosis (cats)	+	+
Biochemical changes consistent with hepatic dysfunction: ↓ albumin, ↓ blood urea nitrogen, ↓ creatinine, ↓ glucose, ↑ bile acids, biurate crystalluria	+	+/−
Hypocholesterolaemia	+	+/−
Serum alanine transferase concentration	Normal to ↑	↑
Serum alkaline phosphatase concentrations	↑	↑
Liver size	Normal to ↓	↑
Abnormal vessel on ultrasonography	Single	Multiple
Portal blood flow	↓, Hepatopedal	↓, Hepatofugal
Gross liver appearance	Normal	Abnormal, nodular, variable
Portal pressure	Normal	↑
Liver biopsy	Hepatocellular atrophy, arteriolar duplication, inconspicuous portal veins	Necrosis, fibrosis, cholestasis

Survey abdominal radiographs reveal bilateral renomegaly and microhepatica which result in an upright gastric shadow close to the diaphragm. Calculi are often radiolucent and may be detected ultrasonographically or using excretory urography.

Abdominal ultrasonography can confirm microhepatica and detect a reduced number and size of intrahepatic branches of the portal and hepatic veins (Wrigley *et al.*, 1987). An intrahepatic shunt within the hepatic parenchyma or an extrahepatic shunt anastomosing with the caudal vena cava just caudal to the liver may be visualized. Other ultrasonographic findings include enlargement of the caudal vena cava, splenomegaly secondary to portal hypertension and Doppler ultrasonographic evidence of portal hypertension and hepatofugal portal blood flow. Multiple acquired shunts may be visualized as an accumulation of tortuous vessels in the splenic or renal hilus or near the colon (Biller and Partington, 1995).

Colonic scintigraphy can be used as a non-invasive screening test for portosystemic shunts (Kobilek *et al.*, 1990) but requires special equipment and facilities for handling radioactive isotopes and is not essential to a diagnosis of portosystemic shunt. A small amount of ^{99m}technetium-pertechnetate is injected into the colon where it is absorbed into the portal circulation. Normally the isotope should proceed directly to the liver where a high number of isotope emissions would be detected. In an animal with a portosystemic shunt, the isotope bypasses the liver and enters the systemic circulation via the heart and lungs where a high count is detected (Fig. 6.17).

(a)

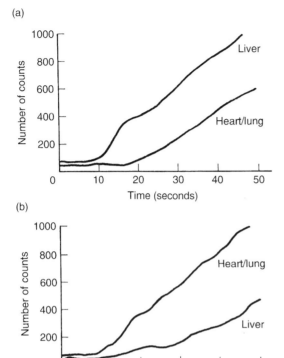

(b)

Figure 6.17 [99m]Technetium-pertechnetate scintigraphy count for (a) a normal dog and (b) a dog with portosystemic shunt. Note that labelled particles reach the liver before the lung in the normal dog but not in the dog with the portosystemic shunt.

Surgical exploration with transsplenic or preferably mesenteric portography (Birchard *et al.*, 1989) and liver biopsy is required for definitive diagnosis and differentiation from microscopic vascular dysplasia (Schermerhorn *et al.*, 1993). Liver biopsy typically shows lobule atrophy, decreased distance between portal triads, narrowed portal venules, proliferation of hepatic arterioles, hepatocellular degeneration and foci of macrophages containing iron-like pigments. Mesenteric portography is performed by catheterizing a jejunal vein and injection of sterile, water-soluble iodinated contrast. Following injection, contrast medium will outline the portal vasculature and opacifies any abnormal vascular connection with the vena cava. If the caudal extent of the portosystemic shunt is cranial to the 13th thoracic vertebra, it is probably intrahepatic, and if it is caudal to the 13th thoracic vertebra, it is probably extrahepatic (Biarchard *et al.*, 1989). The amount of contrast

flow into the liver at the time of portography is not indicative of whether partial or complete attenuation can be performed (Swalec and Smeak, 1990).

Treatment and surgical technique

Animals should be stabilized with medical management prior to surgery (Tables 6.23 and 6.24). Medical management is indicated in animals with shunts not amenable to surgical ligation (Table 6.25). Severely affected animals should be treated with intravenous fluids with dextrose supplementation for hypoglycaemia, and with saline or saline–lactulose enemas. Plasma transfusion or colloid expanders or both are indicated in the severely hypoalbuminaemic animal. Activated charcoal can be administered by stomach tube in the non-responsive animal.

Surgical treatment is the treatment of choice for single congenital shunts. Important pre- and postoperative considerations include measures to prevent hypoglycaemia, hypothermia and overhydration. If necessary, shunts may require partial ligation to prevent portal hypertension. During surgery, the objective is to ligate the shunt without inducing life-threatening portal hypertension. Parameters used to monitor portal hypertension include portal manometry, central venous pressure, splanchnic surface oximetery (Peterson *et al.*, 1991) and visual subjective signs of portal hypertension (Mathews and Gofton, 1988; Table 6.26). Ideally, assessment should involve all parameters. In animals with high splanchnic compliance, portal pressure may not change after ligation and assessment should be based on central venous pressure and subjective signs.

Surgical technique

Preoperative considerations include fluid therapy for hypoglycaemia, plasma expansion or plasma transfusion for hypoproteinaemia and administration of perioperative antibiotics. Cephalosporins are the antibiotic of choice since they have a broad spectrum of activity and are excreted in the bile in high concentrations (Butler *et al.*, 1990). The surgical protocol used for definitive diagnosis and treatment of portosystemic shunts may vary from surgeon to surgeon, depending on the facilities available, surgical experience and status of the animal.

Table 6.23 Medical management strategies for portosystemic shunts

Medical treatment	Comment
Low-protein diet	Require diets with 15–20% protein on a dry matter basis for dogs and 30–35% for cats
	Preferably vegetable and dairy protein over meat protein
	Remainder of caloric requirements met with carbohydrate and fat content
Lactulose	1-4-β-Galactosidofructose; a synthetic disaccharide that is hydrolysed by colonic bacteria to lactic and acetic acids
	Is beneficial by acidifying colonic contents and trapping ammonium ions. It also inhibits ammonia generation by colonic bacteria, decreases colonic transit time due to its cathartic properties and decreases bacterial and intestinal ammonia generation by providing an alternative carbohydrate source
	Desired dose should result in 2–3 soft stools a day. Dose may range from 2.5 to 20 ml given 2–3 times a day for dogs; 2.5 to 5 ml given 2–3 times a day for cats
	As a retention enema for acute hepatic coma, 20–30 ml/kg at 30% concentration (30% lactulose, 70% water) is infused and retained in the colon for 20–30 minutes
Oral antibiotics	Indicated to reduce colonic bacterial load
	Neomycin or metronidazole is commonly used
	Due to side-effects, antibiotic therapy may be indicated for acute exacerbation of hepatoencepholapathy rather than chronic use
	Neomycin is a non-absorbable antibiotic with possible side-effects of diarrhoea, ototoxicity and nephrotoxicity with chronic use
	Metronidazole at 7.5 mg/kg t.i.d. is as effective but can cause neurotoxicity
	Ampicillin is a safe alternative to neomycin, especially in azotaemic animals

Whether complete abdominal exploration is performed at the time of mesenteric portography or after, or whether surgical ligation (if possible) is performed at the time of portography may vary. The following protocol is one used by the author.

A midline exploratory coeliotomy is performed. The entire abdominal cavity is explored to detect any anomalous vessels. A 22- to 20-gauge venous catheter is placed in a jejunal vein, connected to a venous extension and a water manometer. The catheter must be secured in place using sutures through the intestinal segment. Heparinized saline can be used to flush the catheter initially but continual flushing must be performed with extreme care in small animals due to the likelihood of overhydration and systemic heparinization. A measurement of portal pressure can be taken at this time since it may be affected by any subsequent dissection of the vessel which may induce spasm. If an anomalous vessel has been identified, it should be dissected and marked with a loose radiopaque ligature (radiopaque marker from a gauze sponge). Any vein entering the caudal vena cava cranial to the phrenicoabdominal veins may be considered anomalous (Butler *et al.*, 1990). The marker will allow confirmation of the vessel as the shunt during portography. The manometer is disconnected and replaced with a syringe of saline. The abdomen is then closed in a single layer and covered by an adhesive plastic drape, allowing access to the syringe port. The animal can then be transported to radiology or, preferably, intraoperative radiography can be performed. Fluoroscopic capabilities and digital subtraction angiography can enhance the portographic study (Tobias *et al.*, 1996). Portography is performed using water-soluble iodinated contrast material and should demonstrate the shunt.

Table 6.24 Suitable commercial diets for dogs with portosystemic shunts*

Diet
Purina Clinical Nutrition – NF Formula
Hill's Prescription Diet k/d
Waltham medium- and low-protein diets
K:IVD by Innovative Veterinary Diets

*Canine Prescription diet u/d is not suitable for long-term management of growing dogs because of its low protein content (9.3–11.5% protein on a dry matter basis).

Table 6.25 Management options for animals with portosystemic shunts (modified from Bunch, 1995)

Medically manageable; surgical intervention not indicated	Potentially surgically correctable portosystemic shunts	
	Type of portosystemic shunt	*Treatment*
Any congenital anomaly that is inaccessible, or ligation of which causes unacceptable portal hypertension	Single extrahepatic or intrahepatic shunt with normal portal pressure	Surgical ligation +/− ultrasonic aspiration (or transvenous embolization or extravascular ameroid constrictor; Vogt *et al.*, 1994)
Chronic primary hepatobiliary disease with portal hypertension and acquired portosystemic shunting	Poorly defined intrahepatic portal hypertension with acquired portosystemic shunts in young dogs	Caudal vena caval banding (controversial)
Portal vein thrombosis	Intrahepatic arteriovenous fistula with acquired portosystemic shunts	Liver lobectomy
Portal venous atresia	Portal vein obstruction	Removal of extraluminal obstruction
Microvascular dysplasia		

After confirmation of the shunt's location, the animal is returned to surgery and the shunt ligated. For single extrahepatic shunts, ligation should be performed using non-absorbable suture as close to the vascular insertion point in the vena cava as possible. The suture tags are left long to facilitate location of the suture in case reoperation is required. If partial ligation is required, a catheter can be placed alongside the vessel and included in the ligature, subsequently being removed, making the ligature loose. Recently, the use of an ameroid constrictor for gradual occlusion of extrahepatic porto-systemic shunts has been described (Vogt *et al.*, 1996). The ameroid constrictor is a device composed of hygroscopic, compressed casein that rapidly expands when immersed in fluid. Rapid expansion occurs over 14 days, then slow expansion continues for a further two months. Its use in 12 dogs and 2 cats was successful in all but 2 dogs. Those dogs dying initially had greater than 50% reduction in vessel diameter with placement of the constrictor and the authors recommended using a size that resulted in no more than 25% reduction in vessel diameter upon placement (Vogt *et al.*, 1996). The ameroid

Table 6.26 Intraoperative monitoring of portal hypertension

Parameter	Comment
Portal pressure	Normal is 8–13 cmH$_2$O but may be lower (4–8 cmH$_2$O) in dogs with single congenital shunts due to decreased hepatic resistance
	After ligation, portal pressure should be kept below 16–18 cmH$_2$O, result in a less than 10 cmH$_2$O increase or should not double from resting pressure
Central venous pressure	Normal is 2–7 cmH$_2$O
	After ligation, it should not drop more than 1 cmH$_2$O
Splanchnic surface oximetry	Provides objective information about splanchnic blood flow that moderately correlates with portal pressure
	May be a more accurate indicator of lack of splanchnic congestion that portal pressure (Peterson *et al.*, 1991)
Subjective assessment	Signs of increased portal pressure include increased peristalsis, increased intestinal vascular pulsation and pallor and cyanosis of the intestines and pancreas

constrictor has the potential advantage of reducing the risk of acute postoperative portal hypertension through its ability to gradual constrict the shunt vessel. For single intrahepatic shunts, ligation can be performed after visualization of the shunt which may or may not require some dissection and extension of the midline coeliotomy incision through the diaphragm and caudal sternum. Ultrasonographic guidance can be used to facilitate identification of the shunt or, more recently, ultrasonic aspiration of the liver parenchyma has been described (Tobias *et al.*, 1996). Prehepatic intravascular caval approach to occlusion of intrahepatic shunts has been reported (Breznock *et al.*, 1983). This technique requires obvious technical expertise. Recently, placement of a vascular graft (jugular vein) to create an extrahepatic portocaval anastomosis and control postoperative portal hypertension in two dogs was reported (White *et al.*, 1996). Both dogs survived the procedure and showed a reduction in portal shunting postoperative. One dog was clinically normal 8 months after surgery; however, one dog was euthanized 5 months after surgery due to renal failure (White *et al.*, 1996). A non-invasive alternative to surgical ligation is intravascular occlusion of the shunt using a transvenously placed coil (Partington *et al.*, 1993). Alternatively, the left hepatic vein (for left-sided shunts) draining the shunt or the portal branch supplying the shunt (for right-sided shunts) can be ligated.

The application of caudal vena cava banding is controversial for animals with multiple acquired shunts. The caudal vena cava is partially occluded until its pressure is 1.5–2.5 cmH$_2$O greater than the portal pressure. This forces blood to flow through the portal vein. The portal pressure should be kept below 22 cmH$_2$O. Generally, if the multiple acquired shunts are the result of portal hypertension, the pressures will eventually equilibrate and any benefit from banding is lost.

After ligation, the intestines are observed for 10 minutes to monitor for subjective signs of portal hypertension. If these do not develop, the jejunal catheter is removed and the jejunal vein ligated. The abdomen is lavaged with warm saline and a routine three-layer abdominal closure is performed. Consideration of the possibility of delayed healing in hypoproteinaemic animals should influence suture material selection. A monofilament, prolonged absorb-able suture such as polydioxanone or a non-absorbable suture such as nylon or polypropylene should be used in the linea alba.

If cystic calculi are present, they can be removed via cystotomy at the time of shunt ligation or at a subsequent surgery, depending on the status of the animal. Some renal calculi may dissolve after shunt ligation and close monitoring of animals with renal calculi for urinary obstruction is important in the late postoperative period.

Postoperative considerations and prognosis

Immediate postoperative care requires continued supportive therapy and monitoring for portal hypertension and seizures. Signs of portal hypertension include abdominal pain, ascites, progressive hypothermia and hypovolaemic shock. Mild ascites may develop and usually resolves in 1–3 weeks and can be managed with diuretics if drainage of fluid occurs from the incision site or abdominal distension causes discomfort (Butler *et al.*, 1990). Animals that develop severe postoperative portal hypertension require immediate reoperation and ligature removal. Religation may be attempted at a later time. Seizures may occur in up to 11% of animals between 13 and 72 hours after surgery (Hardie *et al.*, 1990; Matushek *et al.*, 1990). Animals over 18 months appear more likely to have intractable seizures and the seizures do not appear to be correlated with ammonia concentrations or degree of shunt ligation (Hardie *et al.*, 1990; Matushek *et al.*, 1990). Treatment requires intravenous mannitol and barbiturates; however, the mortality is 50–80% (Hardie *et al.*, 1990; Hatushek *et al.*, 1990).

The animals will require continuation of a low-protein diet until evidence of improved hepatic function is observed (increased albumin concentrations), usually for 3 months. An adult maintenance diet can then be fed. Serum bile acids continue to be abnormal after shunt ligation: up to 75% of dogs had abnormal concentrations at a median of 18.6 months after ligation (Lawrence and Bellah, 1992). If clinical signs of the shunt recur, scintography or portography is required to assess the success of the ligation and to determine whether other shunts are present or a second ligation is required.

The prognosis depends on the type of shunt and the age of the animal. Animals less than

2 years of age with single extrahepatic shunts that can be completely ligated have the best prognosis and up to a 95% survival rate (Lawrence and Bellah, 1992; Bostwick and Twedt, 1995; Hottinger *et al.*, 1995; Komtebedde *et al.*, 1995). Clinical improvement is usually seen in nearly all dogs with partial or completely occluded shunts and some partially occluded shunts may go on to thrombose and become completely occluded. However, up to 50% of animals with partial ligation will have recurrence of clinical signs and may develop multiple shunts (Hottinger *et al.*, 1995; Komtebedde *et al.*, 1995). Reoperation, as early as 1 month after partial ligation, is recommended to complete shunt attenuation (Hottinger *et al.*, 1995). Prior evaluation, including ultrasonography and transcolonic scintigraphy, is indicated to determine if the shunt is still only partially occluded.The prognosis for cats appears less favourable than dogs (VanGundy *et al.*, 1990; Birchard and Sherding, 1992; Scavelli *et al.*, 1986).

The prognosis for intrahepatic shunts is guarded due to the difficulty in ligating or occluding the shunts. Intraoperative arterial hypotension, haemorrhage and acute hepatic congestion, all requiring intervention, are reported (Komtebedde *et al.*, 1991). However, if surgery is without complication, the prognosis is good, with 10 of 13 dogs alive at 12–46 months after surgery in one study (Komtebedde *et al.*, 1991). Animals with multiple acquired shunts may improve but postoperative morbidity is high, with ascites and leg oedema often persisting for up to 6 weeks.

References

Aller, S. (1989) Basic prophylaxis and home care. *Compendium of Continuing Education for the Practicing Veterinarian*, **11**, 1447–1457.

Attum, A.A., Hankins, J.R., Ngangana, J. and McLaughlin, J.S. (1979) Circular myotomy as an aid to resection and end-to-end anastomosis of the esophagus. *Annals of Thoracic Surgery*, **28**, 126–132.

Basher, A.W.P., Hogan, P.M., Hanna, P.E., Runyon, C.L. and Shaw, D.H. (1991) Surgical treatment of a congenital bronchoesophageal fistula in a dog. *Journal of the American Veterinary Medical Association*, **199**, 479–482.

Bellah, J.R., Spencer, C.P., Brown, D.J. *et al.* (1989) Congenital cranioventral abdominal wall, caudal sternal, diaphragmatic, pericardial and intracardiac defects in Cocker spaniel littermates. *Journal of the American Veterinary Medical Association*, **12**, 1741–1745.

Biller, D.S. and Partington, B.P. (1995) Diagnostic ultrasound of the liver. *Veterinary Previews*, **2**, 14–17.

Birchard, S.J. and Sherding, R.G. (1992) Feline portosystemic shunts. *Compendium of Continuing Education for the Practicing Veterinarian*, **14**, 1295–1301.

Birchard, S.J., Biller, D.S. and Johnson, S.E. (1989) Differentiation of intrahepatic versus extrahepatic portosystemic shunts in dogs using positive-contrast portography. *Journal of the American Animal Hospital Association*, **25**, 13–17.

Bostwick, D.R. and Twedt, D.C. (1995) Intrahepatic and extrahepatic portal venous anomalies in dogs: 52 cases (1982–1992). *Journal of the American Veterinary Medical Association*, **206**, 1181–1185.

Breznock, E.M., Berger, B., Pendray, D. *et al.* (1983) Surgical manipulation of intrahepatic portocaval shunts in dogs. *Journal of American Veterinary Medical Association*, **182**, 798–805.

Bunch, S.E. (1995) Diagnosis and management of portosystemic shunts in dogs and cats. *Veterinary Previews*, **2**, 2–6, 19.

Butler, L.M., Fossum, T.W. and Boothe, H.W. (1990) Surgical management of extrahepatic portosystemic shunts in the dog and cat. *Seminars in Veterinary Medicine and Surgery*, **5**, 127–133.

Dallman, M.J. (1988) Functional suture-holding layer of the esophagus in the dog. *Journal of the American Veterinary Medical Association*, **192**, 638–640.

Dean, P.W., Bojrab, M.J. and Constantinescu, G.M. (1990) Inguinal hernia repair in the dog. In: M.J. Bojrab (ed.) *Current Techniques in Small Animal Surgery*, pp. 439–442. Philadelphia: Lea & Febiger.

Degner, D.A., Lanz, O.I. and Wlashaw, R. (1996) Myoperitoneal microvascular free flaps in dogs: An anatomical study and a clinical case report. *Veterinary Surgery*, **25**, 463–470.

Ellison, G.W., Mulligan, T.W., Fagan, D.A. and Tugend, R.K. (1986) A double reposition flap technique for repair of recurrent oronasal fistulas in dogs. *Journal of the American Animal Hospital Association*, **22**, 803–808.

Evans, S.M. and Biery, D.N. (1980) Congenital peritoneopericardial diaphragmatic hernia in the dog and cat: a literature review and 17 additional case histories. *Veterinary Radiology*, **21**, 108–116.

Fingeroth, J.M. (1993) Surgical diseases of the esophagus. In: Slatter, D.H. (ed.), *Textbook of Small Animal Surgery*, vol. 1, pp. 534–548. Philadelphia: WB Saunders.

Flanders, J.A. (1989) Problems and complications associated with esophageal surgery. *Problems in Veterinary Medicine*, **1**, 183–194.

Fox, M.W. (1963) Inherited inguinal hernia and midline defects in the dog. *Journal of the American Veterinary Medical Association*, **143**, 602–604.

Grauer, G.F. and Pitts, R.P. (1987) Primary polydipsia in three dogs with portosystemic shunts. *Journal of the American Animal Hospital Association*, **23**, 197–200.

Hardie, E.M., Greene, R.T., Ford, R.B., Davidson, M.G. and Herring, M. (1987) Balloon dilatation for treatment of esophageal stricture: a case report. *Journal of the American Animal Hospital Association*, **23**, 547–550.

Hardie, E.M., Kornegay, J.N. and Cullen, J.M. (1990) Status epilepticus after ligation of portosystemic shunts. *Veterinary Surgery*, **19**, 412–417.

Harvey, C.E. (1987) Palate defects in dogs and cats. *Compendium of Continuing Education for the Practicing Veterinary Surgery*, **19**, 412–417.

Harvey, C.E. and Emily, P.P. (1993) Oral surgery. In: C.E. Harvey and P.P. Emily (eds), *Small Animal Dentistry*, pp. 312–377. St Louis: Mosby-Year Books.

Hawkins, J. (1991) Applied dentistry for veterinary technicians: lesson one. *Compendium of Continuing Education for the Practicing Veterinarian*, **13**, 818–838.

Hayes, H.M. (1974) Congenital umbilical and inguinal hernia in cattle, horses, swine, dogs and cats: risk by breed and sex among hospital patients. *American Journal of Veterinary Research*, **35**, 839–842.

Hosgood, G. (1990) The omentum – the forgotten organ: pathophysiology and potential surgical applications in dogs and cats. *Compendium of Continuing Education for the Practicing Veterinarian*, **12**, 45–50.

Hoskins, J.D. and Dimski, D.S. (1995) The digestive system. In: J.D. Hoskins (ed.), *Veterinary Pediatrics*, pp. 133–187. Philadelphia: WB Saunders.

Hottinger, H.A., Walshaw, R. and Hauptman, J.G. (1995) Long-term results of complete and partial ligation of congenital portosystemic shunts in dogs. *Veterinary Surgery*, **24**, 331–336.

Johnson, S.E., Crisp, S.M., Smeak, D.D. and Fingeroth, J.M. (1989) Hepatic encephalopahy in two aged dogs secondary to presumed congenital portal-azygous shunt. *Journal of the American Animal Hospital Association*, **25**, 129–137.

Kirby, B.M. (1990) Oral flaps: principles, problems, and complications of flaps for reconstruction of the oral cavity. *Problems in Veterinary Medicine*, **2**, 494–509.

Kirby, B.M., Bjorling, D.E. and Mixter, R.C. (1988) Surgical repair of a cleft lip in a dog. *Journal of the American Animal Hospital Association*, **24**, 683–687.

Koblik, P.D., Komtebedde, J., Yen, C.-K. and Hornof, W.J. (1990) Use of transcolonic [99m]technetium-pertechnetate as a screening test for portosystemic shunts in dogs. *Journal of the American Veterinary Medical Association*, **196**, 925–930.

Komtebedde, J., Forsyth, S.F., Breznock, E.M. and Koblik, P.D. (1991) Intrahepatic portosystemic venous anomaly in the dog. Perioperative management and complications. *Veterinary Surgery*, **20**, 37–42.

Komtebedde, J., Koblik, P.D., Breznock, E.M., Harb, M. and Garrow, L.A. (1995) Long-term clinical outcome after partial ligation of single extrahepatic vascular anomalies in 20 dogs. *Veterinary Surgery*, **24**, 379–383.

Lawrence, D. and Bellah, J.R. (1992) Results of surgical management of portosystemic shunts in dogs: 20 cases (1985–1990). *Journal of the American Veterinary Medical Association*, **201**, 1730–1753.

Lunney, J. (1992) Congenital peritoneal pericardial diaphragmatic hernia and portocaval shunt in a cat. *Journal of the American Animal Hospital Association*, **28**, 162–166.

Mathews, K. and Gofton, N. (1988) Congenital extrahepatic portosystemic shunt occlusion in the dog: gross observations during surgical correction. *Journal of the American Animal Hospital Association*, **24**, 387–394.

Matushek, K.J., Bjorling, D. and Mathews, K. (1990) Generalized motor seizures after portosystmeic shunt ligation in dogs: five cases (1981–1988). *Journal of the American Veterinary Medical Association*, **196**, 2104–2117.

Oakes, A.B. (1993) Lingually displaced mandibular canine teeth in dogs. *Compendium of Continuing Education for the Practicing Veterinarian*, **15**, 961–968.

Oakes, M.G., Hosgood, G., Snider, T.G., Hedlund, C.S. and Crawford, M.P. (1993) Esophagotomy closure in the dog: a comparison of a double-layer appositional and two single-layer appositional techniques. *Veterinary Surgery*, **22**, 451–456.

Oakes, M.G., Lewis, D.D., Hosgood, G. and Beale, B.S. (1994) Enteroplication for the prevention of intussusception recurrence in dogs: 31 cases (1978–1992). *Journal of American Veterinary Association*, **205**, 72–75.

Parker, N.R., Walter, P.A. and Gay, J. (1989) Diagnosis and surgical management of esophageal perforation. *Journal of the American Animal Hospital Association*, **25**, 587–594.

Partington, B.P., Partington, C.R. and Biller, D.S. (1993) Transvenous coil embolization for treatment of patent ductus venosus in a dog. *Journal of the American Veterinary Medical Association*, **202**, 281–284.

Pearson, H., Gaskell, C.J., Gibbs, C. and Waterman, A. (1974) Pyloric stenosis and oesophageal dysfunction in the cat. *Journal of Small Animal Practice*, **15**, 487–501.

Peddie, J.F. (1980) Inguinal hernia repair in the dog. *Modern Veterinary Practice*, **61**, 859–861.

Peterson, S.L., Gregory, C.R., Snyder, J.R., Whiting, P.G., Strack, D. and Breznock, E.M. (1991) Splanchnic surface oximetery during experimental portal hypertension and surgical manipulation of portosystemic shunts in dogs. *Veterinary Surgery*, **20**, 164–168.

Phillips, L., Tappe, J. and Lyman, R. (1993) Hepatic microvascular dysplasia without demonstrable macroscopic shunts. In: *American College of Veterinary Internal Medicine*, pp. 438–439. Proceedings of 'AM College Vet Int Med' Forum, Washington, DC.

Robinson, R. (1977) Genetic aspects of umbilical hernia incidence in dogs and cats. *Veterinary Record*, **100**, 9–10.

Scavelli, T.D., Hornbuckle, W.E., Roth, L. *et al.* (1986) Portosystemic shunts in cats: seven cases (1976–1984). *Journal of the American Veterinary Medical Association*, **189**, 317–325.

Schermerhorn, T., Center, S.A., Rowland, P.J. *et al.* (1993) Characterization of inherited portovascular dysplasia in Cairn terriers. In: *American College of Veterinary Internal Medicine*. Proceedings of 'Am College Vet Int Med' Forum, Washington, DC.

Smith, B.A. and Clark, W.T. (1992) Post-anesthetic oesophageal stricture in a dog managed by balloon catheter dilation. *Australian Veterinary Practitioner*, **22**, 124–127.

Speilman, B.L., Shaker, E.H. and Garvey, M.S. (1992) Esophageal foreign body in dogs: a retrospective study of 23 cases. *Journal of the American Animal Hospital Association*, **28**, 570–574.

Stickle, R.L. and Love, N.E. (1989) Radiographic diagnosis of esophageal diseases in dogs and cats. *Seminars in Veterinary Medicine and Surgery*, **4**, 179–187.

Strande, A. (1989) Inguinal hernia in dogs. *Journal of Small Animal Practice*, **30**, 520–521.

Swalec, K.M. and Smeak, D.D. (1990) Partial versus complete attentuation of single portosystemic shunts. *Veterinary Surgery*, **19**, 406–411.

Tams, T.R. (1990) Endoscopic removal of gastrointestinal foreign bodies. In: T.R. Tams (ed.), *Small Animal Endoscopy*, pp. 245–255. St Louis: CV Mosby.

Tobias, K.S., Barbee, D. and Pluhar, G.E. (1996) Intraoperative use of subtraction angiography and an ultrasonic aspirator to improve identification and isolation of an intrahepatic portosystemic shunt in a dog. *Journal of the American Veterinary Medical Association*, **208**, 888–890.

Twedt, D.C. (1995) Diseases of the esophagus. In: S.J. Ettinger (ed.), *Textbook of Veterinary Internal Medicine*, vol. 1, pp. 1124–1142. Philadelphia: WB Saunders.

VanGundy, T.E., Boothe, H.W. and Wolf, A. (1990) Results of surgical management of feline portosystemic shunts. *Journal of the American Animal Hospital Association*, **26**, 55–62.

Vogt, J.C., Krahwinkel, D.J., Bright, R.M., Daniel, G.B., Toal, R.L. and Rohrbach, B. (1996) Gradual occlusion of extrahepatic portosystemic shunts in dogs and cats using the ameroid constrictor. *Veterinary Surgery* **25**, 495–502.

Wallace, J., Mullen, H.S. and Lesser, M.B. (1992) A technique for surgical correction of peritoneal pericardial diaphragmatic hernia in dogs and cats. *Journal of the American Animal Hospital Association*, **28**, 503–510.

Waters, D.J., Roy, R.G. and Stone, E.A. (1993) A retrospective study of inguinal hernia in 35 dogs. *Veterinary Surgery*, **22**, 44–49.

White, R.N., Trower, N.D., McEvoy, F.J., Garden, O.A. and Boswood, A. (1996) A method for controlling portal pressure after attenuation of intrahepatic portacaval shunts. *Veterinary Surgery*, **25**, 407–413.

Willard, M.D., Delles, E.K. and Fossum, T.W. (1994) Iatrogenic tears associated with ballooning of esophageal strictures. *Journal of the American Animal Hospital Association*, **30**, 431–435.

Wrigley, R.H., Konde, L.J., Park, R.D. and Lebel, J.L. (1987) Ultrasonographic diagnosis of portocaval shunts in young dogs. *Journal of the American Veterinary Medical Association*, **191**, 421–424.

Wylie, K.B. and Hosgood, G. (1994) Mortality and morbidity of small and large intestinal surgery in dogs and cats. *Journal of the American Animal Hospital Association*, **30**, 469–474.

7

Thoracic cavity and respiratory disorders

The thoracic cavity

Surgical approaches

The surgical approach used to enter the thoracic cavity depends on the lesions and/or anatomical structures that require exposure (Table 7.1). Viewing a lateral thoracic radiograph often facilitates the selection of a surgical approach.

Ventilation during surgery

Thoracotomy causes the normal negative intrathoracic pressure to become positive; therefore, assisted ventilation is required with increased ventilatory pressure (15–20 cmH$_2$O) to avoid atelectasis. As a result of the positive intrathoracic pressure, the tidal volume will be decreased. The decreased tidal volume will be

Table 7.1 Indications for lateral thoracotomy approaches

Thoracic structure	Intercostal space	
	Left	Right
Heart, pericardium*	4, 5	4, 5
Ductus (ligamentous) arteriosus	4, (5)†	4, 5
Pulmonic valve	4	
Lungs		
Exploratory thoracotomy (all lung lobes)	Median sternotomy	
Cranial lobe	4–6	4–6
Middle lobe	(4), 5	(4), 5
Caudal lobe	5, (6)	5, (6)
Caudal vena cava	(6–7)	7–10
Diaphragm	7–10	7–10
Thoracic duct		
Cat	8–10	(8–10)
Dog	(8–10)	8–10
Oesophagus		
Cranial intrathoracic (heart base)		5
Caudal intrathoracic	8–9	8–9
Trachea		
Thoracic inlet	Midline caudal cervical incision combined with median sternotomy	
Thoracic trachea	Right fourth intercostal space combined with median sternotomy	

* An alternative approach is a median sternotomy.
† Numbers in parentheses are alternate sites.

even more pronounced if the lung lobes are collapsed or surgically packed off. The respiratory rate may have to be increased (12–15 breaths/minute) to maintain adequate alveolar minute ventilation. The positive intrathoracic pressure also reduces the thoracic pumping assistance to venous return to the heart.

Analgesia

Spontaneous ventilation during surgical recovery will be impaired by actual or perceived pain, as well as the presence of any air or fluid in the thoracic cavity. Pain can be alleviated by using intercostal nerve blocks, intrapleural regional analgesia, intramuscularly or intravenously administered analgesic agents or epidural analgesia. Intercostal nerve blocks using 0.5% bupivacaine (not to exceed 2 mg/kg body weight as the total dose) are best performed at the time of surgery and injected in the region of the intercostal nerve at the proximal, caudal rib surface. Blocking two or three intercostal nerves on either side of the thoracotomy incision is generally recommended. Intrapleural administration of bupivacaine causes minimal cardiovascular effects and provides prolonged analgesia following surgery. The bupivacaine can also be repeatedly administered through the thoracostomy tube following completion of the surgery.

Intramuscular or intravenous opioids (e.g. morphine, oxymorphone, butorphanol, buprenorphine and meperidine) provide good analgesia; however, they may cause cardiorespiratory depression and subsequently prolong the duration of hypothermia following surgery. Dosages for these analgesic agents should be reduced for puppies and kittens younger than 12 weeks of age (see Chapter 3). Epidural morphine or oxymorphone provides good postoperative analgesia. Epidural oxymorphone is effective for up to 10 hours, as opposed to 2 hours with intramuscular oxymorphone. Cardiorespiratory depression will occur, however. Because of size the epidural technique may only be for puppies weighing more than 5 kg.

Thoracostomy tube

Air and/or fluid accumulation may be removed via a properly positioned thoracostomy tube.

If the tube is placed during surgery, it is important to have an adequate area of the thorax prepared beforehand for aseptic placement, and the fluid and/or air is removed before anaesthesia is terminated. The tube can be aspirated following surgery should air or fluid continue to accumulate. One properly placed thoracostomy tube will drain both hemithoraces in most dogs and cats since their mediastinum is usually incomplete. Diseases that cause loculation within the thoracic cavity (i.e. chylothorax and pyothorax) may require placement of bilateral thoracostomy tubes.

Procedurally, the thoracostomy tube is introduced through the skin at the level of the 10th or 11th rib, in the dorsal one-third of the thorax, passed subcutaneously for two intercostal spaces in a cranioventral direction, then introduced through the intercostal muscles and pleura using a stylet or a large-sized haemostatic forcep (Fig. 7.1). The tube is then sutured to the skin (Fig. 7.2) and supported by bandaging to the thorax with only the free end exposed. Care is required to ensure that the bandaging procedure is not too tight so that is does not interfere with natural respiration.

A continuous suction system may be used for spontaneous pneumothorax or pleural effusions (i.e. chylothorax and pyothorax), using a two- or three-underwater-bottle system (Fig. 7.3). Continuous suction of 8–15 cmH$_2$O is effective for pneumothorax; however, pressure up to 20 cmH$_2$O may be needed to aspirate viscous

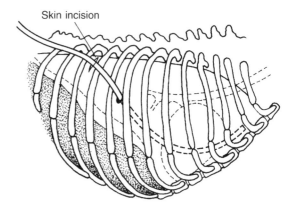

Figure 7.1 Line drawing of the lateral thorax showing proper placement of a thoracostomy tube. The tube penetrates the skin between the 10th and 11th ribs and enters the thoracic cavity between the eighth and ninth ribs. The tube should be placed no further cranial than the second rib.

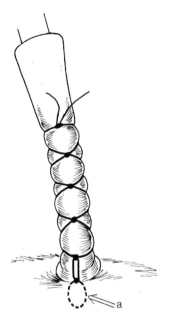

Figure 7.2 The thoracostomy tube (and any tubular drain or catheter) can be sutured to the skin using a Chinese finger trap suture. (a) The suture is first tied to the skin without tension, then (b) repeatedly crossed and tied on the front of the drain with square knot progressing along a length of the drain.

fluid. One-way valves such as the Heimlich valve are usually unsuitable for removal of air in the thoracic cavity of puppies and kittens weighing less than 15 kg.

Intermittent suction using a three-way stopcock valve on the end of the thoracostomy tube is usually adequate for removal of any residual air or fluid following thoracic surgery. A C-clamp should also be used to occlude the thoracostomy tube between aspirations. This is necessary to prevent pneumothorax developing from a leaky stopcock valve connection. Intermittent suction is applied every 15 minutes, lengthening the intervals as the amount of aspirated air or fluid decreases. Care to close the stopcock valve completely, making sure all connections are tight, is imperative.

Lateral thoracotomy

A lateral thoracotomy is the standard approach used when exposure of a known anatomical structure is required. The skin and cutaneous trunci muscle are incised over the selected intercostal space, counted backwards from the 13th rib. The latissimus dorsi is then incised parallel to the skin incision or, if a caudal approach is used, may be elevated to expose the deeper muscles. The intercostal spaces are recounted backwards from the first rib under the latissimus dorsi muscle to confirm the surgical site. The end of the scalenus muscle at its junction with the external abdominal oblique marks the fifth intercostal space. The deeper muscles are incised

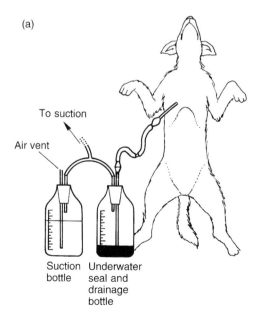

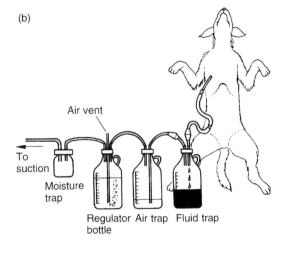

Figure 7.3 (a) Two bottle and (b) three bottle suction systems.

(scalenus, ventral serratus, external abdominal oblique). The muscle bellies of the ventral serratus may be separated rather than incised. The intercostal muscles are incised down the middle of the space to avoid damage to the intercostal blood vessels on the caudal aspect of the ribs.

The ribs are spread with a baby Finochetto rib retractor. The thoracotomy is closed with relatively heavy-gauge (2-0) simple interrupted sutures placed circumferentially around the ribs immediately cranial and caudal to the incision. Each muscle layer is closed separately over the incision to ensure an airtight seal of the thorax.

Rib resection or rib pivot thoracotomy can be performed to gain increased exposure, although the ribs of puppies and kittens are soft and can be retracted easily. Once the ribs are exposed, the periosteum of the rib to be resected is incised over the mid lateral surface of the rib and elevated circumferentially from the rib. The rib is removed with bone cutters. The underlying periosteum is incised to gain access to the thoracic cavity. The thoracotomy is closed similarly to a lateral thoracotomy.

For rib pivot thoracotomy, the rib is exposed and the periosteum elevated as for rib resection. The rib is severed with bone cutters at the costochondral junction and pivoted at the chondrovertebral articulation. The underlying periosteum is incised to gain access to the thoracic cavity. For closure, the rib is reapposed using hemicerclage wires or heavy suture and a routine thoracotomy closure is performed.

Median sternotomy

Median sternotomy is the preferred approach for access to the entire thoracic cavity. It is indicated for exploration of the thoracic cavity and for procedures at the base of the heart (e.g. pericardectomy). Median sternotomy is performed with the puppy or kitten in dorsal recumbency. This will cause the heart to tilt downwards, increasing venous pressure and reducing cardiac output. The skin and subcutaneous tissue are incised along the midline. The pectoral muscles are elevated off the midline of the sternum. The sternum is scored with a scalpel blade, then cut with an osteotome and mallet, oscillating saw or a sternal knife (Lebske sternal knife). In an attempt to reduce postoperative move-

ment and pain, either the manubrium or the xiphoid is left intact. A median sternotomy may be combined with a ventral midline abdominal incision. Incision of the diaphragm may be required to increase exposure. A median sternotomy can be combined with a lateral thoracotomy to create a thoracic wall flap for greater exposure.

The sternum is closed with cruciate (figure-of-eight) circumferential sutures of relatively heavy absorbable suture (2-0) which pass around each costosternal junction. Avoid stainless-steel wire since it cycles and will break. The pectoral muscles, subcutaneous tissue and skin are closed in separate layers using standard technique.

Transsternal thoracotomy will allow for greater exposure than a lateral thoracotomy. A lateral thoracotomy incision is extended across the sternum to incorporate another lateral thoracotomy. The internal thoracic arteries that course along the lateral aspect of the sternum must be ligated. The sternal osteotomy is closed as described for the median sternotomy.

Postoperative considerations

Continuous monitoring of the puppy and kitten is imperative as long as a thoracostomy tube remains in place. Analgesia may need to be repeated, either systemically, locally, or both. Continued intravenous fluid support may be required until the animal is able to eat and drink. Keeping the animal warm is always important. Antimicrobial therapy is indicated if penetrating trauma was the reason for the thoracic surgery. Forelimb lameness may be evident after lateral thoracotomy if the latissimus dorsi muscle was severed.

Thoracic trauma

Trauma to the thoracic wall may be the result of either blunt trauma or a penetrating wound. Blunt trauma usually occurs from being hit by car or a bite wound. Bite wounds often cause a combination of penetrating and crushing injuries. Severe contusion to the internal thoracic organs (heart and lung) may occur during blunt trauma without obvious damage to the external thoracic wall. Penetrating injury often causes haemorrhage or pneumothorax depending on the extent of internal organ damage.

Pneumothorax may also arise in injury to the lung parenchyma or airways within the confines of the ribs. Lung lacerations occur secondary to rib fractures and occasionally from the blunt trauma itself.

Clinical signs

Signs associated with thoracic wall trauma depend on the extent of the trauma. Signs of haemorrhagic shock can occur if haemorrhage is severe and acute. Respiratory distress may be associated with pneumothorax or haemothorax, flail chest or pulmonary contusions. Cardiac dysrhythmias may be associated with myocardial contusion (traumatic myocarditis). Rupture of intercostal muscles by blunt trauma or bite wounds may result in significant herniation of lung lobes. Ruptured intercostal muscles and pneumothorax often cause paradoxical movement of the skin, which should be differentiated from a flail chest segment. If the intercostal muscle tear communicates with a skin wound, a sucking wound may occur, resulting in pneumothorax. Subcutaneous air accumulation usually denotes a disrupted thoracic wall. Respiratory distress is usually associated with haemothorax and pneumothorax, and moist lung sounds are associated with pulmonary haemorrhage or oedema.

Pain or crepitus on palpation may be associated with fractured ribs. Multiple rib fractures that involve both proximal and distal fractures may cause a free segment of thoracic wall that moves paradoxically with respiration (flail chest) and causes a reduction in the animal's ventilation capacity. The veterinarian should be aware that severe pulmonary contusions are also usually present and not overinterpret the effect of the flail segment on ventilation capacity.

Diagnosis

Thoracic radiographs are important for a diagnosis of pneumothorax or pleural fluid (i.e. haemothorax) and associated rib fractures. Oxygen should be available during radiography since the handling may induce life-threatening respiratory distress. Stabilizing the animal before radiography is always advised. If haemothorax or pneumothorax is suspected, this may require thoracocentesis prior to radiography to evacuate some of the air or blood and

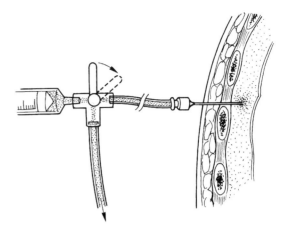

Figure 7.4 Use of a three-way stopcock to facilitate thoracocentesis using an indwelling intravenous catheter and a large syringe.

improve respiration. Thoracocentesis is performed using aseptic technique. An over-the-needle venous catheter of appropriate size for the animal can be used, introducing it through the ventral third of the fourth to seventh intercostal spaces. It can be connected to a three-way stopcock valve to facilitate rapid withdrawal of accumulated fluid or air (Fig. 7.4).

Thoracic radiographs will usually show free air and fluid within the pleural space (Table 7.1). Bronchoscopy may be useful to locate tracheal or mainstem bronchial tears because haemorrhage within a bronchus helps to identify the affected lung lobe.

Diagnosis of haemothorax is made by demonstrating blood within the pleural space via thoracocentesis. Evidence of pleural effusion is observed on the radiographs and aspirated fluid has a packed cell volume, total protein, total cell count and cytological appearance similar to that of peripheral blood. Haemorrhage associated with severe trauma occasionally clots within the pleural space as a result of release of tissue thromboplastin but then undergoes complete fibrinolysis within 7–10 days. In comparison, haemorrhagic effusions usually do not clot within the pleural cavity due to mechanical defibrination and activation of fibrinolytic mechanisms.

Treatment and surgical technique

Initial treatment should always emphasize stabilization of the cardiovascular system and evacuation of pneumothorax or haemothorax. Shock therapy and placement of a thoracotomy tube may be indicated. Isolated rib fractures generally do not require repair; however, stabilization of multiple rib fractures causing a flail segment should be performed. This can be performed percutaneously using a simplified technique (McNulty, 1995) under local anaesthesia with the animal sedated. Blocking one or two ribs cranial to the flail segment is required. Systemic analgesic may also be indicated. A single, non-absorbable monofilament suture swaged to a large tapered needle is passed percutaneously around the centre of each floating rib (Fig. 7.5). Each suture is then tied to the middle of a supporting splint (wooden tongue-depressor) with the splint positioned parallel to the affected rib. Grooving the splint in the region of the suture may improve stability. The splint will be used to apply traction to the ribs.

The length of the splint is not critical but should be about the length of the floating rib segment. Dorsal and ventral countertraction splints are placed perpendicular to the rib axis between the skin and the traction splints and should be extended beyond the flail segment. Padding is laced between the countertraction splint and the traction splints at the point where they overlap and the splints are compressed over the padding and taped in place. This arrangement creates outwards traction on

the rib segments. The entire apparatus is covered with a light bandage for protection.

For penetrating wounds or blunt trauma that have caused considerable intercostal muscle damage, surgical repair may be indicated but should be delayed until the animal is stable. Muscle can be apposed primarily, by circumferential rib sutures or by patching techniques using an omental pedicle or muscle flaps (latissimus dorsi, external abdominal oblique). Concurrent isolated rib fractures are treated conservatively with cage rest. Multiple rib fractures may necessitate primary repair with intramedullary pins and hemicerclage wire. Multiple, staggered, encircling rib sutures using heavy suture material (0-polydioxanine or 0-nylon) can help to stabilize multiple rib fractures and provide a scaffold for soft tissue reconstruction (Shahar *et al.*, 1997). Alternatively, percutaneous encircling sutures can be placed around the ribs and tied to an external splint, as described above.

Conservative therapy with one or two thoracostomy tubes may be useful for traumatic pneumothorax if the site of injury is small. For penetrating wounds or spontaneous pneumothorax, treatment in this manner often results in complications and early surgical intervention is indicated. Surgery intervention is indicated if there is continued evidence of pneumothorax despite treatment or there is evidence

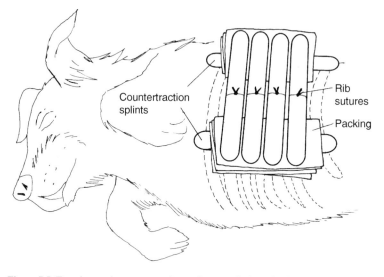

Figure 7.5 Traction and countertraction splints applied to the lateral thorax for treatment of a flail segment. Perpendicular splints are sutured to the ribs and compressed against gauze packing and horizontal splints. Tape is then placed over the ends of the splints to prevent the packing becoming dislodged.

of moderate to severe haemorrhage from the injury. A lateral thoracotomy is performed over the affected lung lobe and the lung laceration is sutured with large horizontal mattress sutures using monofilament absorbable suture on a small tapered swaged needle. In addition, the edges of the laceration can be apposed with a simple continuous or a continuous Lembert suture pattern. If there is a pulmonary lesion such as an air bulla, definitive treatment may require excision of the affected lung lobe.

Treatment of haemothorax depends on the degree of respiratory distress. If respiratory distress is minimal, the blood is not withdrawn from the pleural space because most dogs are capable of absorbing 30% of their blood volume within 90 hours. As 70–100% of the red blood cells are absorbed intact, pleural drainage is only performed if absolutely necessary.

If drainage of haemothorax is necessary, autotransfusion is possible, providing a readily available source of compatible blood. Blood from cats and small dogs can be collected in heparinized syringes; blood from large dogs can be collected with 100 ml citrate-phosphate-dextrose or 60 ml of anticoagulant-citrate-dextrose with 800 ml of blood. Filtration of the blood through a micropore filter before infusion is recommended.

Pectus excavatum

Pectus excavatum, although uncommon, is the most frequently observed congenital malformation of the thoracic wall in young dogs and cats. Pectus excavatum is characterized by concave, inward deformation of the caudal sternum and costal cartilages causing dorsoventral flattening of the thoracic cavity (Shires *et al.*, 1988; Boudrieau, 1990). It may be related to the so-called swimmer syndrome, a poorly described disorder of neonatal dogs and cats where the animal remains in sternal recumbency with the legs splayed outwards. Brachycephalic dog breeds appear to be affected most often.

Clinical signs

Clinical signs include gross deformation of the sternum, stunted growth, exercise intolerance, dyspnoea, cyanosis and vomiting. Cardiac murmurs and dysrhythmias may also occur due to compression of the heart and vessels and not due to congenital anomalies.

Diagnosis

A clinical diagnosis can be confirmed by radiography. The degree of compression can be evaluated from the lateral radiographic projection. It is important to differentiate pectus excavatum from paradoxical movement of the sternum in a young animal with respiratory distress and profound respiratory effort. In distressed animals, the soft cartilage of the sternum will flex with the respiratory effort, but on radiographs it will appear to follow the normal contour. In pectus excavatum, the deformity of the sternum is constant and is revealed on the radiographs.

Treatment and surgical technique

Surgical repair can be attempted if cardiopulmonary compromise is severe or for aesthetic reasons. External splints are useful for most animals younger than 2 or 3 months of age when the sternum is still flexible. Large sutures are placed percutaneously around the sternum, and tied to an external splint (Fig. 7.6; Boudrieau *et al.*, 1990). Internal fixation with intramedullary pins or Kirschner wires may be required in older animals.

Postoperative considerations and prognosis

The splint is left in place for approximately 14 days. A moist contact dermatitis may develop underneath the splint and routine cleansing will usually resolve this and any suture tract wounds after the splint is removed. The thorax should be radiographed at the time of splint removal and again when the animal reaches skeletal maturity to monitor for conformational changes.

Complications during surgery are related to suture placement and include the possibility of laceration of the lungs or internal thoracic vessels (which course on either side of the sternum). Careful placement of the needle, use of a taper point needle and careful attention to the phase of respiration when the needle is placed may help reduce these potential problems. Re-expansion pulmonary oedema may occur in severe cases with significant atelectasis. Fatal re-expansion pulmonary oedema following surgery has recently been reported in an

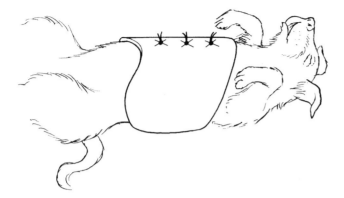

Figure 7.6 Cruciate (figure-of-eight) sutures placed through an external splint and encircling the sternebrae for treatment of pectus excavatum.

8-week-old kitten (Soderstrom *et al.*, 1995). The prognosis is fair if surgical correction is performed early and the deformation is mild.

Other thoracic wall anomalies

Rib deformities or abnormalities are not uncommon and include missing ribs, fused ribs, extra ribs and malformed ribs. Surgical treatment is usually unnecessary.

Mediastinal disorders

Mediastinal disorders usually characterized by a soft-tissue mass include neoplasia, cyst, abscess/granuloma, haematoma, tracheobronchial lymphadenopathy and encapsulated fluid accumulation. The cranial region of the mediastinum is most often affected in young cats. The cranioventral and perihilar mediastinal regions are commonly affected in young dogs. Pneumomediastinum may also occur. Mediastinal disorders affecting the thymus are the most common in paediatric animals.

Thymic haematomas may be a cause of sudden death in puppies. Affected puppies range from 3 to 24 months of age. Most thymic haematomas are associated with automobile-induced and somersaulting leash injuries. The traumatic insult triggers the sudden onset of weakness, dyspnoea, pallor, collapse and death. At necropsy, extensive haemorrhage is noted in the thymus and mediastinum. Haemothorax may be present if mediastinal tissue surrounding the thymus ruptures. Affected puppies are usually found to be undergoing thymic involution with resultant lymphoreticular tissue degeneration and loss of vascular support. This results in thin-walled dilated vessels that are vulnerable to trauma. Thymic haematomas have also been recognized in cases of anticoagulant toxicity.

Clinical signs

Clinical signs associated with a mediastinal mass include respiratory distress, cough associated with tracheal and bronchial compression, and regurgitation and dysphagia associated with oesophageal compression. Head, neck and forelimb oedema may occur due to intrathoracic vein and lymphatic compression. Horner's syndrome (characterized by ptosis, myosis and prolapse of the third eyelid) may occur with compression of the sympathetic ganglion.

Diagnosis

Diagnosis for most mediastinal masses includes radiography, ultrasonography and biopsy. Mediastinal widening, soft-tissue density, tracheal displacement to the right and aortic displacement to the left may be observed. In young cats, the most common mediastinal mass is lymphosarcoma. In young dogs, lymphosarcoma, thymoma and lymphadenopathy are common causes. Hilar and perihilar masses are more common in dogs, usually the result of enlargement of the tracheobronchial lymph nodes. Increased perihilar density, tracheal compression and ventral mainstem bronchi displacement are observed.

Treatment and surgical technique

Treatment is usually based on the diagnosis, either from a fine-needle aspirate biopsy taken by a transthoracic approach, or from a tissue biopsy taken during exploratory thoracotomy. Animals with large mediastinal masses are a poor anaesthetic and surgical risk. However, the prognosis is favourable, should resection be possible (granuloma, cyst, haematoma or thymoma). The treatment of choice for lymphosarcoma is chemotherapy as used for adult dogs and cats.

Pneumomediastinum

Pneumomediastinum is defined as air accumulation around the mediastinal structures and confined by the mediastinal pleura. Pneumomediastinum may be caused by rupture of the thoracic trachea or oesophagus, or from penetrating neck wounds where air dissects along the fascial planes of the neck into the mediastinum.

Clinical signs

Clinical signs may initially include emphysematous head and neck swelling. Respiratory distress is uncommon. Cyanosis is usually only observed in severe cases with rapid air leakage into the mediastinum.

Diagnosis

Diagnosis is by radiography. Unlike their normally indistinct radiographic appearance, the mediastinal structures appear clearly with a distinct outline. Air may be present within the soft tissue of the neck with extension caudally into the retroperitoneal space. In severe cases, the mediastinum may rupture, causing a pneumothorax.

Treatment

Treatment is usually unnecessary, although correction of the inciting cause is required. Air will be resorbed within 2–10 days.

Chylothorax

Chylothorax is an uncommon condition of young dogs and cats characterized by collection of chyle from the chylothoracic duct system in the pleural space. The cause of chylothorax is often unknown (idiopathic) but has been associated with trauma, dirofilariasis, blastomycosis, cardiomyopathy, lung lobe torsion, heart base tumours, thymoma and lymphangiectasia. The Afghan Hound is identified as a breed at higher risk for developing chylothorax. Clinical signs of chylothorax often manifest gradually and include dyspnoea, tachypnoea, exercise intolerance, anorexia, weight loss and dehydration.

Diagnosis

Diagnosis of chylothorax is based on radiographs, pleural fluid analysis and lymphangiography. Radiographic signs are consistent with the presence of pleural fluid (Table 7.2). Evaluation of fluid aspirate from the thoracic cavity is important to differentiate it from other non-chylous effusions (Table 7.3). Thoracic radiographs after evacuation of the pleural fluid may rule out the presence of intrathoracic masses. Cardiac disease should be ruled out with electrocardiographic and echocardiographic examination. Direct lymphangiography using aqueous contrast medium into an ileocolic lymphatic vessel may help elucidate the cause of chylothorax.

Treatment and surgical technique

Treatment of chylothorax may be either medical or surgical. Medical management involves drainage of the thoracic cavity and dietary manipulation to reduce the fat content of the chyle. Drainage of the thorax is performed via thoracostomy tube(s) and preferably by continuous drainage. Feeding a low-fat, high-protein and high-carbohydrate diet is recommended. Addition of medium-chain triglycerides, which are absorbed directly into the portal system, can be made to the diet to increase energy content. Supplementation with fat-soluble vitamins is required. Rutin (50 mg/kg t.i.d. PO), a benzopyrone available from most health food stores in the US, has been used in dogs and cats with chylothorax in conjunction with other medical management. The effects of its use are unknown

Table 7.2 Radiographic signs of fluid and air within the thoracic cavity

	Radiographic sign
Fluid	Partial or complete obliteration of cardiac silhouette
	Visualization of interlobar fissures due to fluid within them
	Homogeneous density of ventral thorax on lateral projection, often with scalloped appearance due to fluid in interlobar fissures
	Loss of normal sharp angles at the costophrenic junction
	Loss of diaphragmatic outline if a lot of fluid is present
Air	Heart elevated from sternum on lateral projection
	Increased radiolucent appearance of thorax
	Edges of caudal lung lobes separated from ventral aspect of thoracic vertebrae or diaphragm
	Increased density of lungs due to collapse
	Air observed in interlobar fissures of the lungs

and results of its use in veterinary patients with chylothorax have not been reported. The authors have not noted any adverse side-effects. Benzopyrones have been used successfully to reduce lymphoedema of the extremities in humans. Minimal side-effects, notably mild nausea and diarrhoea, are reported after its use in humans (Casely-Smith *et al.*, 1993).

Surgical management can involve transthoracic ligation of the caudal thoracic duct, implantation of active pleurovenous shunts or pleuroperitoneal shunts, or creation of passive pleuroperitoneal shunting through fenestrated Silastic sheeting in the diaphragm or transdiaphragmatic tubes. Pleurodesis using intrapleural administration of irritants (e.g. tetracycline) has not been successful.

Despite medical and surgical treatment, the prognosis for an animal with chylothorax is poor. Only about 50% of animals respond to treatment. If treatment for the cause of chylothorax is possible, the prognosis may be more favourable. Pleuroperitoneal or pleuro-venous shunts are used to palliate animals with refractory chylothorax. Constrictive pleuritis is a sequela to chylothorax (and other pleural effusions such as pyothorax, haemothorax and exudative effusion of feline infectious peritonitis). Severe constrictive pleural adhesions develop secondary to the irritation and inflammation associated with chylous accumulation in the pleural space. Constriction of the lung parenchyma can cause significant respiratory compromise.

Table 7.3 Characteristics of chylous effusion

Characteristics of chylous effusion	*Characteristics of non-chylous effusions*
Milky-white appearance, which remains after standing	Milky-white appearance, which may settle out after standing
Total protein concentration ranges from 3 to 5 g/dl	
Demonstration of chylomicrons, either on direct smears, or with vital stains such as Sudan III or IV	
Triglyceride concentrations 12–100 times greater than serum, with cholesterol concentrations similar to that of the serum	High cholesterol with low triglyceride concentrations
Clears after the addition of ether	Does not clear with ether
Cytological examination may show a predominance of small and large lymphocytes. Chronic chylous effusions have progressive increases in neutrophils, macrophages and mesothelial cells	

Pyothorax

Pyothorax is the accumulation of exudate and fluid within the pleural space. Pyothorax may be the result of systemic sepsis, spread from adjacent structures (pneumonia with bronchopneumonic spread, oesophageal rupture or mediastinitis) or by direct introduction of infectious organisms by penetrating trauma, foreign bodies, thoracocentesis or surgery.

Clinical signs

Clinical signs associated with pyothorax include fever, anorexia, weight loss, exercise intolerance and respiratory distress.

Diagnosis

Diagnosis is based on radiographic findings consistent with pleural fluid (Table 7.2) and fluid analysis. A moderate to severe pleural effusion is present – characteristically bilateral – and obscures the cardiac silhouette and some pulmonary detail. Radiographs should be repeated after thoracocentesis. Pulmonary infiltrates or consolidation may be present. The left cranial lung lobe is frequently affected in young dogs and cats. Thoracocentesis and cytological and microbiological evaluation of the pleural fluid is essential to a diagnosis of pyothorax. Gram staining gives initial indications of the type of bacteria present. Anaerobic infections are common, either as a pure infection or combined with aerobic bacteria. Culture and sensitivity testing for both aerobic and anaerobic bacteria are recommended. In affected cats, the immune status of the animal should be questioned and FeLV and FIV testing should be performed. Feline infectious peritonitis should also be ruled out as a cause of pyothorax.

Treatment

Successful treatment requires both fluid removal and appropriate systemic antimicrobial therapy. The necessity for pleural lavage using 20 ml/kg or warm, sterile 0.9% saline solution twice a day is controversial. The addition of antimicrobial agents to the lavage solution is not recommended. Tube thoracostomy should be performed as soon as possible. Usually a single tube is sufficient, although bilateral thoracostomy tubes may be required if fluid is loculated.

Use of continuous suction with a water seal is recommended. Antimicrobial medication should be based on bacterial culture and sensitivity test results. Penicillin remains the antimicrobial of choice for anaerobic infections in which *Bacteroides fragilis* is most commonly isolated. Cytological evaluation of fluid can be used to monitor the effectiveness of the medication. Gram stains should fail to reveal bacteria by 2–3 days after drainage and medication.

Failure to respond to treatment or persistence of a consolidated lung lobe on radiographs may be an indication for exploratory thoracotomy, performed through a median sternotomy. Consolidated lung lobes may require partial or complete lobectomy. The prognosis is fair to good, depending on the chronicity of the problem, the overall health of the animal and its immune status. Early, aggressive treatment in the immune-competent animal carries a good prognosis.

Diaphragmatic hernia

Diaphragmatic hernias may be traumatic, congenital or hiatal. Traumatic diaphragmatic hernias (pleuroperitoneal) are most common. Congenital hernias may be either pleuroperitoneal or, more frequently, peritoneopericardial. Hiatal hernias may be sliding or paraoesophageal and are considered congenital.

Traumatic diaphragmatic hernias

Traumatic diaphragmatic hernias are commonly circumferential, ventral to the oesophagus at the right costomuscular region (Boudrieau and Muir, 1987). Radial tears are less common and the central tendon is rarely affected due to its strength.

Clinical signs

Clinical signs may be inapparent for days or even years after the injury and are usually referable to the respiratory or gastrointestinal tracts. Respiratory compromise exacerbated by stress is the most common sign. Pleural effusion may be detected, especially if liver herniation is present. Haemorrhagic, modified transudate or chyle may be present (Boudrieau and Muir, 1987).

Diagnosis

Diagnosis of traumatic diaphragmatic hernia is usually made with thoracic radiographs (Tables 7.4 and 7.5; Fig. 7.7). Hernias may be inapparent if viscera move freely across the tear. Removing pleural fluid and repeating the radiographs may be useful. Negative-contrast peritoneography can be performed. After aseptic injection of air or carbon dioxide, the animal is held standing on its hind legs and a ventrodorsal radiographic projection is taken using a horizontal beam. Air will normally accumulate between the liver and the diaphragm and outline the diaphragm. If a diaphragmatic tear is present, air will accumulate in the thoracic inlet. If the liver is incarcerated or adhered, an abrupt stop in the outline of the diaphragm will occur in this location. Positive peritoneography may reveal contrast in the thoracic cavity, absence of a normal liver outline and, most often, incomplete visualization of the normal outline of the abdominal surface of the diaphragm. Ultrasound is a non-invasive, quick method for potentially confirming a traumatic diaphragmatic hernia (Fagin, 1989).

Table 7.4 Radiographic characteristics of traumatic diaphragmatic hernia

Interruption of the diaphragmatic outline
Abdominal contents within the thorax
Displacement of thoracic structures
Displacement of abdominal viscera
Pleural effusion and thoracic trauma
Divergence of the diaphragmatic crura
Radiographic evidence of trauma to other tissues

Treatment and surgical technique

Treatment requires surgical repair of the diaphragm. Anaesthetic management of any animal with a diaphragmatic hernia requires minimizing stress. Preanaesthetic tranquillization with an agent that does not severely depress cardiovascular and respiratory function is preferred. Rapid induction with a barbiturate allows the animal to be intubated. If possible, isoflurane is preferred due to its minimal cardiac-depressant and dysrhythmogenic effects. Nitrous oxide should not be used. Controlled ventilation is required immediately after induction: peak airway pressures should not exceed

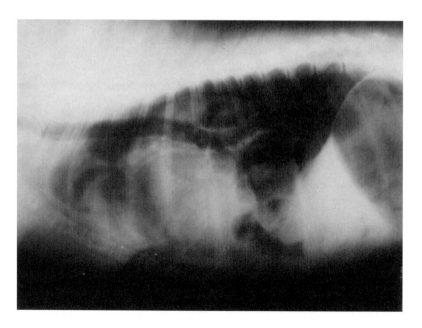

Figure 7.7 Lateral thoracic survey radiograph of traumatic diaphragmatic hernia in a dog. Note the loss of diaphragmatic outline ventrally and the intestinal gas shadows within the thoracic cavity.

Table 7.5 Features of various radiographic techniques to assist in the diagnosis of diaphragmatic hernias

Radiographic technique	Comment
Plain radiographs	Interruption of the diaphragmatic outline may be obvious with increased soft-tissue density in the thorax. Pleural effusion may make discerning detail in the thoracic cavity difficult. Gas-filled intestinal loops cranial to the diaphragm may be observed
Horizontal beam/plain radiographs	Horizontal beam projection with the animal in dorsal recumbency can highlight diaphragm outline if pleural fluid is present
Negative-contrast peritoneography	Air is injected into the abdomen (room air or carbon dioxide). Risk of air embolization is less with carbon dioxide than air since it is more soluble in blood. Ventrodorsal radiographic projection taken using a horizontal beam while the animal is standing on its hind legs. If a diaphragmatic tear is present, air will accumulate in the thoracic inlet
Positive-contrast peritoneography	Water-soluble iodinated contrast is injected into the abdomen (1–2 ml/kg). Positive contrast may move into thoracic cavity. Lateral and ventrodorsal projections are repeated. Incomplete visualization of the normal outline of the abdominal surface of the diaphragm is diagnostic
Positive-contrast gastrointestinal study	Oral administration of barium and subsequent radiography is associated with a high percentage of false negatives due to absence of portions of the gastrointestinal tract in the hernia

$20-30\ cmH_2O$. Overinflation may cause re-expansion pulmonary oedema.

Surgical repair is an emergency if the stomach is entrapped and distended with gas. Emergency decompression of the stomach by percutaneous trocarization may be required. Definitive evidence of incarcerated bowel, obstructed bowel, bowel rupture or ongoing haemorrhage also requires immediate attention. All other diaphragmatic hernias should be repaired only after the animal's condition is stabilized, since the mortality of animals operated in the first 24 hours after injury is significantly higher than animals operated later than 24 hours after injury.

Herniorrhaphy is performed through a midline coeliotomy, with extension of the incision through the xiphoid and sternum if necessary. Once the diaphragm tear is identified, herniated viscera can be returned to the abdominal cavity using gentle traction. The tear can be extended to facilitate reduction of the viscera. The abdominal and thoracic viscera are examined to determine integrity. The diaphragm is examined for other tears. The free edge of a chronic tear should be debrided. The diaphragm margins are approximated using atraumatic (Babcock) forceps. Many suture patterns and materials are suitable. The author prefers short runs of simple continuous or interrupted

mattress sutures using a monofilament non-absorbable suture. Working initially from the least accessible dorsal aspect is advised. Failure to close large defects is rare because the diaphragm is exceptionally mobile and elastic. Reconstructive techniques include use of an omental pedicle based on the left or right gastro-epiploic artery, a fascia lata graft, prosthetic materials or sliding and transpositional abdominal muscle flaps from the transverse abdominal muscle. Air must be removed from the thoracic cavity prior to abdominal closure. Transdiaphragmatic aspiration of air is possible; however, the use of a lateral thoracostomy tube is preferred and provides an access for postoperative assessment of pneumothorax or haemothorax after surgery. The thoracostomy tube is usually removed within a few hours.

Postoperative considerations and prognosis

Thoracic radiographs should be taken several days after herniorrhaphy to examine for pneumothorax and hydrothorax, and to assess lung inflation. A chronic, atelectatic lung is at risk from torsion and may also be a site for development of pneumonia. Consequently, lobectomy may be required. Mortality rates for animals with traumatic diaphragmatic hernia after surgical repair range from 10 to 35%. The prognosis for long-term survival is good if the animal survives the first 24 hours after surgery.

Congenital pleuroperitoneal diaphragmatic hernias

Congenital pleuroperitoneal diaphragmatic hernias have been infrequently reported in the veterinary literature. Large defects in puppies have been described and all the puppies died at birth or shortly thereafter. An 8-month-old cat underwent successful surgical repair of a congenital pleuroperitoneal diaphragmatic hernia in the right crus (Mann *et al.*, 1991).

Congenital peritoneopericardial diaphragmatic hernias

Congenital peritoneopericardial diaphragmatic hernias are not uncommon. The disorder may be more common in Weimaraner dogs and Persian cats. The disorder is due to faulty development of the septum transversum, in combination with incomplete fusion of the caudal pleuropericardial membranes. Other defects associated with congenital peritoneopericardial hernia include cranial abdominal hernia, absence of a xiphoid, ventral diaphragmatic defect and abdominal organs in the caudal mediastinum rather than the pericardium. Concurrent ventricular septal defect, atrial septal defect and pulmonic stenosis have been reported. Malformed sternebrae and umbilical hernias are also reported.

Clinical signs

Clinical signs may be of gastrointestinal, respiratory or cardiac origin.

Diagnosis

Diagnosis is by radiography and ultrasound (Fig. 7.8). Survey radiographs show enlargement of the cardiac silhouette, dorsal displacement of the trachea or interruption of the diaphragmatic outline. Small intestinal gas patterns over the cardiac silhouette are common and considered pathognomonic. In cats, the dorsal peritoneopericardial mesothelial remnant may be identified between the caudal cardiac silhouette and the diaphragm (Berry *et al.*, 1990).

Treatment and surgical technique

Herniorrhaphy is performed through a midline coeliotomy with extension through the xiphoid and sternebrae if necessary. The viscera are reduced and the edges of the diaphragm are debrided and sutured. Separating the pericardium from the diaphragm and closing it separately is unnecessary. Like other diaphragmatic hernias, re-expansion pulmonary oedema is possible if the duration of the hernia is chronic and excessive positive-pressure ventilation is used.

Prognosis

The prognosis is good to excellent for long-term survival.

Respiratory system disorders

General surgical procedures

Tracheostomy

Tracheostomy is a procedure to bypass upper-airway obstruction. It can be performed temporarily with a tube tracheostomy or permanently with creation of a stoma. Tracheostomy may be an elective procedure (preoperative temporary tube tracheostomy or permanent tracheostomy) or an emergency procedure.

Tracheostomy technique

Tube tracheostomy is performed aseptically through a ventral midline incision over the trachea. A transverse incision is made between the third and fourth or fourth and fifth tracheal rings (Fig. 7.9). Other incisions, such as a vertical, elliptical, U and window-type, may also be used. A tube no larger than one-half the diameter of the trachea is inserted to prevent total tracheal obstruction should the tube become occluded. Tracheostomy tubes may be metal or plastic, cuffed or non-cuffed, and cannulated or non-cannulated. Intense care after tube insertion is always required. The tube may need cleaning as often as every 15 minutes using a sterile suction cannula inserted into the tube lumen. Sterile saline solution can be infused into the trachea immediately before suctioning to loosen any secretions (Table 7.1). The tracheostomy tube is removed when an adequate airway is established. Alternatively, smaller

(a)

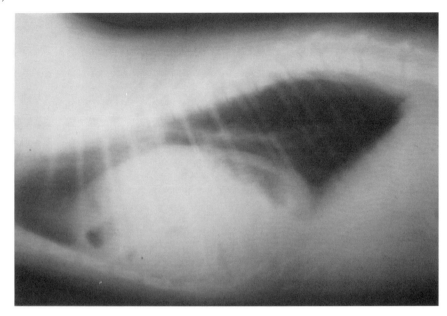

(b)

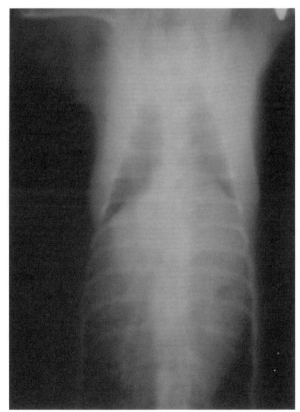

Figure 7.8 (a) Lateral and (b) ventrodorsal survey radiographs of peritoneopericardial hernia in a cat. Note the enlarged cardiac silhouette, loss of diaphragmatic outline ventrally and intestinal gas shadows within the cardiac silhouette.

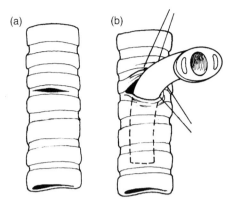

Figure 7.9 Technique for performing a temporary tracheostomy. (a) A transverse incision is made between the third and fourth or fourth and fifth tracheal rings, no more than half the circumference of the trachea. (b) Stay sutures facilitate separation of the incision to allow placement of the tube. A tube no larger than one-half the diameter of the trachea is used to prevent total tracheal obstruction should the tube become occluded.

Table 7.6 Techniques employed for tracheobronchial suction

Technique for tracheobronchial suction
1. Catheter selection – smooth surface, side-holed sterile catheter of sufficient length to reach mainstem bronchi. Diameter not to exceed half the airway diameter
2. Frequency – only when secretions are present; this will decrease over time
3. Preoxygenate animal with 100% oxygen
4. Insert sterile catheter to the level of the carina without suction; avoid contaminating catheter
5. Infuse 2–5 ml of warm sterile saline down catheter, depending on size of animal
6. Apply intermittent suction (while rotating the catheter and withdrawing it). Proper suction levels are –80 to –120 mmHg
7. Total duration of procedure must not exceed 10–15 s
8. Signs of distress or arrhythmias necessitate discontinuing procedure and oxygenating animal
9. Reoxygenate and repeat if necessary

tubes can be gradually replace larger tubes until adequate ventilation is resumed. After tube removal, the incision is allowed to heal by second intention. Complications may include gagging, vomiting, tube obstruction, tube dislodgement, emphysema, tracheal stenosis, tracheocutaneous or tracheo-oesophageal fistula formation and tracheal malacia.

Permanent tracheostomy

Permanent tracheostomy provides relief of upper-airway obstruction which is non-responsive to other methods of medical or surgical management. Permanent tracheostomy is performed at the level of the third to sixth tracheal rings, via a ventral cervical approach (Fig. 7.10; Hedlund *et al.*, 1988). A ventral segment of the tracheal wall is resected, approximately three to four tracheal rings long and one-third of the tracheal circumference in width. An I or H incision is made into the tracheal mucosa and the edges sutured to the edges of the skin to create a tracheostoma.

Immediate postoperative management requires inspection of the tracheostoma every 1–3 hours. Mucus accumulation is gently wiped from the stoma. The distal trachea can be suctioned using sterile equipment. By 7 days, cleansing can be reduced to every 4–6 hours and by the end of the first month cleansing may only

be required twice daily. Hair is kept short around the stoma to prevent matting. Exercise must be limited to clean areas and swimming is prohibited. Complications include stomal occlusion due to skin folds or stenosis.

Brachycephalic syndrome

Brachycephalic syndrome affects brachycephalic breeds of dogs (English Bulldog, French Bulldog, Boxer, Boston Terrier, Pug, Pekinese and Shih Tzu) and other short-nosed dogs or cats, including the Cocker Spaniel and Chinese Shar-Pei dogs and Persian and Himalayan cats (Aron and Crowe, 1985; Wykes, 1991; Hendricks, 1992). Anatomical changes in the skulls of these animals distort the nasopharynx. The three major components of the syndrome include stenotic nares, elongated soft palate and everted laryngeal saccules. Laryngeal and tracheal hypoplasia are often present concurrently.

As the syndrome progresses, associated abnormalities include laryngeal and pharyngeal oedema and collapse. The pathophysiology of the syndrome is based on stenotic nares and an elongated soft palate causing increased airflow resistance which requires increased inspiratory effort. This generates an increased negative pressure during each respiratory cycle which leads to

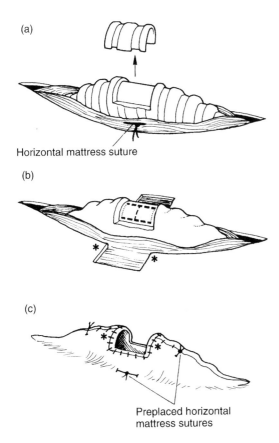

(a)

Horizontal mattress suture

(b)

(c)

Preplaced horizontal
mattress sutures

Figure 7.10 (a) Permanent tracheostomy through a ventral approach with horizontal mattress sutures placed through the sternohyoid muscles to elevate the trachea and resection of a portion of the ventral trachea without entering the mucosa. (b) Lateral sections of skin are excised. The mucosa is incised in an H-shaped incision and a portion is excised, leaving a rim of mucosa. (c) The stoma is created by apposition of the rim of mucosa and skin with simple interrupted sutures. Note that four large horizontal mattress sutures are preplaced through the trachea and skin before the mucosal sutures are placed to bring the skin into position (note location of *) and to reduce tension on the stomal closure.

eversion of the laryngeal saccules, oedema and thickening of the laryngeal and pharyngeal mucosa and collapse of the cuneiform and corniculate processes of the arytenoid cartilages. Non-cardiogenic pulmonary oedema may also develop. Rarely, is laryngeal paralysis present.

Clinical signs

Clinical signs include respiratory distress, stridor, mouth-breathing, gagging, cyanosis and collapse and are exacerbated by exercise, excitement or high ambient temperatures.

Diagnosis

Diagnosis is based on history, profile, clinical signs, physical examination, airway endoscopy and radiography.

Treatment and surgical technique

Treatment requires surgical correction of the stenotic nares, resection of a portion of the elongated soft palate, resection of the everted laryngeal saccules and possibly laryngeal abduction techniques if laryngeal paralysis is present. Permanent tracheostomy may be indicated in severe cases. To avoid severe postoperative oedema, perioperative corticosteroids should be administered. All brachycephalic animals are high-anaesthetic-risk patients. Preoxygenation, rapid anaesthetic induction, immediate intubation, assisted intraoperative ventilation and postoperative administration of oxygen are required.

Stenotic nares correction is often performed at the same time as shortening of the elongated soft palate and resection of everted laryngeal saccules. However, it is a relatively simple procedure and may be of more benefit if performed early (for example, at the time of elective castration or ovariohysterectomy). The nasal cavity accounts for 70% of normal upper-airway resistance; hence, early nares correction may slow the development of changes secondary to brachycephalic syndrome. Surgical correction requires resection of a wedge of tissue; this may be a vertical wedge from the wing of the nostril that extends caudally to include a portion of the alar cartilage (Fig. 7.11). Alternatively, a horizontal wedge from the wing of the nostril can be resected. Third, a lateral wedge from the caudolateral border of the wing of the nostril and a triangle of skin adjacent to it can be resected. This technique is useful in very small animals where the wing of the nostril is tiny.

For all techniques, the edges of the cut tissue edges are sutured using simple interrupted, fine absorbable sutures. Using a reverse cutting or a taper-cut needle facilitates suture placement. Haemorrhage becomes readily controlled once sutures are placed. Electrosurgery or laser resection may result in considerable swelling and dehiscence due to excessive tissue destruction.

Elongated soft-palate correction requires resection (staphylectomy) of excessive length and suturing of the oral and nasal mucosa at

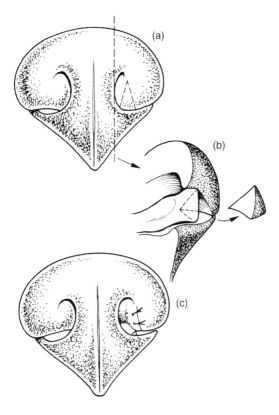

Figure 7.11 (a) Resection of a vertical wedge of tissue for stenotic nares. (b) The depth of the wedge must extend to the alar cartilage. (c) The defect is closed with absorbable, simple interrupted sutures.

is grasped with forceps and cut with scissors or biopsy forceps. No sutures are required.

Laryngeal collapse is characterized by medial and rostral collapse of the arytenoid cartilages and aryepiglottic folds. It can result from trauma or loss of supporting function of the cartilages but usually occurs secondary to brachycephalic syndrome disease. Laryngeal collapse occurs in stages characterized by laryngeal saccule eversion (stage 1), medial collapse of the cuneiform process (stage 2) and medial collapse of the corniculate process (stage 3). Signs may be similar to those of laryngeal paralysis. Conservative treatment (medication and rest) may help some animals, although surgery can provide more reliable relief of clinical signs. In brachycephalic breeds, resection of nares, soft palate and everted saccules is performed. A permanent tracheostomy may be indicated in

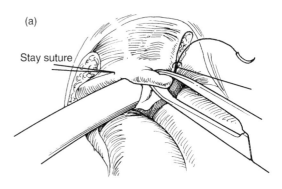

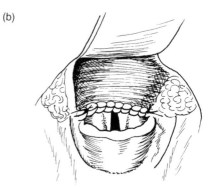

Figure 7.12 Staphylectomy. (a) A stay suture is placed on one side, at the level of resection determined by the caudal extent of the tonsillar crypts. A second suture is tied at the opposite side; the needle is left attached. A portion of the soft palate is cut and sutured using absorbable sutures in a simple continuous pattern. The nasal and pharyngeal mucosa is apposed. (b) The remainder of the palate is cut and sutured, the continuous suture being tied to the stay suture at that side.

the cut edge using a simple continuous, absorbable suture. This is performed through an oral approach. The normal soft palate should overlap the epiglottis by 1–2 mm. Since endotracheal intubation distorts this relationship, the landmarks for correct length are the caudal margins of the tonsillar crypts. A suture is first placed at this landmark on one edge of the soft palate (Fig. 7.12). This helps identify the line of the cut in the soft palate and the ends of the suture are used for traction. A second suture is tied at the opposite side; the needle is left attached. The soft palate is cut approximately halfway. This portion of palate is then sutured using the second suture. The remainder of the palate is then cut and sutured; the last bite is tied to the first stay suture. Electrosurgical or laser resection is possible but may result in considerable swelling.

Eversion of the laryngeal saccules is the first stage of laryngeal collapse. The everted tissue severe disease. In other breeds, a permanent tracheostomy only, is indicated.

Postoperative considerations and prognosis

Prognosis depends on the age of the animal and the severity of the disease. Postoperative complications include oedema, haemorrhage and nasal regurgitation if excessive palatal tissue is removed.

Nasopharyngeal polyps

Inflammatory polyps may occur in the nasopharynx, middle ear or external ear canal of cats. Typically, they affect young cats, younger than 2 years of age, with clinical signs occurring as young as 2–6 months (Pope, 1990). A nasopharyngeal polyp has also been reported in a 7-month-old Chinese Shar-Pei (Fingland *et al.*, 1993). The cause of inflammatory polyps is unclear. Development of the polyps secondary to bacterial or viral (calicivirus) infections is a likely cause.

Clinical signs

Typical clinical signs include stertorous respiration, chronic nasal discharge, sneezing, voice change, dyspnoea and dysphagia. Polyps that are lodged within the external ear canal are often associated with an otitis externa with exudative discharge and head shaking. Middle-ear involvement may cause a head tilt, nystagmus and disequilibrium.

Diagnosis

Diagnosis is based on the history and physical examination findings, laboratory test evaluation and upper-airway and otic examination performed under general anaesthesia. The diagnosis is confirmed by histological examination of the polyp. Laboratory evaluation should include determination of the FeLV and FIV status of the animal. Radiographs should be performed to evaluate the nasal passages, nasopharynx and tympanic bullae. Soft-tissue density may be observed in the region of the nasopharynx with ventral displacement of the soft palate. Fluid/soft-tissue density may also

be observed in the tympanic bullae with osseous thickening or irregularity consistent with chronic disease. Involvement of the nasopharynx and external ear canal can be confirmed by visual examination under general anaesthesia. The soft palate may be obviously depressed and the polyp can be palpated through the soft palate. The polyp may be obvious or may be visualized by gentle retraction of the soft palate with a blunt instrument such as a spay hook. Otic examination may reveal a glistening, pink mass filling the lumen of the canal. Apart from a ceruminous exudate, the ear canal generally does not appear inflamed.

Treatment and surgical technique

Treatment requires removal of the polyp and tympanic bulla osteotomy. Since the polyps are thought to originate in the tympanic bullae, a ventral bulla osteotomy is performed first, to free the stalk of the polyp. With the animal in dorsal recumbency and the head stretched to expose the laryngeal area, a paramedian incision between the midline and the angle of the mandible is made. The bulla of a cat is prominent and should be palpable in the depression between the angle of the mandible and the larynx. The subcutaneous tissue is bluntly dissected and the platysma muscle incised to reveal the lingual vein, which is retracted. Dissection continues in the deep tissue between the digastricus muscle laterally and the hyoglossus and styloglossus muscles medially. The hypoglossal nerve and linguofacial artery will be observed running across the lateral surface of these muscles and should be retracted medially. The bulla should be palpable just cranial to the hyoid apparatus.

A self-retaining retractor can be placed and the bulla is cleared of surrounding tissue and periosteum using periosteal elevators. Using a small Steinmann pin or K-wire, a hole is drilled into the base of the bulla, and repeated with a larger pin until a hole big enough to place rongeurs is achieved. Rongeurs are then used to remove a portion of the base of the bulla. In the cat, the bulla is compartmentalized by a transverse septum. Access to the bulla ventrally typically opens the ventromedial compartment. Since the polyps most often involve the dorsolateral compartment (since this contains both the external auditory meatus and the auditory os of the eustachian tube), the dorsolateral compartment must also be opened to achieve adequate drainage. This can be performed using the pins and rongeurs as described.

A bacterial culture is taken from the bulla before curettage. The inside of the bulla is gently curetted to remove any granulation tissue and the epithelial lining of the bulla. Curettage near the dorsomedial aspect of the bulla should be minimal to avoid damage to the auditory ossicles and the bony labyrinth of the inner ear. In the cat, sympathetic nerve fibres enter the bulla at the ventromedial compartment, pass through fissures in the septum and through the dorsolateral compartment to exit near the auditory os of the eustachian tube. Damage to these may result in Horner's syndrome (ptosis of eyelid, myosis and prolapse of the third eyelid) after surgery. These are very difficult to visualize in the bulla. Any tissue removed from the bulla should be submitted for histopathologic examination. The polyps are typically made up of fibrous tissue with plasmacytic and lymphocytic cellular infiltrates.

The bulla is lavaged and a drain should be placed in the bulla to allow for collection of fluid after surgery. A closed-suction drain works best. The author avoids using ingress/egress drains entering through the external ear canal and exiting the bulla and does not flush the ears after surgery. Irritation and inflammation can result from lavage solutions and, if curettage of the bullae and cleansing of the external ear canal at surgery are adequate, ingress/egress lavage should not be required. A closed-suction drain can be fashioned from a butterfly catheter and an evacuated blood collection tube (Fig. 7.13). This allows non-dependent drainage easy replacement of the collection tube for accurate monitoring of fluid volume and nature.

The polyp is then removed from its location. For a polyp within the external ear canal, it can usually be pulled from the ear canal using Allis tissue forceps or alligator forceps; however, lateralization of the ear canal may be required if it cannot be removed in this manner. For polyps in the nasopharynx, again, they can be pulled free after retraction of the soft palate with a atraumatic instrument such as a spay hook. However, incision of the soft palate may be required if the polyp is large and wedged firmly.

If incision of the soft palate is required, stay sutures are placed on both lateral aspects of the soft palate and a midline incision is made along the soft palate. This allows the corners

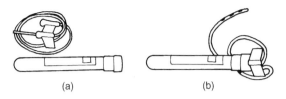

Figure 7.13 Creation of an active suction drain from (a) an intravenous butterfly catheter, and (b) evacuated blood collection tube. The needle port has been cut from the catheter and the multiple fenestrations have been made.

of the cut edge to be reflected laterally, exposing the caudal nasal cavity. The polyp is then removed and the palate sutured in three layers: the nasal mucosa, submucosal tissue and oral mucosa, using a simple continuous suture of fine monofilament absorbable material (4-0 to 5-0).

Postoperative considerations and prognosis

The most common complication is associated with the bulla osteotomy and is Horner's syndrome. The complication may not be a permanent change. If damage has occurred to the auditory ossicles or the labyrinth of the inner ear, deafness and vestibular signs may be present after surgery. The overall prognosis is good, although recurrence of an inflammatory polyp is not uncommon, particularly if bulla osteotomy was not performed.

Pneumonia

Pneumonia generally represents a primary lung disorder, extension of an existing tracheobronchial disease, opportunistic invasion or the spread of a systemic disease to the lungs.

Aetiology

Bacterial pneumonia (i.e. *Bordetella bronchiseptica*, *Streptococcus zooepidemicus* and other Gram-negative bacteria) is more common in puppies than in kittens. In kittens, *B. bronchiseptica* and *Pasteurella* spp. are the most likely bacteria causing a primary pneumonia. However, bacterial pneumonias are often secondary, following viral infection or in animals with pre-existing upper-airway anomalies, immunocompromise or gastrointestinal disease that results in dysphagia, regurgitation or vomiting and sub-sequent aspiration. *Toxoplasma gondii* and, rarely, *Pneumocystis carinii* infections can cause pneumonia in puppies and kittens. Infections with *Aelurostrongylus abstrusus* in cats, *Paragonimus kellicotti* in dogs and cats, and *Filaroides hirthi* in dogs are the most common pulmonary parasitic causes of pneumonia, but are uncommon in animals younger than 6 months of age. Pulmonary migration of larval stages of *Toxocara canis* may infrequently produce a verminous pneumonia. Fungal pneumonia rarely occurs in dogs or cats younger than 6 months of age.

Clinical signs

Typically, puppies or kittens with primary or secondary bacterial pneumonia will show tachypnoea, respiratory distress, fever and a productive cough. Lung sounds are often normal but may reveal an increased intensity of normal lung sounds.

Diagnosis

Diagnosis is based on clinical signs and radiographs. Radiographs may demonstrate an interstitial and alveolar lung pattern with a cranioventral distribution, typical of bacterial pneumonia; a diffuse interstitial lung pattern, typical of viral pneumonia; or a mixed lung pattern (i.e. a combination of alveolar, interstitial and peribronchial lung patterns) such as seen in pulmonary toxoplasmosis, *Aelurostrongylus* pneumonia or secondary bacterial pneumonia.

Treatment

Antimicrobial agents are the mainstay of medical therapy for bacterial pneumonia. The choice of an antimicrobial agent should be based on bacterial culture and sensitivity test results. However, therapy should be commenced before the culture results are available. The antimicrobial agents generally preferred for the initial treatment of an uncomplicated bacterial pneumonia are amoxycillin–clavulanate or trimethoprim-sulphonamide combinations in dogs or a first-generation cephalosporin in cats. Chloramphenicol or amoxycillin–clavulanate combinations should be used in dogs or cats with suspected *Bordetella* infections. In severe cases, gentamicin or amikacin and a first-generation cephalosporin are usually effective when used in combination. Antimicrobial therapy should be modified based on culture results and continued for at least 4 weeks. Alternatively, antimicrobial therapy may be continued for at least 1 week beyond radiographic resolution.

Attention to the animal's hydration is important to ensure adequate mucociliary clearance. Crystalloid solutions should be given intravenously or subcutaneously to prevent dehydration. Additionally, airway hydration can be maximized by nebulization with normal saline solution. Oxygen and bronchodilator therapy may be needed in hypoxaemic animals. Cough suppressants should not be used in animals with pneumonia. *Aelurostrongylus* and *Paragonimus* infections can be treated successfully with fenbendazole at 50 mg/kg orally once a day for 10–14 days. Fenbendazole therapy is terminated when larvae or eggs are not found in the faeces or when anorexia develops. Other therapies for *Aelurostrongylus* infection include ivermectin (400 g/kg subcutaneously once). *Paragonimus* can also be treated with praziquantel (25 mg/kg orally three times a day for 3 days). Toxoplasmosis can be effectively treated with clindamycin at a total daily dosage of 25 mg/kg divided twice a day for 4 weeks.

Aspiration pneumonia

Aspiration pneumonia occurs more frequently in puppies than in kittens; most often it is associated with congenital megaoesophagus or improper feeding of milk replacer. Aspiration may also result from oesophageal or pharyngeal dysfunction, chronic vomiting or depressed state of consciousness. Anaesthesia is always a risk factor for aspiration pneumonia that may regurgitate gastric contents into the pharynx during general anaesthesia or cause vomiting during recovery.

Clinical signs

Typically, once a significant quantity of material is aspirated, rapid onset of clinical signs occurs. The signs are similar to those observed with a bacterial pneumonia; the severity depends on the amount and content of the aspirated material. Aspiration of acidic gastric contents will cause the most severe damage.

Diagnosis

Radiographic abnormalities may not be apparent until 12–24 h after aspiration and include consolidation and alveolar and interstitial infiltration of dependent lung lobes. The right cranial and middle lung lobes are most commonly affected in animals that aspirate while in a sternal position while other lung lobes are probably affected in animals that are in prone positions.

Treatment

Aspiration pneumonia should be treated similarly to other types of pneumonia. On immediate aspiration, mechanical suction of the airways should be attempted.

References

Aron, D.N. and Crowe, D.T. (1985) Upper airway obstruction: general principles and selected conditions in the dog and cat. *Veterinary Clinics of North America [Small Animal Practice]*, **15**, 891–917.

Berry, C.R., Koblik, P.D. and Ticer, J.W. (1990) Dorsal peritoneopericardial mesothelial remnant as an aid to the diagnosis of feline congenital peritoneopericardial diaphragmatic hernia. *Veterinary Radiology*, **31**, 239–245.

Boudrieau, R.J., Fossum, T.W., Hartsfield, S.M., Hobson, P.H. and Rudy, R.L. (1990). Pectus excavatum in dogs and cats. *Compendium of Continuing Education for the Practicing Veterinarian*, **12**, 341–355.

Boudrieau, R.J. and Muir W.M. (1987) Pathophysiology of traumatic diaphragmatic hernia in dogs. *Compendium of Continuing Education for the Practicing Veterinarian*, **9**, 379–385.

Casely-Smith, J.R., Morgan, R.G. and Piller, N.B. (1993) Treatment of lymphedema of the arms and legs with 5,6 benzo[alpha]pyrone. *New England Journal of Medicine*, **329**, 1158–1163.

Fagin, B. (1989) Using radiography to diagnose traumatic diaphragmatic hernia. *Veterinary Medicine*, **July**, 662–672.

Fingland, R.B., Gratzek, A., Worhies, M.W. and Kirpenstein, J. (1993) Nasopharyngeral polyp in a dog. *Journal of the American Animal Hospital Association*, **29**, 311–314.

Hedlun, C.S., Tangner, C.H., Waldron, D.R. and Hobson, H.P. (1988) Permanent tracheostomy: perioperative and long-term data from 34 cases. *Journal of the American Animal Hospital Association*, **24**, 585–591.

Hendricks, J.C. (1992) Brachycephalic airway syndrome. *Veterinary Clinics of North America [Small Animal Practice]*, **22**, 1145–1153.

Mann, F.A., Aronson, E. and Keller, G. (1991) Surgical correction of a true congenital pleuroperitoneal diaphragmatic hernia in a cat. *Journal of the American Animal Hospital Association*, **27**, 501–507.

McNulty, J. (1995) A simplified method for stabilization of flail chest injuries in small animals. *Journal of the American Animal Hospital Association*, **31**, 137–141.

Pope, E.R. (1990) Feline inflammatory polyps. *Friskies Veterinary Journal*, 18–20.

Shahar, R., Shamir, M. and Johnston, D.E. (1997) A technique for management of bite wounds of the thoracic wall in small dogs. *Veterinary Surgery*, **26**, 45–50.

Shires, P.K., Waldron, D.R. and Payne, J. (1988) Pectus excavatum in three kittens. *Journal of the American Animal Hospital Association*, **24**, 203.

Soderstrom, M.J., Gilson, S.D. and Gulbas, N. (1995) Fatal reexpansion pulmonary edema in a kitten following surgical correction of pectus excavatum. *Journal of the American Animal Hospital Association*, **31**, 133–136.

Wykes, P.M. (1991) Brachycephalic airway obstructive syndrome. *Problems in Veterinary Medicine*, **3**, 188–197.

8
Cardiovascular disorders

Congenital cardiac disorders requiring surgery

Common congenital cardiac defects that are amenable to surgical treatment in the puppy include patent ductus arteriosus (PDA), pulmonic stenosis, subaortic stenosis and persistent right aortic arch (PRAA). Tetralogy of Fallot and atrial or ventricular septal defects (VSDs) are less common and require considerable surgical expertise for correction.

Patent ductus arteriosus

Patent ductus arteriosus is the most common congenital cardiac defect in dogs and is occasionally seen in cats (Bonagura, 1989; Goodwin and Lombard, 1992; Table 8.1). The ductus arteriosus is the normal foetal communication between the aorta and pulmonary artery and should close within the first 2–3 days after birth in the dog and cat (Fig. 8.1). Failure of closure of the ductus arteriosus results in left-to-right shunting of blood from the aorta to the pulmonary artery.

Table 8.1 Order of frequency of congenital cardiac defects in the dog and cat

Dog	Cat
Patent ductus arteriosus	Mitral/tricuspid malformations
Pulmonic stenosis	Ventricular septal defect
Aortic stenosis	
Persistent right aortic arch	

Certain breeds are predisposed to PDA (Table 8.2), especially the collie, Shetland Sheepdog, Miniature Poodle, Pomeranian and German Shepherd Dog.

Clinical signs

Clinical signs are usually not noticeable until the defect and the resulting pathology have progressed, and the puppy has developed left-sided congestive heart failure. In most puppies the characteristic heart murmur should be discerned before this time. Pulmonary hypertension may develop in some animals and cause right-to-left shunting of blood.

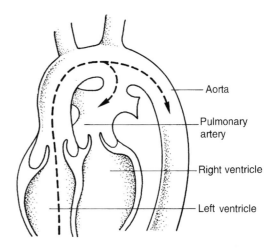

Figure 8.1 The blood flow pattern in a left-to-right shunting patent ductus arteriosus with left ventricular ejection of blood into the aorta. A portion of the aortic blood flow is diverted to the pulmonary artery and lungs through the ductus arteriosus.

Table 8.2 Dog breeds predisposed to congenital heart defects

Congenital defect	Breed predisposition
Atrial septal defect	Boxer
	Old English Sheepdog
Patent ductus arteriosus	Brittany Spaniel
	Cocker Spaniel
	Collie
	German Shepherd Dog
	Keeshond
	Pomeranian
	Miniature Poodle
	Shetland Sheepdog
Persistent right aortic arch	Dobermann
	German Shepherd Dog
	Great Dane
	Irish Setter
	Weimaraner
Pulmonic stenosis	Beagle
	Chihuahua
	English Bulldog
	German Shepherd Dog
	Giant Schnauzer
	Keeshond
	Miniature Schnauzer
	Samoyed
	Terriers
Subaortic stenosis	Boxer
	German Shepherd Dog
	German Shorthair Pointer
	Golden Retriever
	Newfoundland
Tetralogy of Fallot	Keeshond
	Miniature Poodle
	Miniature Schnauzer
	Terriers
	Wire-haired Fox Terrier
Valve dysplasia	Chihuahua
	English Bulldog
	Great Dane
	Weimaraner
Ventricular septal defect	Beagle
	English Bulldog
	German Shepherd Dog
	Keeshond
	Mastiff
	Miniature Poodle
	Siberian Husky

Diagnosis

Diagnosis is by thoracic auscultation, electrocardiography, radiography and, if necessary, echocardiography and contrast angiography. Characteristic thoracic auscultation findings include a continuous murmur over the left heart base, often associated with a palpable cardiac thrill. Femoral pulses are hyperkinetic (water-hammer) because of diastolic run-off of blood through the ductus arteriosus. Mucous membrane colour is normal. In puppies that develop right-to-left shunting, caudal mucous membranes (vulva and prepuce) will be cyanotic and the puppies have polycythaemia. No cardiac murmur is discerned and the femoral pulse is normal.

Electrocardiography shows tall R waves (> 2.5 mV) in leads II and aVF. In leads I and aVF, deep Q waves may be present. Thoracic radiographs show left atrial and ventricular enlargement, enlargement of pulmonary vessels, often described as overcirculation of the lungs, and dilatation of the descending aorta. On the dorsoventral view, these changes represent the characteristic four bulges on the left side of the heart. Echocardiography may confirm the cardiac changes but rarely actually identifies the shunt. With Doppler echocardiography, pressure changes characteristic of PDA may be assessed indirectly by measurement of blood flow velocity.

Although usually unnecessary, selective angiography can be used to confirm PDA and rule out other congenital heart defects with similar presentation, including aortic-pulmonary window (a communication in the ascending aorta) and VSD. Selective angiography should be performed in cats since the presence of multiple congenital heart defects is common. Cardiac catheterization is performed via the femoral or carotid arteries with injection of contrast medium into the ascending aorta.

Treatment and surgical technique

Surgical treatment should be performed as soon as possible after diagnosis. However, puppies younger than 6 weeks of age or less than 500 g are a greater anaesthetic risk. If the puppy is otherwise clinically asymptomatic, apart from the murmur, delaying the surgery until this age or size is attained is desirable. Ligation of the left-to-right PDA is performed through a left lateral thoracotomy at the fourth intercostal space (Birchard *et al.*, 1990; Fig. 8.2). Ligation is contraindicated in right-to-left shunts because the cardiac and pulmonary changes are irreversible and rapid: fatal heart failure and pulmonary oedema would occur. Puppies presented with pulmonary oedema should be pretreated with furosemide before surgery.

The pericardium is incised over the region of the PDA and retracted using stay sutures. This helps retract the left vagus nerve dorsally or ventrally, away from the PDA. The PDA is bluntly dissected with right-angle forceps; dissection should be performed primarily at the caudal aspect against the tougher aorta. The region of the junction of the PDA and pulmonary artery is fragile and dissection should be directed away from this area. A loop of non-absorbable

suture is passed below the ductus from cranial to caudal, cut in half and the ductus is double-ligated. The PDA is slowly ligated with the arterial ligature tightened first. The heart rate may slow (Branham's sign) during ligation due to a sudden increase in arterial blood pressure. The PDA is not severed due to its limited length. The pericardium is left open and thoracotomy closure is routine. A thoracostomy tube should be placed.

An alternative non-surgical technique for certain PDAs is the percutaneous placement of intravascular embolization coils (Snaps *et al.*, 1995). The helical coils are introduced via the femoral artery and placed so that they lodge in the PDA. These are applicable for cone or funnel-shaped PDAs which allow easy lodgement of the coil. They also have application

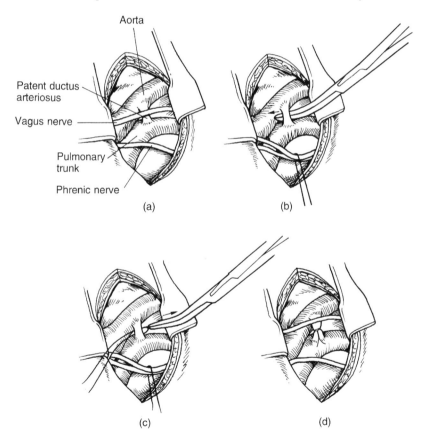

Figure 8.2 Ligation of patent ductus arteriosus. (a) A left lateral thoracotomy is performed through the fourth intercostal space, exposing the patent ductus arteriosus. Note the location of the vagus and phrenic nerves. (b) The pericardium is incised over the ductus arteriosus and retracted, in this case, retracting the vagus nerve ventrally. (c) The ductus arteriosus is dissected from the caudal aspect. (d) A non-absorbable double ligature is passed around the ductus arteriosus and each is tied separately; the ligature closest to the aorta is tied first.

for the retreatment of surgically ligated PDAs that have residual blood flow. Up to 30% of surgically ligated PDAs at one institution were found to have residual blood flow through the PDA (Miller *et al.*, 1995). The coils are Dacron-coated and have a fringe of filamentous Dacron fibres. The coils are extremely thrombogenic and cause almost immediate obstruction of the PDA (Miller *et al.*, 1995). Disadvantages of the technique are that candidates require a selective angiogram to determine their suitability, and that special equipment is required to perform and evaluate the procedure. The cost of the coils themselves is not prohibitive. Complications include dislodgement of the coils, which may require retrieval using a special percutaneous basket-retrieval device (Miller *et al.*, 1995).

Postoperative considerations and prognosis

Postoperative management is as for any animal undergoing thoracic surgery – close monitoring and management of a thoracotomy tube. The tube can be removed within a few hours of surgery. Profound hypothermia may be present since these animals are small and the thoracic cavity has been exposed. A continuous murmur should no longer be auscultated after PDA ligation; however, a systolic murmur may be present if left ventricular dilation has caused mitral insufficiency. The murmur should resolve as cardiac changes will reverse after ligation of the PDA. The prognosis for long-term survival is excellent if heart failure has not occurred (Birchard *et al.*, 1990).

Pulmonic stenosis

Pulmonic stenosis is the second most common congenital cardiac defect in puppies. It is rare in cats. Pulmonic stenosis may be supravalvular, valvular or subvalvular: valvular stenosis is the most common (Eyster *et al.*, 1993). Valvular stenosis may be simple, characterized by incomplete separation of the valve leaflets, or dysplastic, characterized by a narrow valve annulus and thickened valve leaflets. Pulmonic stenosis results in right ventricular hypertrophy to compensate for the increased pressure required for pulmonary outflow. Right ventricular hypertrophy may exacerbate the stenosis by narrowing the right ventricular outflow tract at the level of the infundibulum. This is especially apparent during systole and causes dynamic stenosis.

Clinical signs

Most dogs are asymptomatic at the time of diagnosis; however, some dogs will present with clinical signs consistent with right-sided heart failure.

Diagnosis

Diagnosis is by thoracic auscultation, electrocardiography, radiography, echocardiography and indirect pressure evaluation. Contrast angiography and direct-pressure evaluation may also be required. Characteristic thoracic auscultation finding includes a systolic murmur over the left heart base. A second systolic murmur may be heard over the right hemithorax due to tricuspid insufficiency. Electrocardiographic findings on lead I show a deep S wave, indicative of right ventricular enlargement and right axis deviation. Tall P waves on leads I, II, III and aVF indicate right atrial enlargement. Leads II and aVF may also show deep S waves.

Right ventricular and poststenotic pulmonary enlargement are observed on the thoracic radiographs. Echocardiography findings include right ventricular hypertrophy and high blood flow velocity in the pulmonary outflow tract. Blood pressure gradients across the pulmonic valve can be measured indirectly by assessment of blood flow velocity using Doppler echocardiography. Cardiac catheterization can be performed to measure the blood pressure gradient directly across the pulmonic valve and to perform contrast angiography. The catheter is passed down a jugular vein into the right ventricle with injection of contrast medium into the right ventricle.

Treatment and surgical technique

The decision to perform surgery is based on the age and clinical findings of the puppy and the blood pressure gradient across the pulmonic valve (Fingland *et al.*, Table 8.3).

Techniques for correction of pulmonic stenosis include balloon valvuloplasty, valvuloplasty, valvulectomy and patch grafting (Table 8.4).

Table 8.3 Recommendation for surgery of puppies with pulmonic stenosis

Clinical findings and blood pressure gradient	Recommendation
Pulmonary blood pressure gradients > 50 mmHg	Surgery indicated
Right ventricular pressures > 70 mmHg	Surgery indicated
Severe right ventricular hypertrophy	Surgery indicated
Puppies that are asymptomatic with right ventricular pressures < 70 mmHg	Treated conservatively
Asymptomatic or symptomatic puppies with right ventricular pressures > 70 mmHg	Surgery indicated
Symptomatic, puppies older than 6 months of age with right ventricular pressures > 70 mmHg	Poor candidates for surgery; best treated conservatively

Table 8.4 Comparison of techniques available for correction or treatment of pulmonic stenosis

Technique	Comment
Balloon valvuloplasty	Relatively non-invasive; indicated for valvular stenosis; results give the greatest immediate and long-term survival rates
Valvuloplasty	Indicated for valvular stenosis; requires least surgical expertise
Valvulectomy	Requires cardiac venous inflow occlusion; indicated for valvular stenosis
Patch grafting	Useful technique that manages valvular stenosis and infundibular hypertrophy; technically more difficult

Balloon valvuloplasty is performed percutaneously (Bright *et al.*, 1987). The catheter is introduced through a jugular vein, passed into the right ventricle and across the pulmonic valve. The catheter is filled with contrast medium to facilitate monitoring its position fluoroscopically. The balloon is inflated to dilate the valve and the systolic blood pressure is monitored to evaluate the effectiveness of the dilation and the change in systolic pulmonic blood pressure gradient.

Blind valvuloplasty (Brock procedure) is indicated for simple valve stenosis without infundibular (subvalvular) stenosis (Eyster, 1993). Blind valvuloplasty is performed via a lateral thoracotomy at the fourth intercostal space. A pursestring suture is placed at the base of the pulmonary outflow tract in the right ventricle. A valve dilator is placed through a stab incision in the middle of the pursestring suture and passed through the valve. The pursestring is tightened around the instrument to prevent haemorrhage. The pulmonic valve is dilated several times by opening the instrument. The instrument is then withdrawn and the pursestring suture tied.

Valvulectomy is indicated for valvular pulmonic stenosis. Cardiac venous inflow occlusion is performed; temporary ligatures are placed around the cranial and caudal vena cavae and the azygous vein. The venous inflow is occluded and the heart is allowed to beat once or twice to empty the ventricles. A pulmonary arteriotomy is performed directly over the valve and the valve leaflets are resected. A Satinsky clamp is placed on the arteriotomy incision to allow closure of the arteriotomy without occlusion of the pulmonary artery and to allow release of the venous inflow occlusion. Venous inflow occlusion should be for no longer than 2 minutes. However, it can be released and re-occluded several times.

Patch grafting is indicated for severe valvular stenosis with infundibular hypertrophy (subvalvular). Patch grafting can be performed open with venous inflow occlusion or closed without venous inflow occlusion. A patch of pericardium or synthetic material (polytetrafluorethylene; Dacron®) is placed over the pulmonary outflow tract, extending from the ventricle to the supravalvular area. Some redundancy in the patch is required, especially for young, growing puppies.

In open grafting, venous inflow occlusion is performed to allow incision into the right ventricular outflow tract and valvulectomy. The patch is then sutured to the epicardium to cover the area of the open incision. For closed grafting, a cutting wire is initially preplaced in the pulmonary outflow tract through a hole in the pulmonary artery above the pulmonic valve, emerging from a hole in the right lateral ventricular wall (Fig. 8.3). The graft is sutured over the pulmonary outflow tract; the last two sutures at the distal aspect of the patch are left open to allow for removal of the cutting wire. The wire is pulled through the lateral wall of the pulmonary outflow tract and the sutures in the graft are quickly tied once the wire is pulled free.

Postoperative considerations and prognosis

Postoperative management is as for any animal undergoing thoracic surgery – close monitoring and management of a thoracostomy tube. The tube can be removed within a few hours of surgery. Profound hypothermia may be present since these animals are small and the thoracic cavity has been exposed. Palliative therapy with diuretics and vasodilators should be initiated if right-sided congestive heart failure is present.

Puppies with moderate or severe pulmonic stenosis will benefit from balloon valvuloplasty or surgical resection. The prognosis for puppies varies according to severity. Dogs with right ventricular blood pressures less than 70 mmHg or a pulmonic blood pressure gradient less than 50 mmHg may be asymptomatic. The prognosis for dogs that are asymptomatic until adulthood and undergo surgery for valvular or subvalvular stenosis is good. Young symptomatic dogs and dogs with severe muscular hypertrophy have a poor prognosis.

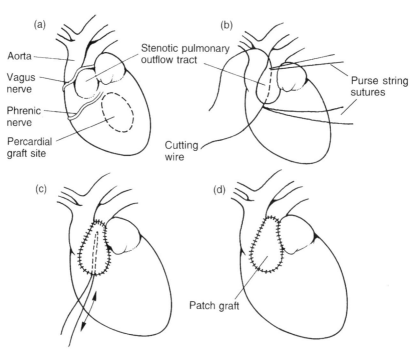

Figure 8.3 Closed patch graft placement for pulmonic stenosis. (a) A left lateral thoracotomy through the fourth intercostal space (dog) or sixth intercostal space (cat) is performed. A pericardial patch is harvested. (b) The cutting wire is preplaced in the pulmonary outflow tract. (c) The pericardial patch is sutured over the pulmonary outflow tract, leaving a small section open at the bottom to allow exit of the cutting wire. (d) The wire is pulled and the patch graft completely closed.

Aortic stenosis

Aortic stenosis is the third most common congenital heart defect in dogs and the most common congenital heart defect of large-breed dogs. The lesion is usually a subvalvular ring or ridge of fibrocartilaginous tissue, hence, the disorder is referred to as subaortic stenosis (Komtebedde *et al.*, 1993). Supravalvular and valvular disease can also occur. Subaortic stenosis results in pressure overload of the left ventricle causing hypertrophy without dilation.

Clinical signs

Tachydysrhythmias and sudden death can occur in severely affected animals. On thoracic auscultation, a systolic murmur is heard that is loudest at the base of the heart; it may radiate towards the thoracic inlet. The murmur may radiate up the neck and across to the right hemithorax. A palpable thrill over the left hemithorax may be present. Femoral pulses are weak.

Diagnosis

Diagnosis is by thoracic auscultation, electrocardiography, radiography, echocardiography and indirect pressure evaluation. Contrast angiography and direct-pressure evaluation may also be required. Electrocardiography may be normal in puppies or may show tall R waves, depression of the ST segment and arrhythmias, especially premature ventricular contractions. Thoracic radiography may be within normal limits or show slight ventricular enlargement with tracheal elevation on the lateral projection, and dilation of the ascending aorta and loss of the cardiac waist on the dorsoventral projection. Echocardiography shows thickening of the left ventricular wall and inter-ventricular septum with narrowing of the ventricular lumen. Doppler echocardiography can be used to measure the systolic pressure gradient indirectly. Dogs with systolic aortic blood pressure gradients greater than 70 mmHg have a poor prognosis. Contrast angiography is usually unnecessary to obtain a diagnosis; however, cardiac catheterization can be performed by passage of a catheter into the left ventricle via the femoral or carotid artery.

Treatment and surgical technique

Surgical correction is indicated in puppies with systolic aortic blood pressure gradients greater than 70 mmHg. Puppies with gradients less than this should be re-evaluated and those developing clinical signs, progressive left ventricular hypertrophy or increases in the gradient may require surgery. Surgical options available include blind valvulotomy, open arteriotomy and valvulectomy or conduit placement (Table 8.5).

Blind valvulotomy is performed through a median sternotomy. The technique is similar to the procedure for pulmonic stenosis. A valve-dilating instrument is passed through a stab incision in the left ventricle into the aortic outflow tract. The instrument is then passed across the aortic valve, opened to dilate the valve and withdrawn. A suture is tied over the stab incision. Long-term results of this surgery are discouraging and sustained reductions in systolic aortic blood pressure gradients are not achieved.

Open arteriotomy during extracorporeal cardiopulmonary bypass appears more useful for discrete subvalvular lesions. During cardiopulmonary bypass, the aorta is opened and the subvalvular lesion is excised. Alternatively, a prosthetic conduit can be placed to bypass the

Table 8.5 Surgical options for correction or treatment of aortic stenosis

Surgical technique	Comment
Blind valvulotomy	Requires the least surgical expertise but shows poor results. Since in most cases stenosis is subaortic, technique does not really address the site of stenosis
Open arteriotomy and valvulectomy	Requires extracorporeal cardiopulmonary bypass; useful for discrete valvular lesions
Conduit placement	Conduit placed from left ventricle to aorta to bypass valve; technical expertise required

aortic valve. The conduit passes from the left ventricle to the descending aorta.

Postoperative considerations and prognosis

The prognosis for dogs with severe subaortic stenosis without surgery is poor; sudden death is possible. The prognosis after effective surgery is good; however, treated dogs are at risk of developing cardiomyopathy within 5–7 years due to underlying muscular disease.

Persistent right aortic arch

Persistent right aortic arch is the most common vascular ring anomaly. This congenital defect, because of the abnormal positioning of the vascular structures, causes mostly extracardiac problems, namely regurgitation. It is commonly seen in German Shepherd Dogs and Irish Setters. Kittens are less commonly affected. It is, however, an uncommon cause of regurgitation in puppies; idiopathic megaoesophagus is the most common. PRAA is the result of the aorta developing from the right fourth aortic arch rather than the left. The persistent left ligamentum arteriosus connecting the left pulmonary artery to the descending aorta forms a ring around the oesophagus which is completed by the base of the heart (Fig. 8.4). Occasionally there is a PDA. Persistent left vena cava occurs with PRAA approximately 40% of the time. Other much less common vascular ring anomalies include PRAA with persistent left subclavian artery, PRAA with persistent left subclavian artery and persistent left ligamentum arteriosus, double aortic arch, normal left aortic arch with persistent right ligamentum arteriosus, normal left aortic arch with persistent right subclavian artery, and normal left aortic arch with persistent right ligamentum arteriosus and right subclavian artery.

Clinical signs

Clinical signs become evident after weaning when the puppies or kittens begin eating solid food. Postprandial regurgitation occurs and the oesophagus dilates proximal to the vascular ring. Animals often aspirate food during regurgitation and develop aspiration pneumonia. The physical appearance is typically a stunted animal in poor body condition. An oesophageal bulge may be present at the thoracic inlet. Murmurs are typically not present. Other concurrent congenital anomalies are rare. Clinical signs consistent with aspiration pneumonia, such as cough, pyrexia and rales, or absence of lung sounds, may be apparent.

Diagnosis

Diagnosis is based on history and profile, physical examination findings and radiography. Thoracic radiographs reveal a dilated oesophagus cranial to the heart which usually contains large amounts of food and/or air. Evidence of pneumonia may be present, especially in the right middle lung lobe. Positive-contrast radiography using an oral barium suspension will demonstrate an oesophageal constriction at the base of the heart with varying degrees of oesophageal dilation cranial to this. The constriction must be in this location for a diagnosis of PRAA. Oesophagitis and idiopathic megaoesophagus can cause varying degrees of oesophageal dilation but a definite stricture in the region of the base of the heart is not evident. Fluoroscopy may confirm the constriction and evaluate the oesophageal motility, which is often abnormal.

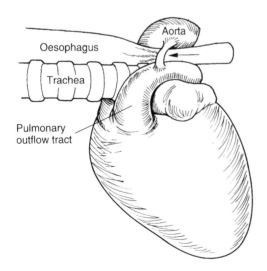

Figure 8.4 Persistent right aortic arch. The dilated oesophagus is seen anterior to the heart. The oesophagus and trachea are constricted by the ligamentum arteriosus (arrow), aorta, pulmonary artery and the base of the heart.

Treatment and surgical technique

Surgery is indicated to free constriction of the ligamentum arteriosus around the oesophagus. The procedure is performed through a left lateral thoracotomy at the fourth intercostal space. The ligamentum arteriosus is dissected free, double-ligated and severed between the ligatures. Constricting perioesophageal fibres should also be dissected free. A balloon catheter passed down the oesophagus intraoperatively and dilated at the site of the constriction helps identify constricting fibres. Imbrication of the dilated oesophagus is not recommended because it does not reduce postoperative regurgitation and may increase the risk of postoperative complications such as mediastinitis, pyothorax and broncho-oesophageal fistulation.

Postoperative considerations and prognosis

Immediate postoperative management is similar to that for animals undergoing other thoracic procedures. The postoperative prognosis is guarded. Oesophageal motility is often abnormal and long-term elevated feeding and diet manipulation may still be required; feeding soft food or gruels may be necessary. Medical management of aspiration pneumonia may be required (see Chapter 7). Surgery on very young animals carries the best prognosis.

Tetralogy of Fallot

Tetralogy of Fallot involves four combined congenital heart defects, including VSD, pulmonic stenosis, right ventricular hypertrophy and dextropositioning or overriding of the aorta which accepts blood from both ventricles (Eyster *et al.*, 1993; Fig. 8.5). Right ventricular hypertrophy is secondary to pulmonic stenosis. As blood pressure increases in the right ventricle, right-to-left shunting of blood causes mixing of blood in the aorta. Chronic hypoxia will cause polycythaemia.

Clinical signs

Clinical signs include exercise intolerance and cyanosis that is unresponsive to oxygen therapy. Tachypnoea and syncope may be present. Physical examination findings include a systolic murmur that is heard over the left heart base;

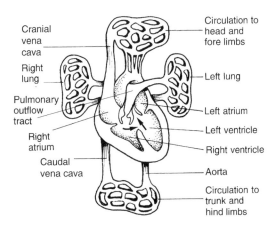

Figure 8.5 Tetralogy of Fallot. Obstruction at the pulmonary artery causes increased pressure in the right ventricle and secondary muscular hypertrophy. The ventricular septal defect allows blood to exit from the high-pressure right ventricle and the overridden aorta allows diversion of low-oxygen-tension blood to the systemic circulation (arrows).

however, marked polycythaemia may cause the murmur to be inaudible.

Diagnosis

Diagnosis is based on physical examination findings, electrocardiography and radiography. Electrocardiography reveals evidence of right ventricular hypertrophy, including deep S waves in leads I, II, III and aVF, and right axis deviation. Thoracic radiographs show right ventricular hypertrophy and a hyperlucent lung field due to attenuation of the pulmonary vasculature. Positive-contrast angiography after cardiac catheterization of a jugular vein and injection of contrast medium into the right ventricle can be used for definitive diagnosis and direct assessment of heart chamber blood pressures.

Treatment and surgical technique

Medical treatment includes phlebotomy to maintain the packed cell volume between 62 and 68%. Blood volume should be replaced with crystalloid fluids. Treatment with a β-blocker, such as atenolol and propranolol, may be beneficial for reducing muscular contractility and muscular constriction. Use of drugs causing systemic vasodilation should be avoided. Definitive surgical repair of tetralogy of Fallot requires closure of the VSD and correction of the pulmonic stenosis during cardiopulmonary bypass. Palliative surgical procedures are designed to increase pulmonary blood flow by shunting blood from the aorta to the pulmonary artery. A modified Blalock–Taussig procedure uses a harvested subclavian artery as a free graft conduit between the aorta and pulmonary artery. A Pott's anastomosis can be performed, creating a direct communication between the aorta and pulmonary artery. This procedure, however, may overload the pulmonary circulation (Eyster, 1993).

Postoperative considerations and prognosis

The prognosis for untreated tetralogy of Fallot is poor. Many animals may die suddenly. Surgical palliation may result in postoperative survival up to 4 years.

Atrial septal defect

Atrial septal defect causes left-to-right shunting with overloading of the right ventricle and eventual right-sided congestive heart failure. Pulmonary hypertension may occur. If right atrial pressures become elevated during heart failure, right-to-left shunting may result.

Clinical signs

Clinical signs include a systolic murmur over the left heart base caused by increased blood flow through the pulmonic valve (a relative pulmonic stenosis).

Diagnosis

Diagnosis is based on clinical signs and results of electrocardiography, radiographs and echocardiography. Electrocardiography reveals evidence of right ventricular hypertrophy. Thoracic radiographs show right ventricular hypertrophy and overcirculation of the pulmonary vasculature. Echocardiography can confirm these findings and may isolate the septal defect.

Treatment and surgical technique

Surgical repair requires an open-heart procedure to suture or patch the defect during cardiopulmonary bypass.

Ventricular septal defect

VSD is more common than atrial septal defect and is not an uncommon congenital heart defect in cats. The VSD causes left-to-right shunting which overloads both the left and right ventricles. A large VSD essentially creates a common ventricle and cause significant right ventricular dilation and hypertrophy. If pulmonary hypertension develops, right-to-left shunting can occur (Eisenmenger's syndrome).

Clinical signs

Clinical signs vary depending on the size of the defect. Animals with a small VSD may be asymptomatic and it may close as the animal gets older. Clinical signs otherwise include a cough, exercise intolerance and stunted growth. If right-to-left shunting has occurred, cyanosis, exercise intolerance and polycythaemia are evident.

Diagnosis

Diagnosis is based on physical examination findings, electrocardiography, radiography and electrocardiography. Thoracic auscultation reveals a holosystolic murmur loudest at the cranial sternal border. A diastolic murmur at the left heart base may also be present due to aortic regurgitation. Thoracic radiographs show left and right ventricular enlargement, left atrial enlargement and pulmonary over-circulation. Positive-contrast angiography after cardiac catheterization through a femoral or carotid artery and injection of contrast medium into the left ventricle can be used to determine a definitive diagnosis and rule out PDA as the cause of the murmur. Electrocardiography is often normal, although left or right ventricular hypertrophy may be evident. Echocardiography can confirm ventricular enlargement. Doppler echocardiography can be used to identify the septal defect and determine the shunt blood flow velocity. A high shunt velocity represents a small defect which carries a good prognosis.

Treatment and surgical technique

Definitive surgical correction of the VSD requires open-heart surgery to suture or patch the defect during cardiopulmonary bypass. Palliative surgical procedures include pulmonary arterial banding to decrease pulmonary blood flow. Reducing the pulmonary artery by two-thirds or doubling the right ventricular pressure is desired. Surgical correction of the VSD in an animal with right-to-left shunting is contraindicated due to irreversible cardiac changes. The prognosis for a large, untreated VSD is poor.

Cor triatriatum dexter

Cor triatriatum is an infrequent congenital defect that results from persistence of the embryological right sinus venosus valve. This defect causes a partitioning of the right atrium into two chambers separated by a perforate or imperforate muscular septum. It has been reported in several breeds and mixed-bred dogs (Miller *et al.*, 1989; Jevens *et al.*, 1993; Tobias *et al.*, 1993; Brayley *et al.*, 1994; Kaufman *et al.*, 1994). Cor triatriatum sinister (partitioning of the left atrium) has been reported in cats. Concurrent cardiac anomalies are reported in humans but have not been reported in dogs.

The cranial right atrial chamber communicates normally with the right ventricle via the tricuspid valve. However, the anomalous membrane obstructs blood flow from the caudal to cranial right atrial chamber. Dogs usually present in right heart failure with ascites and portal hypertension.

Clinical signs

The most common clinical sign is abdominal distension in a puppy usually less than a year of age. Physical examination reveals ascites and systemic venous distension of the caudal half of the body. Abdominal fluid is high in protein (> 3.0 g/dl), compatible with postsinusoidal obstruction. Jugular distension is characteristically absent.

Diagnosis

Diagnosis is by physical examination, thoracic radiographs and echocardiography. Thoracic radiographs are usually unremarkable except for enlargement of the caudal vena cava. Echocardiography can demonstrate the intra-atrial septum caudal to the tricuspid valve. Non-selective angiography can be used if echocardiography is non-diagnostic. Differential diagnosis should include heartworm-related caval syndrome, Budd–Chiari-type lesions such as hepatic cirrhosis, hepatic veno-occlusive disease, hepatic vein or caudal vena cava obstruction due to thrombosis, constrictive pericardial disease, hepatic arteriovenous fistula or right-heart defects resulting in congestive heart failure.

Treatment and surgical technique

Surgery is the definitive treatment of the condition; however, stabilization of the animal prior to surgery is indicated. Plasma transfusion or administration of colloid expanders is indicated in the hypoproteinaemic/hypoalbuminaemic animal.

Vascular inflow occlusion with right atriotomy and septectomy is successful in treating the disease (Tobias *et al.*, 1993; Kaufman *et al.*, 1994) although dilation of the septum has also been reported (Miller *et al.*, 1989; Jevens *et al.*, 1993). Surgery is performed through a right lateral thoracotomy. Inflow occlusion should be limited to less than 4 minutes in the normothermic animal. Moderate hypothermia (28° C) allows prolongation of venous inflow occlusion to 8–10 minutes.

Postoperative considerations and prognosis

Postoperative considerations include those for thoracic surgery. In addition, the protein status of the animal should be monitored and support given as necessary. The prognosis for return to normal function after successful surgical correction is excellent (Jevens *et al.*, 1993; Tobias *et al.*, 1993; Kaufman *et al.*, 1994).

Cardiac medication

The normal rhythm of the heart in puppies and kittens is a regular sinus rhythm. In young animals there is little to no variation in cardiac rhythm associated with breathing. The absence of a respiratory arrhythmia is consistent with the fact that vagal reflexes responsible for cardiac inhibition during expiration are immature at birth and develop shortly after 8 weeks of age in the dog. The vagal-mediated rhythm changes are unusual and usually pathological in young cats.

As in adults, arrhythmias can occur in puppies and kittens from a variety of cardiac and extracardiac abnormalities. Ventricular extrasystoles and tachycardias commonly occur secondary to inflammation, stretching or hypoxia of the myocardium in animals with myocarditis or congenital heart disease. The treatment of arrhythmias in puppies and kittens is similar to treatment in adults. It is important to note, however, the difference in responsiveness of the immature myocardium to many antiarrhythmic agents. Both increased and decreased sensitivities to antiarrhythmic agents have been demon-

strated in hearts of young animals, depending on the agent used. Puppies younger than 6 weeks of age have a paradoxical negative chronotropic response to atropine and a marked sensitivity to the depressant effects of propranolol on the sinus node.

A list of common antiarrhythmic agents with suggested dosages for puppies and kittens is presented in Table 8.6. It should be mentioned that the pharmacokinetic and toxicologic data that are needed to administer antiarrhythmic agents optimally to puppies and kittens are not available. The listed dosages in Table 8.6 have, therefore, been extrapolated from pharmacodynamic studies and from experience with these agents in older animals.

Table 8.6 Cardiac agents – suggested dosages and indications in young animals

Drug	Dosage*	Indications	Comments
Atropine	Dog and cat: 0.01–0.02 mg/kg IV, IM 0.02–0.04 mg/kg SC	Vagally induced bradyarrhythmias and atrioventricular block	Do not use in animals younger than 8 weeks
Isoproterenol	Dog and cat: 0.4 mg in 250 ml isotonic dextrose, drip slowly to effect IV	Sinus bradycardia, sinoatrial arrest, atrioventricular block, cardiac arrest with asystole	May induce tachycardia, ventricular extrasystoles and hypotension
Digoxin	Dog: 0.01 mg/kg PO divided b.i.d. 0.005 mg/kg IV, repeat with half this dose in 30–60 minutes if necessary Cat: 0.01 mg/kg PO q 48 hours	Supraventricular tachycardia, atrial fibrillation	
Propranolol	Dog and cat: 0.02–0.06 mg/kg IV 0.2–1.0 mg/kg PO q 48 hours	Supraventricular tachycardia, atrial fibrillation, premature ventricular contractions	Do not use in animals younger than 40 days
Lignocaine	Dog: 2–4 mg/kg IV bolus followed by 25–75 g/kg per minute infusion Cat: 0.25 mg/kg slowly IV	Premature ventricular contractions, ventricular tachycardia	May cause seizures, emesis
Procainamide	Dog: 3–6 mg/kg slowly IV 10 mg/kg IM every 4–6 hours 10 mg/kg PO q.i.d.–t.i.d.	Premature ventricular contractions, ventricular tachycardia	May cause hypotension, gastrointestinal upset, prolonged QRS duration and prolonged QT interval
Quinidine	Dog: 10 mg/kg IM or PO q.i.d.	Premature ventricular contractions, ventricular and supraventricular tachycardias	
Verapamil	Dog and cat: 0.05–0.15 mg/kg slowly IV	Supraventricular tachycardias	May cause bradycardia, hypotension and atrioventricular block

* IV = Intravenous administration; IM = intramuscular administration; SC = subcutaneous administration; PO = oral administration; b.i.d. = twice a day; t.i.d. = three times a day; q.i.d. = four times a day.

Vascular disorders

Arteriovenous fistulas

Peripheral arteriovenous fistulas are uncommon congenital or acquired defects of the vasculature in puppies and kittens. An arteriovenous fistula is an abnormal direct communication between an artery and vein which results in left-to-right shunting of blood away from the capillary bed (Hosgood, 1989; Litwalk, 1993). The haemodynamic effects of the arteriovenous fistula depends on the size of the fistula. The most common congenital arteriovenous fistula is a PDA. Other congenital arteriovenous fistulas most commonly involve the extremities, although they have been reported in the temporal region, eye, flank, tongue and liver. Congenital arteriovenous fistulas are often multiple and extensive.

Acquired arteriovenous fistulas are most frequently caused by trauma, including penetrating injury, venepuncture, extravascular injection of irritants, mass ligation of arteries and veins and aneurysm rupture. However, a history of trauma is not always apparent. Neoplasia and ischaemia create extensive collateral circulation which may include arteriovenous fistulas. Surgically created arteriovenous fistulas are created for venous access. Acquired arteriovenous fistulas are usually single and direct, although extensive collateral circulation can develop.

Clinical signs

Clinical signs of arteriovenous fistulas of the extremities include painless swelling of the extremity, bleeding from that site, hypertrophy of the limb, lameness and possibly ulceration of the distal limb. Physical examination reveals a localized swelling at the site and distal to the arteriovenous fistula. The area may be hyperthermic, with the distal limb hypothermic. Dilated tortuous vessels may be apparent at the site. A continuous bruit (murmur) over the site may be auscultated and a palpable thrill may be present. Occlusion of the proximal artery may cause a sudden decrease in heart rate (Branham's sign) due to a sudden increase in blood pressure.

Diagnosis

Diagnosis is by clinical signs (Table 8.7) and possibly radiography. Survey radiographs are usually unremarkable, although periosteal proliferation, limb length discrepancy in young dogs or cortical rarefication or thickening may be seen. Contrast angiography is most useful, although ultrasonography may also demonstrate the arteriovenous fistula. Assessment of cardiovascular function by thoracic radiographs, electrocardiography and echocardiography is indicated for large arteriovenous fistulas since high-output cardiac failure can develop.

Table 8.7 Characteristic clinical signs of an arteriovenous fistula used to make a diagnosis

Painless swelling of the extremity

Bleeding from that site

Hypertrophy of the bone and soft tissue of the limb

Lameness and possible ulceration of the distal limb

Region of suspected fisula may be hyperthermic, while the distal limb may be hypothermic

Dilated tortuous vessels at site

Auscultation of a continuous bruit (murmur) over the site. A palpable thrill may be present

Occlusion of the proximal artery causes a sudden decrease in heart rate (Branham's sign)

Treatment and surgical technique

Treatment for single arteriovenous fistulas is most often surgery to separate the artery and vein. If possible, the region of the fistula is removed. For large arteriovenous fistulas, the arterial supply should be slowly ligated to allow monitoring for bradycardia. Treatment of multiple arteriovenous fistulas is generally palliative (bandaging in association with partial fistula resection) since separation or resection of all the fistulas is impossible. Arterial embolization may be attempted. Multiple arteriovenous fistulas involved in a body organ (liver) are often totally resectable.

Postoperative considerations and prognosis

The prognosis for recovery for single fistulas amenable to surgery or totally excised multiple fistulas (liver lobe) is good.

The prognosis for multiple, congenital fistulas is poor if the entire region cannot be excised.

References

Birchard, S.J., Bonagura, J.D. and Fingland, R.B. (1990) Results of ligation of patent ductus arteriosus in dogs: 201 cases (1969–1988). *Journal of the American Veterinary Medical Association*, **196**, 2011–2013.

Bonagura, J.D. (1989) Congenital heart disease. In: Ettinger, S.J. (ed.), *Textbook of Veterinary Internal Medicine*, vol. 1, pp. 976–1030. Philadelphia: W.B. Saunders.

Brayley, K.A., Lunney, J. and Ettinger, S.J. (1994) Cor triatriatum dexter in a dog. *Journal of the American Animal Hospital Association*, **30**, 153–156.

Bright, J.M., Jennings, J., Toal R. and Hood, M.E. (1987) Percutaneous balloon valvuloplasty for treatment of pulmonic stenosis in a dog. *Journal of the American Veterinary Medical Association*, **191**, 995–996.

Eyster, G.E. (1993) Basic cardiac procedures. In: Slatter, D.H. (ed.), *Textbook of Small Animal Surgery*, vol. 1, pp. 893–918. Philadelphia: W.B. Saunders.

Eyster, G.E., Gaber, C.E. and Probst, M. (1993) Cardiac disorders. In: Slatter, D.H. (ed.), *Textbook of Small Animal Surgery*, vol. 1, pp. 856–889. Philadelphia: W.B. Saunders.

Fingland, R.B., Bonagura, J.D. and Myer, W. (1986) Pulmonic stenosis in the dog: 29 cases (1975–1984). *Journal of the American Veterinary Medical Association*, **189**, 218–226.

Goodwin, J.K. and Lombard, C.W. (1992) Patent ductus arteriosus in adults dogs: clinical features of 14 cases. *Journal of the American Animal Association*, **28**, 350–354.

Hosgood, G. (1989) Arteriovenous fistulas: pathophysiology, diagnosis and treatment. *Compendium of Continuing Education for the Practicing Veterinarian*, **11**, 625–637.

Jevens, D.J., Johnston, S.A., Jones, C.A., Anderson, L.K., Bergener, D.C. and Eyster, G.E. (1993) Cor triatriatum dexter in two dogs. *Journal of the American Animal Hospital Association*, **29**, 289–293.

Kaufman, A.C., Swalec, K.M. and Mahaffey, M.B. (1994) Surgical correction of cor triatriatum dexter in a puppy. *Journal of the American Animal Hospital Association*, **30**, 157–161.

Komtebedde, J., Ilkiw, J.E., Follette, D.M., Breznock, E.M. and Tobias, A.H. (1993) Resection of subvalvular aortic stenosis: surgical and perioperative management in seven dogs. *Veterinary Surgery*, **22**, 419–430.

Litwalk, P. (1993) Peripheral vascular procedures and disorders. In: Slatter, D.H. (ed.), *Textbook of Small Animal Surgery*, vol. 1, pp. 922–929. Philadelphia: W.B. Saunders.

Miller, M.W., Bonagura, J.D., Dibartola, S.P. and Fossum, T.W. (1989) Budd–Chiari-like syndrome in two dogs. *Journal of the American Animal Hospital Association*, **25**, 277–283.

Miller, M.W., Bonagura, J.D., Meurs, K.M. and Lehmkuhl, L.B. (1995) Percutaneous catheter occlusion of patent ductus arteriosus. In: 'Am College Vet Int Med' Forum, *American College of Veterinary Internal Medicine*, pp. 308–310. Lake Buena Vista, Florida.

Snaps, F.R., McEntee, K., Saunders, J.H. and Dondelinger, R.F. (1995) Treatment of patent ductus arteriosus by placement of intravascular coils in a pup. *Journal of the American Veterinary Medical Association*, **207**, 724–725.

Tobias, A.H., Thomas, W.P., Kittleson, M.D. and Komtebedde, J. (1993) Cor triatriatum dexter in two dogs. *Journal of the American Veterinary Medical Association*, **202**, 285–290.

The urinary system

Disorders of the kidney

Congenital disorders of the kidney fall into two categories: anomalies that cause kidney dysfunction (glomerulopathies) and result in renal failure, and structural changes that have no effect on function and are usually an incidental finding (Table 9.1). The pattern of inheritance has been identified for some anomalies, but others remain best described as familial with the mode of inheritance yet to be determined. Treatment of dysfunctional anomalies is directed at supportive care, but all of these diseases are terminal.

Disorders of the ureter

Occasional congenital anomalies of the ureter such as agenesis or duplication can occur. Ureteral agenesis is usually associated with ipsilateral renal aplasia. Ureteral duplication has been reported in the dog but not in the cat.

Ureteroceles are rare congenital anomalies characterized by dilation of the intravesical and intramural position of the ureter which then extends into the lumen of the urinary bladder. The ureters may be normal or ectopic. This results in partial or complete obstruction of the ureter, causing hydroureter and hydronephrosis. Clinical signs vary but may be associated with urinary tract infection (and urolithiasis) or renal compromise in bilateral disease. Diagnosis is made by documenting a filling defect at the site of the ureteral openings in the urinary bladder using positive-contrast cystography or by direct visualization in large dogs using cystoscopy. Treatment is based on surgical excision of the mucosal surface of the distended ureter with apposition of the ureteral and urinary bladder mucosa. Urine should be submitted for bacterial culture and sensitivity testing. The prognosis is fair, depending on the degree of hydronephrosis and hydroureter present, whether the urinary tract infection can be controlled, and whether other anomalies are present.

Ectopic ureters

The most common congenital anomaly of the ureter is ectopia. The ureters typically enter the urinary bladder on the dorsal aspect of the trigone. Faulty differentiation or migration of the mesonephric and metanephric ducts causes abnormal routing of the ureters. Breeds most frequently affected include the Siberian Husky, West Highland White Terrier, Collie, Fox Terrier, Labrador Retriever, Golden Retriever, Welsh Corgi and Miniature and Toy Poodle. Females are affected much more commonly than males (20:1). Breed predisposition is apparent but the mode of inheritance is unclear.

In the female dog, the ureter terminates in the vagina approximately 70% of the time, the urethra 20%, urinary bladder neck 8% and uterus 3%. In the male dog, the ureter usually terminates in the cranial portion of the pelvic urethra. Slightly more than 60% of females with ectopic

Table 9.1 Congenital anomalies of the kidney in dogs and cats

Anomaly	Breed or familial predisposition	Comments
Renal agenesis	Dog: Beagle, Shetland Sheepdog, Dobermann	Complete absence of one or both kidneys
		Unilateral disease more common and may be associated with ipsilateral vas deferens, epididymis or uterine anomalies
		Unilateral disease often an incidental finding. Bilateral disease obviously fatal
Renal hypoplasia		Rare
		Kidney is apparently normal but small. Histology shows reduced number of normal nephrons
		Unilateral disease often undetected. Bilateral disease may lead to renal failure
Renal dysplasia and aplasia	Dog: lhasa Apso, Shih Tzu, Soft-coated Wheaten Terrier, Keeshond, Chow, Standard Poodle, Miniature Schnauzer, Airedale, Alaskan Malamute, Beagle, Boxer, Bulldog, Great Dane, Great Pyrenees, Golden Retriever, Irish Wolfhound, King Charles Spaniel, Old English Sheepdog, Pekinese, Swedish Foxhound, Yorkshire Terrier Cat: Persian	Dysplasia characterized by focal areas of disorganized parenchymal development with immature or anomalous structures in otherwise normal kidney
		Aplasia characterized by changes throughout kidney
		Manifests as chronic renal failure, varying from 4 weeks to 5 years at age of onset (Autran de Morais *et al.*, 1996)
Glomerulopathies	Dog: Samoyed, Dobermann, Bull Terriers, Cocker Spaniels, Newfoundland (single case) and Rottweiler	Associated with abnormalities in the glomerular basement membrane causing clinical signs of mild to severe proteinuria, microscopic haematuria and occasionally glycosuria at 6 weeks to 2 months of age and eventually chronic renal failure near 6–10 months of age
		Samoyed glomerulopathy results from inheritance of abnormal X-linked dominant gene resulting in alteration of type IV collagen (major component of glomerular capillary basement membrane). Males are more severely affected and develop overt chronic renal failure by 8–16 months of age. Affected females show less severe clinical signs and usually do not develop overt chronic renal failure
		Bull terrier nephritis appears to be inherited as an autosomal dominant gene with males and females affected similarly
		Dobermann familial glomerulonephritis affects males and females similarly
		Cocker Spaniel familial nephropathy affects males and females similarly. Characterized by glomerular changes and interstitial fibrosis and inflammatory cell infiltration. Rottweiler atrophic glomerulopathy affects males and females similarly
Tubulointerstitial nephropathy	Dog: Norwegian Elkhound	Familial disease characterized by periglomerular fibrosis, parietal cell hyperplasia and eventually severe, corticomedullary interstitial fibrosis. Males and females affected similarly with clinical signs (isothenuria, proteinuria, azotaemia) and development of chronic renal failure as early as 3 months of age

Table 9.1 (continued)

Anomaly	Breed or familial predisposition	Comments
Polycystic renal disease	Dog: Beagle Cairn Terriers Cats: Domestic Longhair, Himalayan	Characterized by formation of multiple, variable-sized cysts throughout the medulla and cortex. Clinical signs of renomegaly may be observed as early as 2–6 weeks of age, although signs of renomegaly and chronic renal failure may not be apparent until middle age. Cystic alterations of the biliary tree are also reported in affected Cairn Terriers
Amyloidosis	Dog: Shar-Pei Cat: Abyssinian	Familial amyloidosis is characterized by medullary interstitial deposits of amyloid resulting in eventual renal failure and is usually recognized by 1 year of age (in contrast to non-familial amyloidosis)
Renal ectopia and fusion		Ectopia refers to congenital malposition of one or both kidneys Fusion results in malshaped kidneys, the result of congenital union of normal kidneys. Not all ectopic kidneys show fusion
Supernumerary and duplex kidneys		The presence of one or more additional kidneys (supernumerary) or an enlarged kidney with two renal pelves and ureters (duplex) Usually an incidental finding
Fanconi-like syndrome	Dog: Basenji, Miniature Schnauzer, Norwegian Elkhound, Shetland Sheepdog	A functional abnormality resulting in impaired proximal tubular resorption of amino acids, glucose, phosphate, sodium, potassium and uric acid. Clinical signs develop by about 1 year of age, characterized by polyuria, polydipsia, low urine specific gravity, normoglycaemia with glycosuria, aminoaciduria, non-anion gap metabolic acidosis and hypokalaemia
Cystinuria	Dog: Dachshund	Also reported less frequently in several breeds. Inherited defect in renal tubular transport of cystine and dibasic amino acids. Some dogs will develop cystine urolithiasis
Hyperuricuria	Dog: Dalmatian	Recessive, non-sex-linked mode of inheritance resulting in impaired hepatic conversion of uric acid to allantoin by the enzyme uricase and enhanced renal tubular secretion of uric acid. Results in urate uroliths in animals usually older than 2 years of age and males often develop urethral obstruction

ureters have unilateral ectopia. Approximately 50% of males have unilateral ectopia. Ectopic ureter is diagnosed infrequently in cats but is reported in both males and females. All ectopias were bilateral and the ureters terminated in the urethra.

The morphological types of ectopic ureters described in dogs include: intramural with distal ureteral orifice, intramural with no distal ureteral orifice and ureteral troughs, bilateral double ureteral openings, and extramural (Stone and Mason, 1990; Fig. 9.1). Intramural ectopic ureters are most common and dogs

with this type of ectopic ureter have a better prognosis for surgical correction and postoperative continence than dogs with ureteral troughs (Stone and Mason, 1990). Extramural ectopic ureter is the only type reported in the cat.

Clinical signs

Clinical signs include continuous or intermittent urinary incontinence since birth, with wetness and urine scald apparent around the perineum. Both unilaterally and bilaterally affected animals may be capable of normal micturition.

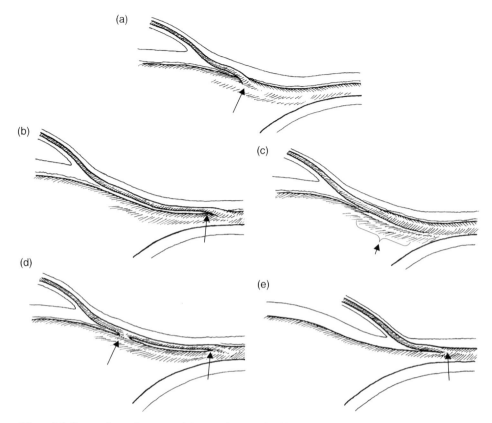

Figure 9.1 Types of ectopic ureters: (a) normal ureteral orifice (arrow); (b) intramural ureter with distal ureteral orifice (arrow); (c) ureteral trough (arrow); (d) double ureteral openings (arrows); (e) extramural ureter with distal ectopic opening (arrow).

Diagnosis

Diagnosis is based on radiographic assessment of positive- and negative-contrast studies, usually an excretory urogram with a negative contrast pneumocystogram. The ureters can be observed to pass the normal entry point in the urinary bladder, although definitive location of their site of entry into the urogenital tract may be difficult. Assessment of hydroureter and evaluation of kidney function can be made from these studies. Establishment of contralateral kidney function is important for unilateral disease since nephroureterotomy may be considered as treatment. Ultrasonographic assessment of the kidneys and ureters may also be useful to establish a diagnosis. Definitive determination of the type of ectopic ureter is best performed at coeliotomy and cystotomy, although preoperative cystoscopy in larger dogs can be useful.

Preoperative work-up to establish the status of the animal and rule out other causes of urinary incontinence must include urine specific gravity, serum creatinine and urea nitrogen to determine the presence of renal compromise (Stone and Barsanti, 1992a). Dogs with ectopic ureters frequently have urinary tract infection. Urine collected via cystocentesis should be submitted for analysis and bacterial culture and sensitivity testing.

Urethral sphincter incompetence is often associated with ectopic ureter and affects the postoperative prognosis. A crude assessment of urethral function can be determined by the ease with which the urinary bladder can be expressed (Stone and Barsanti, 1992a). Urethral pressure profilometry can be performed to assess urethral function more accurately; however, this test may be affected by the presence of an intramural ectopic ureter. Abnormal urethral function is not a contraindication for surgery as some animals respond to postoperative medication; however, assessment is important in establishing the prognosis and for client education.

Vaginal anomalies have been noted concurrently with ectopic ureter (persistent hymen), hence vaginal examination is important in animals with ectopic ureters.

Treatment and surgical technique

Preoperative considerations include stabilization of renal compromise (diuresis) and perioperative and postoperative administration of appropriate antimicrobials if urinary tract infection is present.

The animal is prepared for aseptic abdominal surgery and a ventral midline coeliotomy is performed. The kidneys and ureters are grossly assessed and apparent or inapparent entry of the ureters into the urinary bladder is observed. If it has been predetermined that one kidney is non-functional, severely hydronephrotic or infected, nephroureterectomy is performed (Fig. 9.2). It is important in nephroureterectomy that the entire ureter is excised to avoid vesicoureteral reflux causing the ureteral remnant being a site of residual infection.

The urinary bladder is isolated from the abdominal cavity using moistened laparotomy sponges; stay sutures are placed at the apex and vesicourethral junction, and a ventral cystotomy is performed. The trigone should be examined for normal ureteral openings. Determination of the type of ectopic ureter will decide the treatment necessary (Table 9.2).

Intramural ectopic ureters can be treated by creation of a neoureterocystostomy. An incision is made over the submucosal ridge at the site of a normal ureteral opening. The incision must not completely penetrate the ureter. A small section of urinary bladder and ureteral mucosa is excised and the ureteral mucosal is sutured to the urinary bladder mucosa using 4-0 to 7-0 monofilament absorbable suture in a simple interrupted pattern (Fig. 9.3). The distal ureter

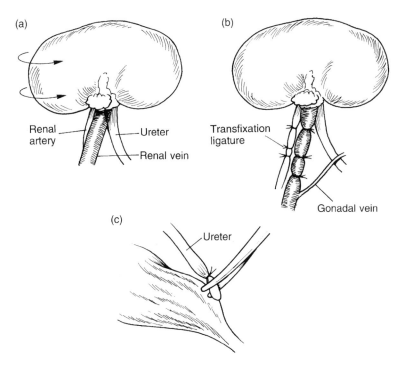

Figure 9.2 Nephroureterectomy. (a) The kidney is dissected from its peritoneal attachments and the cranial pole of the kidney is rotated to reveal the renal artery(s) located on the cranial dorsal surface of the renal vein. The renal artery is triple-ligated first, including a transfixation ligature distal to the proximal ligature. (b) The renal vein is triple-ligated distal to the gonadal venous branch. (c) The ureter is dissected free and ligated and severed at the level of the urinary bladder or its most distal point of entry into the urinary tract.

Table 9.2 Visual characteristics of ureteral ectopia

Type of ectopic ureter	Characteristic appearance intraoperatively
Intramural ureter	Identified by absence of an ureteral opening in the normal location with a submucosal ridge observed over the pathway of the ureter, particularly when the distal ureter (proximal urethra) is occluded
Ureteral trough	Ureteral opening in the normal position but a trough continues distally
Double ureteral openings	Identified by catheterizing normal ureteral opening and being able to pass catheter distally
Extramural ureter	No ureteral opening in trigone, no submucosal bulge after occlusion of the proximal urethra. The ureter is observed to course external to urinary bladder and can be followed distal to trigone

is incised and the incised ureter is sutured to the urinary bladder wall to occlude the distal segment. This is preferred to simply suturing the region of the distal ureter, since recanalization has been observed (Stone and Barsanti, 1992c).

Ureteral troughs are treated by excising a strip of mucosa from each side of the trough and the base if possible, and closing the trough with a simple continuous suture pattern of monofilament absorbable 4-0 to 5-0 suture

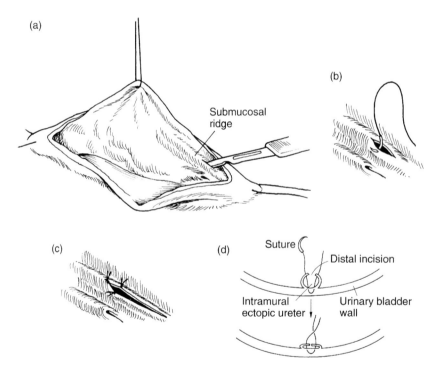

Figure 9.3 Creation of a neouretercystostomy for an intramural ectopic ureter. (a) An incision is made over the submucosal ridge at the site of a normal ureteral opening. The incision must only penetrate the upper wall of ureter. (b) A small section of urinary bladder and ureteral mucosa is excised and the ureteral mucosal is sutured to the urinary bladder mucosa using 4-0 to 7-0 monofilament absorbable suture in a simple interrupted pattern. (c, d) The distal ureter is incised and sutured to the urinary bladder wall, the suturing passing from one side of the incised ureter, to the urinary bladder wall, and then to the other incised ureter. Excising a portion of ureteral mucosa from this section of intramural ureter may facilitate fibrosis and occlusion.

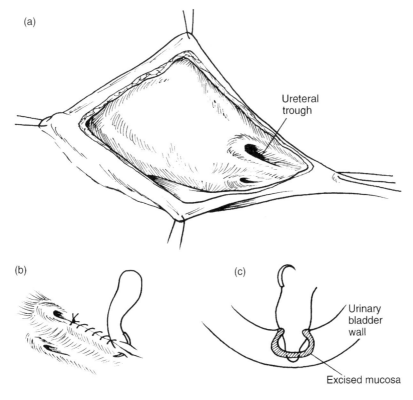

Figure 9.4 (a) Surgical correction of a ureteral trough. Mucosa is excised from each side and the base of the trough if possible. (b, c) The trough is closed in a simple continuous pattern, the needle passing through one side, the dorsal aspect of the trough and the other side of the trough.

with bites engaging both sides of the trough and the base of the trough (Fig. 9.4).

Double ureteral openings are treated by occluding the distal portion of the ureter with sutures, as described for intramural ureters. With a catheter in this distal position, the ureter is incised over the catheter and a portion of ureteral mucosa is excised to facilitate fibrosis. Interrupted sutures are preplaced through the urinary bladder wall and around the catheter, and tied as the catheter is removed.

Extramural ureters must be reimplanted into the urinary bladder in the normal position (Fig. 9.5). The ureter is double-ligated and severed as close to its ectopic entrance as possible. The distal ureter is mobilized only enough to allow its repositioning. Excessive dissection is avoided as this may impair the neurovascular innervation of the ureter. A small circular piece of urinary bladder mucosa is excised from the new stoma site and an oblique tunnel is made from the urinary bladder lumen to the outside using a haemostatic forceps. The ligature on the distal ureter is grasped and pulled through the tunnel. The end of the ureter is severed proximal to the ligature and the ureteral end is spatulated to increase its luminal diameter. A distal retention suture passing through the ureter and the urinary bladder muscle and mucosa is placed to hold the ureter in place. Two lateral retention sutures can also be placed. The remaining ureteral mucosa is then sutured to the urinary bladder mucosa using simple interrupted, monofilament absorbable sutures (5-0 or 6-0). The use of ureteral stenting is controversial and not recommended due to the risk of irritation, inducing stenosis of the stoma. Cystotomy closure is by a single layer of simple interrupted sutures.

Postoperative considerations and prognosis

Gross haematuria is expected for the first 24 hours postoperatively and microscopic

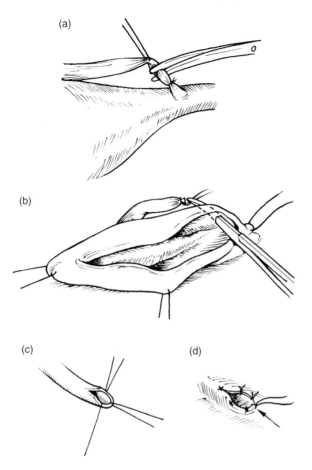

Figure 9.5 Ureteral transplantation. (a) The ureter is double-ligated and severed as close to its ectopic entrance as possible. A small circular piece of urinary bladder mucosa is excised from the new stoma site and an oblique tunnel is made from the urinary bladder lumen to the outside using haemostatic forceps. (b) The ligature on the distal ureter is grasped and pulled through the tunnel. (c) The end of the ureter is severed proximal to the ligature and the ureteral end is spatulated to increase its luminal diameter. (d) A single distal retention suture passing through the ureter and the urinary bladder muscle and mucosa is placed to hold the ureter in place (arrow). Two lateral retention sutures can also be placed. The remaining ureteral mucosa is then sutured to the urinary bladder mucosa using simple interrupted, monofilament absorbable sutures (5-0 or 6-0).

haematuria may persist for a further 12–24 hours. Frequent micturition is encouraged to keep the urinary bladder decompressed. Diuresis may be indicated to encourage urine flow through the ureters. The animals should be monitored for urination. Excretory urography should be performed 4–6 weeks postoperatively to monitor stoma function. Hydroureter should be resolving at this time. An increase in the severity of hydroureter indicates stenosis of the stoma. Reoperation is indicated for revision of the stoma. It is imperative that postoperative excretory urography be performed since by the time a unilateral stenosis becomes obvious, salvage of the kidney is usually not possible.

The overall prognosis for postoperative urinary continence is fair. Up to 50% of dogs have persistent urinary incontinence, possibly due to urethral sphincter incompetence or hypoplastic urinary bladders. Incontinence appeared to be more of a problem in dogs with ureteral troughs

(Stone and Mason, 1990). Careful re-evaluation of animals that show postoperative incontinence is important and obvious causes of incontinence such as vaginal abnormalities or persistent cystitis should be ruled out before oestrogen or α-adrenergic therapy is recommended. Vaginography or vaginourethrography may be useful in evaluating the shape and size of the vagina to determine if vaginal pooling of urine is a cause of postoperative incontinence, or if ureteral reflux is occurring due to inadequate ligation of the distal ectopic ureter. Urethral pressure-profile evaluation of urethral tone is useful to assess urethral sphincter function. If urethral sphincter incompetence appears to be a problem, α-adrenergic receptor agonists such as phenylpropanolamine (1.5 mg/kg t.i.d. or 3 mg/kg b.i.d. PO for dogs) or pseudoephedrine (4–5 mg/kg t.i.d. PO or b.i.d. for sustained-release formula for dogs) may control incontinence in some dogs. Alternatively, imipramine (0.5–

Table 9.3 Surgical techniques for correcting urethral incompetence

Surgical technique	Function
Transurethral Teflon or collagen injection	Teflon or collagen injected into wall of vesicourethral junction provides physical constriction
Vesicourethral sling	Use of prosthetic materials (Teflon, silicone, polypropylene mesh) to provide physical constriction at vesicourethral junction
Sling urethroplasty	Creates a vesicourethral sling from seromuscular flaps from the trigone. Provides physical constriction of vesicourethral junction
Perineal fascial sling	Described for male dogs. An autogenous fascial strip provides physical constriction of perineal urethra
Colposuspension	Permanently suspends urinary bladder (and vesicourethral junction) in abdomen. Increases in abdominal pressure facilitates closure of vesicourethral junction
Urethral extension	Reconstruction techniques that extend the length of the urethra to facilitate positioning of the urinary bladder in the abdomen

1.0 mg/kg t.i.d. PO for dogs), a tricyclic antidepressant that increases urinary bladder capacity as well as increasing urethral sphincter tone, may be used (Stone and Barsanti, 1992b). The recommendation not to ovariohysterectomize female dogs with urethral sphincter incompetence in order to maintain oestrogen levels, based on the theory that oestrogen increases the sensitivity of α-receptors, has not shown benefit in the author's experience. In fact, several reports have noted that some dogs developed incontinence postoperatively, only during oestrus (Stone and Mason, 1990). Thus ovariohysterectomy is recommended in dogs with ectopic ureters since breeding should be avoided. Surgical methods to improve urethral competence have been reported (Table 9.3).

Disorders of the urinary bladder

Agenesis of the urinary bladder has been reported in a 4-month-old dog with urinary incontinence. Hypoplasia of the urinary bladder is a poorly defined condition possibly associated with ectopic ureters. It is thought to contribute to postoperative urinary incontinence in dogs with ectopic ureters.

Exstrophy of the urinary bladder occurs with ventral abdominal defects and may be associated with other urogenital and intestinal defects. Correction requires reconstructive surgery and the prognosis depends on the presence of other defects.

Urolithiasis is uncommon in the puppy or kitten. Struvite calculi are most common, usually associated with urinary tract infection.

Renal, ureteral, cystic and urethral calculi have been reported. The presence of calculi in an animal less than 6 months of age should alert the clinician to look for other problems that would predispose this animal to urinary tract infection (e.g. urethrorectal fistulas, vaginal anomalies, ectopic ureters).

Urachal abnormalities

The urachus is a tubular structure that connects the lumen of the urinary bladder with the allantois and should close shortly after birth. Anomalies may be of four types (Fig. 9.6).

A patent urachus connects the urinary bladder and the umbilicus. Clinical signs include persistent wetness around the umbilicus with urine scald. The animal can still urinate normally through the urethra.

A urachal diverticulum is that portion of the urachus that fails to close completely at the urinary bladder. This is the most common urachal abnormality seen in the dog and cat. It may exist for many years before a problem is apparent. The presence of a urachal diverticulum has been associated with chronic, non-responsive cystitis (haematuria, pollakiuria, dysuria) and may lead to urolith formation. Surgical excision is indicated if urinary tract infection does not respond to appropriate antimicrobial therapy.

A urachal sinus is that portion of the urachus that fails to close at the umbilicus. This causes omphalitis with swelling and discharge at the umbilicus. The sinus may be obvious externally or contained internally. It is seen most often in calves.

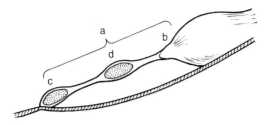

Figure 9.6 Different types of urachal abnormalities: (a) patent urachus; (b) urachal diverticulum; (c) urachal sinus; (d) urachal cyst.

A urachal cyst is a blind cyst that develops anywhere along the urachus. It is associated with variable clinical signs depending on location and size and whether the cystic fluid is sterile or infected. The cysts fill with fluid secreted from the epithelial lining. Large sterile cysts may cause abdominal distension, and peritonitis if it is infected and subsequently ruptures.

Diagnosis

Diagnosis is based on clinical signs, physical examination findings and the results of abdominal radiographs and ultrasound. Even in the case of a persistent urachus, where the diagnosis is obvious on physical examination, radiographic and ultrasonographic evaluation of the entire urinary tract is advised. Excretory urography and positive-contrast cystography may be indicated in addition to plain radiographs and ultrasonographic evaluation. Preoperative documentation of urinary tract infection will allow the use of appropriate perioperative and postoperative antimicrobial therapy. Ultrasound-guided cystocentesis or aspiration of cyst contents can be used to obtain fluid for cytology and bacterial culture and sensitivity testing.

Treatment and surgical technique

Regardless of the type of defect, the principles of treatment are the same. The animal should be stabilized haemodynamically prior to surgical excision of the urachus. A ventral midline coeliotomy is performed. The urachus is excised by making an elliptical incision around the umbilicus and at the apex of urinary bladder. The contents of the urachus should be cultured. The urinary bladder is closed using simple interrupted sutures of 4-0 monofilament absorbable suture with sutures engaging the submucosa but not penetrating the mucosa. The body wall at the region of the umbilicus is closed as for an umbilical hernia. The remainder of the abdominal closure is routine.

Postoperative considerations and prognosis

Treatment for renal compromise should continue if this was present preoperatively. Antimicrobial treatment for 3–4 weeks is indicated if urinary tract infection is present. Reculture of urine 1 week after antimicrobial treatment is completed is indicated to monitor for persistent infection. Overall, if there are minimal secondary changes to the urinary tract, the prognosis for normal function is good.

Disorders of the urethra

Urethral prolapse

Urethral prolapse is an infrequent but not rare problem seen most commonly in young intact male brachycephalic dogs. The exact aetiology is unclear but it is thought to be linked to repeated sexual excitement. In addition, it may be seen associated with straining due to urogenital infection or the presence of urethral calculi.

Clinical signs and diagnosis

Clinical signs include excessive licking of the penis and prepuce by the dog, blood dripping from the end of the penis and the characteristic appearance of the prolapsed urethral mucosa as a 'red doughnut' at the end of the penis (Fig. 9.7).

Treatment and surgical technique

Conservative management can be used for a small acute prolapse. General anaesthesia is usually required. A well-lubricated urinary catheter is inserted into the urethra which reduces the prolapse as it is inserted. A purse-string suture (5-0 or 6-0 monofilament non-absorbable suture) is placed around the tip of the penis to maintain reduction of the prolapse. The catheter is sutured to the prepuce and left in place for 5–7 days.

Do not apply chemical or electrocautery to the urethral mucosa to stop bleeding. This can severely damage the mucosa and may predispose to urethral stricture.

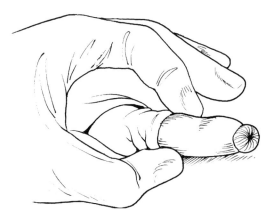

Figure 9.7 Clinical appearance of urethral prolapse.

Recurrence is likely after conservative treatment and there is a risk of ascending urinary tract infection due to the presence of an indwelling catheter. In addition, there is the risk of premature dislodgement of the catheter.

Definitive treatment requires surgical amputation of the prolapsed mucosa. General anaesthesia is required. A well-lubricated urinary catheter is inserted through the prolapse into the urinary bladder. Two to four stay sutures are placed equidistant around the tip of the penis through the urethral mucosa (Fig. 9.8). The prolapsed mucosa is incised over the catheter at the penile margin and the urethral mucosa is sutured to the tip of the penis with simple interrupted 5-0 or 6-0 monofilament absorbable sutures. Usually, a portion of mucosa is incised and sutured in turn until the entire prolapsed

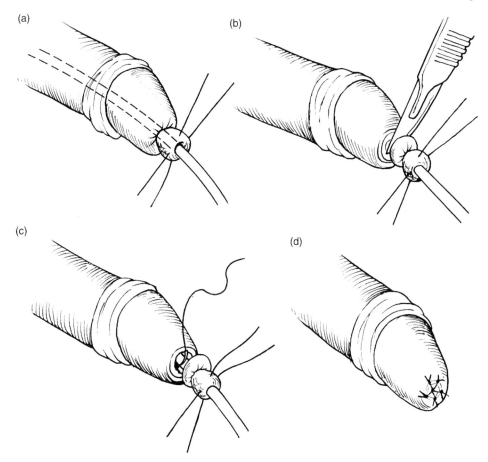

Figure 9.8 Surgical amputation of urethral prolapse. (a) A well-lubricated urinary catheter is inserted through the prolapse into the urinary bladder and two to four stay sutures are placed equidistant around the tip of the penis through the prolapsed urethral mucosa. (b) The base of the prolapsed mucosa is incised and (c) the urethral mucosa is sutured to the penile mucosa. (d) The catheter is then removed.

mucosa has been excised. The catheter is removed.

Castration is recommended. Recurrence is likely in dogs that remain intact. If recurrence of the prolapse occurs, reoperation is indicated, although for complicated cases with continual recurrence, partial penile amputation may be indicated. Treatment of any underlying problem such as urinary tract infection should be addressed.

Postoperative considerations and prognosis

Prevention of self-trauma is imperative and use of an Elizabethan collar is indicated for at least 2 weeks. Intermittent haemorrhage from the penis for the first week after surgery is likely, especially if the dog becomes excited. The dog should be re-evaluated 2 weeks after surgery. The prognosis is fair. Recurrence is most likely if castration is not performed.

The genital system

Prepubertal gonadectomy

There is considerable controversy over the indications and consequences of gonadectomy in very young, prepubescent puppies and kittens. Prepubertal gonadectomy refers to ovariohysterectomy or castration of puppies and kittens younger than 4 months of age, typically performed at 6–12 weeks of age. Recent investigation into the indications and consequences of prepubertal gonadectomy originates from the need for an effective pet population control method. Animal shelters currently experience very poor public compliance: typically only 40–60% of owners who adopt very young animals subsequently have their pets sterilized (Moulton, 1990; Alexander, 1994). From the breeders' perspective, prepubertal gonadectomy may be beneficial in controlling indiscriminate breeding of animals. The purchase of young, sterile, pet-quality animals may be especially attractive to the general public.

It must be remembered that there are health benefits of gonadectomy in addition to reproductive sterilization. Female dogs ovariohysterectomized before their first heat gain considerable protective benefit against the development of mammary neoplasia (Schneider *et al.*, 1969). This protective benefit is considerably reduced when ovariohysterectomy is delayed. Dogs ovariohysterectomized before their first heat have 0.5% the risk of an intact female dog for developing mammary cancer, after their first heat have 8% the risk, after two to three heats have 26% of the risk; and dogs ovariohysterectomized after four or more heats (or after 2.5 years of age) have the same risk as an intact female dog (Schneider *et al.*, 1969). Overall, a sexually intact female dog has three to seven times the risk of developing mammary cancer than an ovariohysterectomized dog (Johnston, 1991). Ovariohysterectomized females obviously have no risk of developing ovarian or uterine disease such as neoplasia or infection (pyometra).

Mammary tumours are the third most common tumour of the female cat, with nearly 90% of them malignant and often already spread to other body organs at the time of presentation to the veterinarian (Johnston, 1991). Although the protective effect of ovariohysterectomy is not as clear as it is in the dog, sexually intact female cats appear to be at seven times the risk of developing mammary cancer than the ovariohysterectomized cat.

In the male dog, the risk of developing prostatic disease, such as benign prostatic hypertrophy, prostatitis and cystic disease, is reduced by early castration. Treatment of prostatic disease is difficult and often associated with complications. Testicular tumours are the second most common tumour in the male dog. After neutering, the risk of testicular disease such as orchitis and neoplasia is obviously zero. For both the male and the female dog, the risk of transmitted venereal diseases such as transmissible venereal tumour and brucellosis (which affects other body systems besides the reproductive system) is reduced as sexual behaviour is reduced.

Purported contraindications for prepubertal gonadectomy include stunted growth, obesity, perivulval dermatitis, vaginitis, endocrine and dermatological changes, immunoincompetence, urethral obstruction, behavioural changes and anaesthetic risk (Bloomberg, 1996). It is important to realize that, while some of these conditions are related to gonadectomy, there is no evidence in the literature that prepubertal gonadectomy increases the risk of these conditions developing. In fact, several studies have shown that these problems are not related to prepubertal gonadectomy (Salmeri *et al.*, 1991a; 1991b; Bloomberg, 1996; Table 9.4).

Table 9.4 Considerations for prepubertal gonadectomy in the cat and dog

Purported contraindication	*Fact or fiction; advantage*	*Comment*
Anaesthetic risk greater in a young puppy or kitten	Fiction. There is minimal risk with appropriate precautions Advantages include shorter operative time, improved visibility of abdominal structures due to absence of fat and small size of organs, and rapid anaesthetic recovery (Bloomberg, 1996)	With consideration of physiological differences in the immature animal, surgery can be performed on young puppies and kittens with minimal risk (Grandy and Dunclop, 1991; Salmeri *et al.*, 1991a; Hosgood, 1992; Arohnson and Fagella, 1993; Fagella and Arohnson, 1993). Remember it is an elective procedure and should not be performed on a sick animal
Skeletal growth will be stunted	Fiction. Due to delayed physeal closure, bone length may be increased (Salmeri *et al.*, 1991a)	Testosterone and oestrogen, although not required, influence growth, maintenance and ageing of the skeleton (Salmeri *et al.*, 1991b). A deficiency of these hormones will delay growth-plate closure in dogs by an average of 9 weeks (Salmeri *et al.*, 1991a) and also delays closure in male and female cats (Bloomberg, 1996). Increased bone length was observed in male and female dogs gonadectomized at 7 weeks compared with dogs gonadectomized at 7 months. No difference was observed in cats (Bloomberg, 1996; Salmeri *et al.*, 1991a)
Early-gonadectomized animals are predisposed to obesity	Fiction. Clinically, ovariohysterectomized females and neutered males are apparently observed more often to be obese (Edney and Smith, 1986). Some experimental studies support this (Root *et al.*, 1996). However, the age of gonadectomy for dogs and cats does not appear to be a factor (Salmeri *et al.*, 1991a; Root and Johnston, 1995; Bloomberg, 1996; Root *et al.*, 1996) and obesity can be controlled by moderation of food intake (Le Roux, 1983)	Ovariohysterectomized dogs appear to be more likely to have indiscriminate appetite and will gain weight if fed ad lib (Houpt *et al.*, 1979; O'Farrell and Peachey, 1990). However, if fed a set amount, ovariohysterectomized dogs did not show any difference in food consumption or weight gain compared to intact female dogs (Le Roux, 1983). Gonadectomized male and female cats do show a decrease in metabolic rate compared with intact male and female cats (Root *et al.*, 1996) and may be at risk of obesity if fed indiscriminately (Root and Johnston, 1995; Root *et al.*, 1996).
Early-gonadectomized animals are less active and will change personality	Fiction. Studies report conflicting results. Activity and behaviour may be more influenced by environmental factors. Again, there is no evidence to support whether prepubertal gonadectomy increases the likelihood of changes	Dogs gonadectomized at 7 weeks and 7 months of age are equally as active as intact dogs, if not more so (Salmeri *et al.*, 1991a). Some investigators report gonadectomized animals actually retain immature puppy- or kitten-like behaviour which is obviously not consistent with inactivity (Lieberman, 1987). Trained ovariohysterectomized female police dogs were less aggressive than intact female dogs; however, their obedience, learning and skills were not changed (Le Roux, 1977). Other studies have found an increase in aggressive behaviour in ovariohysterectomized dogs (O'Farrell and Peachey, 1990).

Table 9.4 (continued)

Purported contraindication	Fact or fiction; advantage	Comment
		Prepubertal castration of the male dog usually eliminates mounting and copulatory behaviour (Johnston, 1991); however, it may not be totally eliminated. Castration after puberty will also reduce this behaviour but mounting and urine marking can still be noted
		Intact female dogs and cats show behavioural changes during whelping and kittening; however, there is no evidence that this makes them a better, more docile pet (Johnston, 1991)
		Prepubertal castration of male cats will reduce urine-spraying behaviour; however, approximately 10% of such cats may still spray urine, especially if housed with female cats (Hart and Cooper, 1984). Castrating adult cats reduces the behaviour also, with a similar percentage retaining the spraying behaviour. Approximately 5% of ovariohysterectomized cats will show urine-spraying behaviour, especially if housed with other cats. Age at ovariohysterectomy does not appear to be a factor (Hart and Cooper, 1984)
External genitalia will be underdeveloped	Fact. The vulva and mammary glands in female dogs and cats ovariohysterectomized at 7 months of age or earlier will be smaller. The penis and prepuce of male dogs and cats castrated at 7 months of age or earlier will be smaller. No clinical significance of these changes is reported. Prepubertal gonadectomy does not appear to cause greater changes in the female dog or cat, but does in the male dog and cat	Female dogs and cats that are ovariohysterectomized at 7 weeks and 7 months of age have a small, infantile vulva and smaller mammary glands and nipples compared with that of intact female dogs (Salmeri *et al.*, 1991a; Bloomberg, 1996). Castration at 7 weeks of age causes the most dramatic effect, with the prepuce, penis and os penis being much smaller than that of the intact male dog. Male dogs castrated at 7 months of age are less affected but the prepuce, penis and os penis are still smaller than those of intact male dogs (Salmeri *et al.*, 1991a). In the male cat, castration at 7 weeks of age causes an infantile appearance to the penis and prepuce with absence of penile spines. Castration at 7 months of age causes a similar infantile penis and prepuce but small penile spines are present (Bloomberg, 1996). The size of the penile urethra in the prepubertal castrated male cat is not different from that of the intact male cat and there is no predisposition to calculus formation or urethral obstruction

Table 9.4 (continued)

Purported contraindication	Fact or fiction; advantage	Comment
Gonadectomized animals will be urine-incontinent	Unclear. Hormone-responsive or stress-induced urinary incontinence is seen in gonadectomized dogs, weeks to years after surgery. While these animals may respond to oestrogen or testosterone supplementation, it has not been proven that hypo-oestrogenism or hypotestosteronism is actually the cause of the problem. Prepubertal gonadectomy does not appear to increase the risk of this problem (Salmeri *et al.*, 1991b)	In the male cat, there is no difference in urethral pressure profile parameters for intact cats or cats castrated at 7 weeks or 7 months of age (Bloomberg, 1996)
Early gonadectomy will stress the animal and reduce its immunological response to disease	Fiction. It must be remembered that gonadectomy is an elective procedure and can be delayed if an infectious challenge is present	There is no prospective study on this issue, however; anaesthesia and surgery will not affect the ability of a puppy to mount a good response to vaccination (Kelly, 1980)

Surgical technique

Ovariohysterectomy in the dog and cat (Table 9.5)

Table 9.5 Review of the surgical anatomy pertaining to ovariohysterectomy

Surgical anatomy
Each ovary lies caudal to a kidney, thus the right ovary is more cranial and more difficult to exteriorize
The suspensory ligament attaches the ovary to the body wall and courses craniodorsally from the ovary. It must be broken down in most dogs to allow adequate exposure of the ovary
The proper ligament of the ovary attaches it to the uterus. It is strong enough to be clamped with a haemostat and used to manipulate the ovary
The ovarian artery and vein are delicate and easily torn. They may be obscured by fat in older animals. They course almost straight dorsally from the exteriorized ovary
The broad ligament attaches the uterus to the dorsolateral body wall and the round ligament runs within the broad ligament. Caudally the round ligaments must be distinguished from the ureters
The uterine artery and vein lie lateral to the uterine body within the broad ligament
The ovarian pedicle includes the ovarian vessels and the fatty part of the broad ligament associated with the ovary

The animal should be prepared for aseptic abdominal surgery. The urinary bladder should be expressed prior to surgery. There are many ways to perform an ovariohysterectomy. The following description is one method preferred by the author using a midline coeliotomy approach. Many European veterinarians use a flank laparotomy approach which will not be described here. Ovariohysterectomy is performed through a midline coeliotomy with the skin incision made 1–2 centimetres caudal to the umbilicus, in the middle third of the distance between the xiphoid and pubis. In cats, the incision should be more caudal than for dogs because the uterine body is more caudal. The abdomen is entered through the linea alba. If the bladder has refilled, it should be emptied at this time by manual expression or cystocentesis. A large bladder obscures the field and increases the risk of ureteral trauma.

A uterine horn is most easily located by retracting the urinary bladder caudally and looking for the uterine horns dorsal to it. Once viewed, the uterus is retracted using a uterine hook. Alternatively, use of the uterine hook in a blinded fashion can be attempted by running it down the body wall, then turning the hooked end towards the midline once you reach the lumbar region. The hook is then withdrawn. This method does risk intestinal and ureteral trauma.

The uterine horn is followed cranially to the ovary. A haemostat can be placed on the proper ligament of the ovary to manipulate the ovary and its pedicle. Traction is placed on the ovary (or haemostat) to aid in identifying the suspensory ligament cranial to the ovary. The index finger is used to stretch the ligament laterally and caudally, forcing the ligament to tear as far as possible from the ovary. This should be controlled traction. Once the support of the suspensory ligament is gone, excessive traction on the ovarian pedicle is avoided. The artery and vein in the ligament may require ligation in dogs or cats in heat.

The ovary is exteriorized, the ovarian vessels are identified within the fat of the broad ligament and a window is made in the mesovarium, just caudal to the vessels using a finger or closed forceps. In very young animals, it is preferable to ligate the pedicle without forceps, placing a forcep across the pedicle only prior to severing it. Forceps are bulky and there is a temptation to use haemostats because the pedicles are small; haemostats should not be used as they are traumatic forceps and will tear the pedicle. For larger animals, a three-forceps technique can be used (Fig. 9.9). Two Carmalt forceps are placed across the ovarian pedicle, perpen-

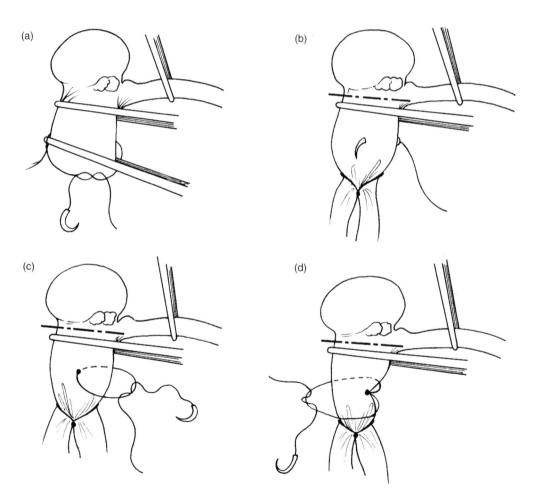

Figure 9.9 Three-clamp technique for ligation of the ovarian pedicle. Two Carmalt forceps are placed across the ovarian pedicle, perpendicular to the vessels, a third across the proximal uterine horn. (a) An encircling ligature is preplaced and then tied into the crushed tissue under the most proximal (bottom) ovarian forceps as the forceps is removed. (b–d) The second ligature is placed distal to (above) the first and, for larger animals, should be a transfixation ligature with two throws on the first side and four throws on the second. The ovarian pedicle is severed above the second forceps (d) and grasped with thumb forceps before release of the Carmalt forceps to allow observance for bleeding.

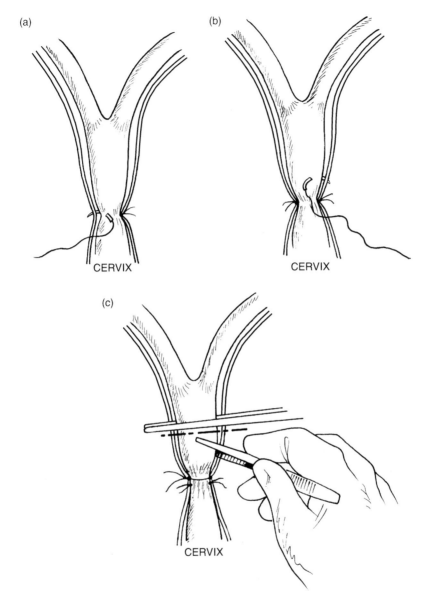

Figure 9.10 Transfixation ligation of the uterine body. (a) A needle is passed through the uterine body so that about one-quarter to one-third of the uterine body is incorporated in the ligature that then encircles the artery. This is repeated on the opposite side. (b) A transfixation ligature is then placed on the entire uterus, distal to the arterial ligatures. The needle is passed through the middle of the uterine body; two throws are tied on one side, the suture is then passed around the uterine body and four throws are tied on the other side. (c) Forceps are placed on the uterus prior to severance. The uterine body is grasped with thumb forceps and severed between the sutures and the clamp.

dicular to the vessels. One Carmalt is placed as low as practical and the second Carmalt is placed about 5–7 mm above the first, ensuring it is below the entire ovary. The haemostat on the proper ligament is replaced by a third Car-

malt that is placed across the proximal uterine horn. This forceps can be used for traction.

In very small animals a second encircling ligature can be placed distal to (above) the first ligature, below the second forceps. For larger animals, the second ligature should be a transfixation ligature. The ovarian pedicle is severed above the second forceps. The pedicle is grasped with thumb forceps before release of the Carmalt forceps and the pedicle is observed for bleeding as the tension is released and the pedicle is placed back in the abdomen. Once in the abdomen, the pedicle is released from the thumb forceps.

The uterine horn is held to identify the uterine artery in the broad ligament. The broad ligament is broken down digitally lateral to the artery to the level of the uterine body. From the uterine bifurcation, the other uterine horn can be identified and exteriorized. The ovarian pedicle is ligated as described.

The entire uterine body is then exteriorized until the bifurcation and cervix are visualized. The uterine ligatures are placed immediately proximal (above) to the cervix. In very small animals, one or two encircling ligatures will suffice. Forceps are not necessary. For larger animals, the uterine arteries are transfixed separately (Fig. 9.10). A needle is passed through the uterine body so that about one-quarter to one-third of the uterine body is incorporated in the ligature that then encircles the artery. A transfixation ligature is then placed on the entire uterus, distal to (above) the arterial ligatures. The needle is passed through the middle of the uterine body; two throws are tied on one side, the suture is then passed around the uterine body and four throws are tied on the other side. Forceps are placed on the uterus prior to severance. The uterine body is grasped with thumb forceps and severed between the sutures and the clamp. The stump is observed for haemorrhage and then released into the abdomen.

All pedicles should then be inspected for bleeding. Retract the duodenum to inspect the right paralumbar fossa. Retract the colon to inspect the left paralumbar fossa. Retract the urinary bladder to inspect the caudal abdomen. Place additional ligatures if needed. The abdomen is closed routinely.

Orchiectomy in the dog (Table 9.6)

Orchiectomy can be performed using an open or closed technique, that is, with the tunica vaginalis opened or left intact. For very young animals, the closed technique is appropriate. A potential complication of this technique is internal retraction of the testicular artery within the tunic so

Table 9.6 Review of the surgical anatomy pertaining to orchiectomy

Surgical anatomy
The testicle is immediately surrounded by the tunica albuginea, then the visceral and parietal vaginal tunics
The ligament of the tail of the epididymis attaches the testicular tunics to the scrotum caudally. It must be broken down with either open or closed castration to gain adequate exposure of the testis
The spermatic cord contains the ductus deferens, deferent artery and vein, testicular artery, pampiniform plexus, testicular nerve and lymphatics and is surrounded by the visceral and parietal tunics
The cremaster muscle is firmly attached to the outside of the parietal tunic of the spermatic cord

that it slips out of the ligature. The use of transfixation ligatures prevents this. For larger puppies and kittens, the open technique should be used to enable accurate and tight placement of ligatures on the spermatic vessels.

The prescrotal area is clipped and prepared for aseptic surgery. It is unnecessary to clip and prepare the scrotum (unless a scrotal ablation is being performed, which is rarely indicated in a prepubertal puppy). This avoids inducing scrotal dermatitis. Long scrotal hairs can be trimmed to avoid contamination of the surgical field.

One testicle is pushed from the scrotum into the prescrotal area. With the testicle held in place, an incision is made through the skin directly over the testicle on the ventral midline. Cutting over the testicle avoids inadvertently cutting into the penis if the skin incision is too deep. Once through the skin, the scalpel is lightly stroked through the subcutaneous tissue and spermatic fascia until the white fibrous parietal vaginal tunic is observed. Pressure is applied on either side of the testicle to force it through the incision and exteriorize it. A dry gauze sponge can be used to strip the ligament of the tail of the epididymis gently and to push fat and fascia around the spermatic cord proximally. The testicle and spermatic cord should then be completely exteriorized.

For a closed castration, an encircling ligature is placed around the spermatic cord, followed by a transfixation ligature 2 mm distal to it (Fig. 9.11). Carmalt forceps are placed at the level of transection, immediately distal to the

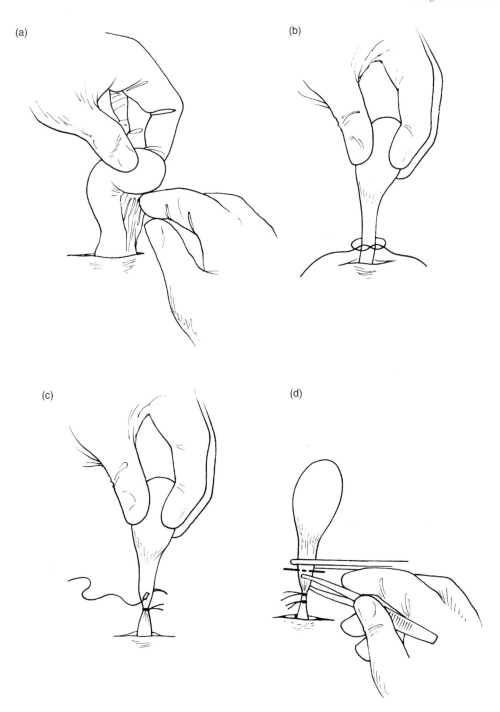

Figure 9.11 Closed castration technique. (a) After exposure of the testicle (without incision into the tunic vaginalis) through a midline, prescrotal incision, the ligament of the tail of the epididymis and any fat present is stripped from the spermatic cord to exteriorize the testicle. (b, c) An encircling ligature is placed around the spermatic cord, followed by a transfixation ligature 2 mm distal to it. Carmalt forceps are placed at the level of transection, immediately distal to the ligatures. (d) The spermatic cord is grasped with thumb forceps and severed distal to the sutures, against the forceps. The spermatic cord is observed for bleeding and gently replaced into the incision.

ligatures. The spermatic cord is grasped with thumb forceps and severed distal to the sutures, against the forceps.

For an open castration, the parietal tunic is opened and the structures to be ligated are identified (Fig. 9.12).

After ligation, the severed spermatic cord is replaced into the incision and the opposite testicle is now pushed into the skin incision. The procedure is repeated.

The subcutaneous tissue is closed, followed by an intradermal or subcuticular closure. Skin sutures are usually unnecessary and this avoids postoperative irritation.

Orchiectomy in the cat

There are multiple techniques for performing castration in the cat. The method described is that favoured by the author. The cat is anaesthetized and placed in dorsal or lateral recumbency. The hair on the scrotum is plucked. The region is prepared for aseptic surgery and the area is draped off to prevent contamination of surgical instruments or suture. A sterile latex glove with a small hole cut in it works well. The base of the scrotum is grasped to pull the testicle caudally. Two skin incisions are made, one over each testicle, in a ventrodorsal orientation and the

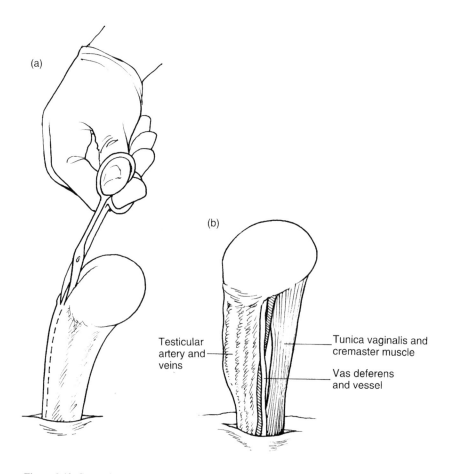

Figure 9.12 Castration using an open technique requires that the parietal tunic is incised with a scalpel over the body of the testicle after exteriorization of the testicle. (a) The incision in the parietal tunic is continued down the spermatic cord using Metzenbaum scissors. (b) The spermatic cord is then laid open and the testicular artery and vein (pampiniform plexus), the vas deferens and its vessels, and the tunic and the closely associated cremaster muscle are separated out, producing three structures that require ligation. Generally two ligatures are required for the spermatic artery and veins and one each for the vas deferens and associated vessel, and the tunica vaginalis and cremaster muscle.

testicle is popped out. Avoid cutting through the parietal tunic into the testicle. The testicle is exteriorized by stripping the spermatic fascia and fat from the parietal tunic as far cranially as possible. This allows the testicle to be pulled several centimetres from the body.

For closed orchiectomy, the testicle is held to keep the spermatic cord taut and a pair of closed curved haemostats held in the palm of the other hand are laid with the tips on top of the cord, pointing to one side (Fig. 9.13). The tips are then moved under the cord and tipped in the air as the testicle is passed underneath the haemostats and brought through the open tips of the haemostats. The spermatic cord is cut close to the edge of the haemostat, allowing remaining cord and testicle to be discarded. With the haemostat clamped, it is turned over and holding it by the box-locks (do not engage the rings of the forceps for risk of inadvertently releasing the spermatic cord), the loop of spermatic cord is slid off the tips of the haemostat to create a knot. The knot is pulled tight and the knotted spermatic cord is placed in the scrotum.

For open castration, the parietal tunic is incised and the ligament of the tail of the epididymis is bluntly separated. This allows the tunic to be detached from the testicle and replaced in the scrotal incision. The spermatic vessels and vas deferens can then be tied as one structure, as described in Figure 9.13. Alternatively, the ductus deferens is cut just proximal to the epididymis. The ductus and spermatic vessels are separated and tied to each other in two square knots (four throws). The spermatic cord distal to the knot is severed. This technique may risk tearing of the vessels in very young animals and is not recommended. The scrotum is allowed to heal by second intention.

After any technique, the scrotal incisions are left to heal by second intention.

Alternative methods for orchiectomy in the cat include using the haemostat to make a figure-of-eight knot or use of ligatures.

Hermaphroditism

Hermaphroditism or intersexuality is a disorder of sexual differentiation involving the chromosomes, gonads and phenotype (Table 9.7).

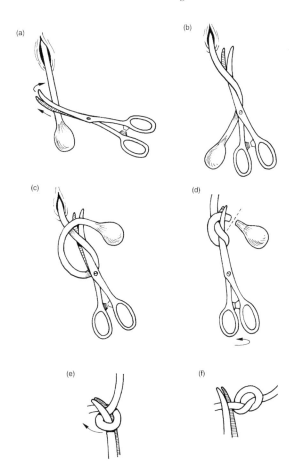

Figure 9.13 Closed castration of the cat. (a) After exteriorization of the testicle (within its tunic), the testicle is held to keep the spermatic cord taut and a pair of closed curved haemostats held in the palm of the other hand are laid with the tips pointing upward, on top of the cord, directed to one side. (b) The tips are then moved under the cord and tipped in the air. (c) The testicle is passed underneath the haemostats, over the spermatic cord and brought through the open tips of the haemostats. (d) The spermatic cord is cut close to the edge of the haemostat, allowing remaining cord and testicle to be discarded. With the haemostat clamped, it is turned over so the tips are pointing down (anti-clockwise). (e) Holding the haemostat by the fulcrum, the loop of spermatic cord is slid off the tips of the haemostat (arrow) to create a knot. (f) The knot is pulled tight and the knotted spermatic cord is placed in the scrotum.

Table 9.7 Disorders of sexual development in dogs (Meyers-Wallen and Patterson, 1989)

Abnormality	Comment
Abnormality of chromosomal sex	Usually not inherited
Abnormal number or structure of chromosomes	Abnormal chromosome number; XXY, XXX, XO syndromes
	Chimeras and mosaics (XX/XY, XX/XXY)
Abnormality of gonadal sex	XX Sex reversal is inherited as an autosomal recessive trait in American Cocker Spaniels; familial in Pugs, Beagles, Kerry Blue Terriers and Weimaraners, English Cocker Spaniels, German Short-haired Pointers
Sex reversal: chromosomal and gonadal sex disagree	
	XX sex reversal = XX Male (testis)
	XX sex reversal = XX True hermaphrodite (ovotestis)
	XY Sex reversal is not reported in dog
Abnormality of phenotypic sex	Female pseudohermaphrodite disorders in dog are usually of iatrogenic origin (exogenous androgens)
Chromosomal and gonadal sex agree but genitalia are ambiguous	
	Male pseudohermaphrodite disorders are frequently inherited
	(1) Persistent Müllerian duct syndrome inherited in Miniature Schnauzers
	(2) Defects in androgen-dependent masculinization e.g. hypospadias, suspected to be inherited in dogs
	Cryptorchidism. The mechanisms of inheritance are unclear but it is possibly a sex-limited autosomal recessive trait

Clinical signs and diagnosis

Intersex animals are usually recognized because of abnormalities in phenotypic sex or external genitalia. Animals with abnormalities of chromosomal sex often have other congenital anomalies and may not survive. With the exception of chimeras and mosaics (which have different tissues exhibiting different karyotypes: XX/XY or XX/XXY), the external genitalia may be underdeveloped but are usually phenotypically male or female. The animals are sterile (Meyers-Wallen and Patterson, 1989). The XXY syndrome is readily recognized in the tortoiseshell cat since the genes for orange and non-orange (black) are X-linked and usually only occur together in the normal female (Meyers-Wallen *et al.*, 1989). Hence a male tortoiseshell cat with both black and orange must be XXY. Definitive diagnosis of chromosomal abnormalities is based on examination of chromosomes and construction of a karyotype. The normal female dog has a 78,XX chromosome constitution, the normal male dog 78,XY. The normal female cat has 38,XX, the normal male cat 38,XY (Chastain, 1992). Karyotype testing can be performed on cultures of circulating lymphocytes, splenic lymphocytes, dermal fibroblasts or bone marrow (Chastain, 1992). Lymphocytes are most commonly used in the dog and cultured dermal fibroblasts are preferred for the cat (Chastain, 1992).

Animals with chromosomal sex and gonadal sex that do not agree are called sex-reversed. Only XX sex reversal is reported in the dog. Affected individuals have a 78,XX (female) chromosome pattern with testicular tissue and are termed XX males or XX true hermaphrodites. A true hermaphrodite has both ovarian and testicular tissue present in the gonads. The animals appear phenotypically as females with varying degrees of masculinization that is correlated with the amount of testicular tissue in the gonads. True hermaphrodites may have unilateral or bilateral ovotestes, oviducts or epididymes and normal or masculinized external genitalia (enlarged, protruding clitoris). They can sometimes reproduce as females. XX males have bilateral testes with epididymes, prostate and male external genitalia that is abnormal (hypoplastic penis, hypospadias, one or both testicles retained; Meyers-Wallen and Patterson, 1989).

A diagnosis of XX sex-reversed animals is usually suspected based on breed and physical findings of abnormal genitalia. Definitive diagnosis is based on chromosomal determination and histological examination of the internal genital tract (Sommer and Meyers-Wallen, 1991).

Animals with abnormalities of phenotypic sex have normal chromosomal and corresponding gonadal sex but the genitalia are ambiguous. Female pseudohermaphrodites are XX and have ovaries but the internal and external genitalia are masculinized, usually as a result of endogenous or exogenous androgen exposure. Female pseudohermaphroditism has been reported in the dog (Meyers-Wallen and Patterson, 1989; Olson *et al.*, 1989; Nemzek *et al.*, 1992). Clinical signs vary but the anogenital distance is generally elongated. The external genitalia may resemble a vulva but are ventral and cranial to the pubic symphysis or may resemble a prepuce but appear hypoplastic. A phallic-like structure is present and an os may be present. A scrotum may be present but is empty. The vagina/vestibule is usually abnormal but the urogenital tract proximal to the vaginovestibular junction can be normal. A prostate-like structure has been observed in some dogs, as has varying degrees of uterine fluid accumulation. Cystic ovaries and evidence of hyperoestrogenisim have been reported in one dog (Nemzek *et al.*, 1992). Although conception may be possible in these dogs, natural mating is impossible.

The male pseudohermaphrodite has testes but the internal and external genitalia are essentially female. This must be differentiated from XX sex reversal. Male pseudohermaphrodites include males with failure of Müllerian duct regression and males with insufficient androgen-dependent masculinization (hypospadias with hypoplasia of the penis, prepuce and scrotum and testicular feminization syndrome; Meyers-Wallen *et al.*, 1989). Persistent Müllerian duct syndrome is an inherited condition in Miniature Schnauzers (Marshall *et al.*, 1982). These dogs are XY males with bilateral testes and a complete uterus (Müllerian duct derivatives). The cranial horns are attached to the testes, which may be inguinal, scrotal or abdominal. The entire Wolffian duct system and prostate are present. The dogs are often cryptorchid but externally otherwise appear as males. Diagnosis is based on chromosomal determination and histological evaluation of the genital tract. The condition is usually not noticed until the dog develops Sertoli cell tumour or pyometra.

Male pseudohermaphrodites with defects in androgen-dependent masculinization include animals with hypospadias, testicular feminization syndrome and cryptorchidism.

Testicular feminization syndrome has been reported in the cat (Meyers-Wallen *et al.*, 1989). The case reported clearly characterizes the features of the syndrome. The cat appeared externally as a female but failed to develop signs of oestrus and was a normal 38,XY male. Although not performed, normal levels of serum testosterone for a male cat were expected. At ovariohysterectomy, two gonads, deemed histologically as testes, were located at the caudal poles of the kidneys but no uterus was found. Defective androgen receptors were demonstrated in fibroblast cultures from external genitalia skin. Although these animals are sterile and exhibit no clinical problems, testicular neoplasia can occur and gonadectomy is recommended (Meyers-Wallen *et al.*, 1989).

Cryptorchidism is also included as a defect of androgen-dependent masculinization since the mechanisms are poorly understood. Cryptorchidism is the most common developmental abnormality in the male dog (up to 13% of dogs) and is also recognized in the cat, although reported to a lesser degree (1.7–3.8%; Millis *et al.*, 1992; Richardson and Mullen, 1993).

In the dog, testicles should be within the scrotum by 10 days after birth. If the testicles are not within the scrotum by 8 weeks of age, a diagnosis of cryptorchidism is warranted. Toy and miniature dog breeds appear overrepresented, including the Miniature and Toy Poodle, Yorkshire Terrier, Pomeranian, Miniature Dachshund, Shetland Sheepdog, English Bulldog, Miniature Schnauzer, Pekinese, Cairn Terrier, Chihuahua and Maltese Terrier (Meyers-Wallen and Patterson, 1989). It appears to be an inherited condition, possibly by sex-limited autosomal recessive inheritance. Affected dogs are carriers and should not be bred (Meyers-Wallen and Patterson, 1989). Carrier parents (heterozygous) and littermates should be removed from the breeding population also.

In the cat, the testicles should be in the scrotum at birth, although they may move up and down the inguinal ring until they remain permanently in the scrotum by 10–14 weeks of age. Mixed-bred cats are presented with cryptorchidism most often, however; the Persian breed appears overrepresented (Millis *et al.*, 1992; Richardson and Mullen, 1993). Cryptorchidism in cats is thought to be of a sex-linked inheritance.

Diagnosis of cryptorchidism is made on physical examination. Despite the unlikelihood of descent after 8–14 weeks, definitive diagnosis is often left until 6 months of age. If one or both testicles are absent from the scrotum, a thorough palpation of the inguinal regions should be made. This is best performed with the animal on its back. Cryptorchidism and monorchidism (absence of one testicle in the scrotum) have been reported in the cat (Millis *et al.*, 1992; Richardson and Mullen, 1993). The apparent absence of testicles (questionable previous castration) in a male cat that has penile spines should arouse suspicion of cryptorchidism (Richardson and Mullen, 1993). If the testicles cannot be palpated, abdominal retention is suspected. Abdominal testicles cannot be detected (unless significantly enlarged by neoplasia in an older dog) by abdominal palpation. Inguinal palpation can be unreliable due to presence of fat in the area (especially cats) and the occasion that the inguinal testicle lies within the inguinal ring itself (Richardson and Mullen, 1993).

Human chorionic gonadotrophin stimulation test can be used to detect elevated testosterone levels in animals where cryptorchidism is suspected but a testicle is not palpated or the history of the animal is unknown. However, plasma concentrations of testosterone and oestradiol do not differ among unilateral inguinal cryptorchids, unilateral abdominal cryptorchids and normal dogs (Romagnoli, 1991).

Treatment and surgical technique

The treatment of choice for any animal with sexual ambiguity is neutering; for XX sex-reversed animals, female pseudohermaphrodites and male pseudohermaphrodites with abdominal gonads, this requires gonadectomy and excision of the genital tract to the level of the cervix in the effort to reduce the chance of infection of any remaining tract. If the genital tract appears pus- or fluid-filled at the time of surgery, the genital tract should be removed below the level of the cervix to avoid leaving an infected segment proximal to a closed cervix. The cut edge of the genital tract should not be oversewn but should be lavaged with normal saline before abdominal closure. For male pseudohermaphrodites with external gonads, routine castration can be performed.

Medical (human chorionic gonadotrophin or gonadotrophin-releasing hormone) and surgical (orchiopexy) attempts to induce testicular descent in cryptorchid animals should be discouraged and is ethically questionable since these animals are carriers of a genetic flaw. The efficacy of medical attempts is questionable anyway (Romagnoli, 1991). Castration is indicated, not only to prevent breeding but also to reduce the risk of later disease. Retained testicles have a greater likelihood of neoplastic development and associated secondary changes (skin changes, bone marrow suppression) and testicular torsion (Romagnoli, 1991). No cryptorchid has been reported as fertile and monorchid dogs, while fertile, probably have reduced fertility.

For castration of cryptorchid males, both testes should be removed. For obvious inguinal testes, two small inguinal incisions can be made to access the testes or, not infrequently, they can be manipulated to the midline location for a routine approach. The recommended surgical approach in animals in which the location of the testicles is uncertain is initially a caudal ventral midline skin incision to expose both inguinal rings. If the spermatic cord is seen exiting the inguinal ring, it can be traced to the location of the testicle. If no spermatic cord is visualized, the abdomen is opened via a caudal midline incision in the linea alba. The incision must be large enough to visualize the location of the testicle; blind fishing with a spay hook may risk ureteral damage.

The testicles will be located somewhere between the kidney and the inguinal ring. Look for the spermatic cord. The vas deferens is the most obvious part of the spermatic cord since the vessels originate at the kidney and can be more confusing to trace. The vas deferens is easiest to trace back from the prostate. The testicles are often located near the urinary bladder. Occasionally a testicle cannot be found external to the inguinal ring but it appears to enter the internal inguinal ring. Gently pull on

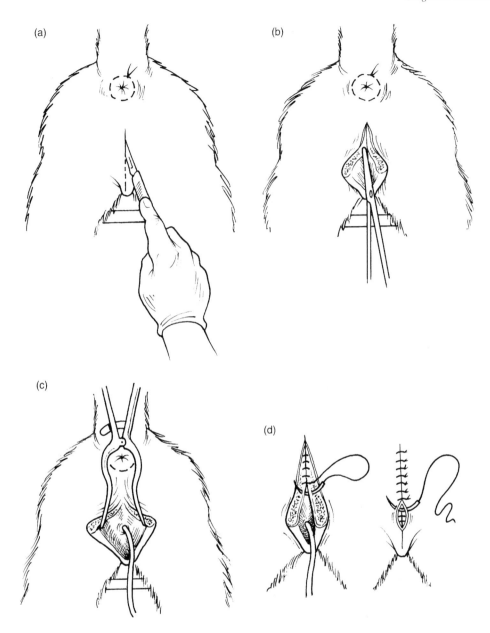

Figure 9.14 Episiotomy. (a) A midline, full-thickness skin incision through the perineal skin ventral to the anus. (b) The vaginal mucosa and muscle are then cut using scissors, from the ventral to the dorsal aspect. (c) The urethral meatus should now be identified and catheterized with a sterile cuffed urethral catheter. (d) The episiotomy is closed in three layers – the vaginal mucosa, the vaginal muscle and the skin. Interrupted or continuous suture patterns are acceptable.

the spermatic cord as the testicle may be lodged within the ring. These testicles are often small and misshapen and easily missed. Always submit the testicles for histological examination to confirm their identity and evaluate for pathology. Ligation of the spermatic cord and closure

of the abdominal and skin incisions are routine.

No initial surgical treatment is indicated for XX sex-reversed dogs or female pseudohermaphrodites with a protruding enlarged clitoris. The clitoris will usually regress after gonadectomy. In the meantime, it should be protected from self-trauma and kept clean and moist to prevent desiccation. At least 4–6 weeks should be allowed to observe for regression. Occasionally regression is not adequate, especially if an os is present, or trauma occurs such that clitorectomy is required. Episiotomy may facilitate exposure of the clitoris as visualization of the urethral orifice is imperative during the procedure to prevent inadvertent trauma.

For episiotomy, the dog is prepared for aseptic perineal surgery. The vagina is lavaged prior to surgery. A midline, full-thickness incision through the perineal skin and vaginal muscle and mucosa is performed at the dorsal aspect of the vagina, ventral to the anus (Fig. 9.14). The length of this incision should only be adequate to expose the clitoris. Haemorrhage is often profuse from this area and electrocoagulation may facilitate haemostasis and visualization. The urethral meatus should now be identified and catheterized with a sterile cuffed urethral catheter. An elliptical incision is made around the base of the clitoris and it is dissected free. The vaginal mucosa is sutured closed using 4-0 monofilament absorbable sutures. The episiotomy is closed in three layers – the vaginal mucosa and vaginal muscle using 4-0 monofilament absorbable suture in a continuous pattern, and the skin using 4-0 or 5-0 monofilament non-absorbable suture.

Postoperative considerations and complications

Prevention of self-trauma is necessary in some animals, especially for those requiring clitorectomy. The prognosis for normal function for animals after gonadectomy is excellent.

Persistent penile frenulum

In the immature dog, the penis and prepuce are joined ventrally by a fine band of connective tissue (frenulum) which normally ruptures by puberty. Occasionally, the separation may be incomplete and the frenulum persists.

Clinical signs and diagnosis

Pain may be evident during sexual excitement or when an attempt is made to extrude the penis. Ventral deviation and observation of the frenulum are made during attempted extrusion.

Treatment and surgical technique

Surgical excision of the frenulum is indicated.

Postoperative considerations and prognosis

The prognosis is excellent.

Hypospadias

Hypospadias is the most common developmental anomaly of the male dog external genitalia and is the result of failure of fusion of the urogenital folds with incomplete formation of the penis and penile urethra. This results in the external urethral orifice opening on the ventral surface of the penis anywhere between the ischial arch and the normal opening. Classification can be made according to the location of the urethral opening: glandular, penile, scrotal and perineal (Ader and Hobson, 1978; Fig. 9.15). Occasionally preputial hypoplasia may occur without any penile anomaly (Pope and Swaim, 1986).

Clinical signs

Generally, the anomaly is obvious. In addition, there may be urine soaking of the hair and skin on the ventrum which may be associated

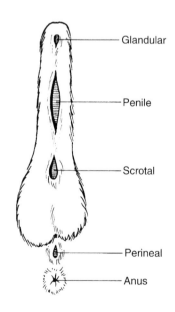

Figure 9.15 Types of hypospadias.

with a foul odour. Urinary incontinence is not usually a clinical feature.

Diagnosis

Diagnosis is by visual inspection of the penis. It is important to examine the animal for the presence of other concurrent anomalies.

Treatment and surgical technique

The surgical technique required depends on the degree of hypospadias. Preputial reconstruction may be indicated in glandular hypospadias or preputial hypoplasia (Ader and Hobson, 1978; Pope and Swaim, 1986). Preputial reconstruction has also been reported for traumatic loss of the cranial portion of the prepuce (Fig. 9.16) (Smith and Gourley, 1990). It is important in the reconstruction of the prepuce that the mucosal integrity of the lining of the prepuce is preserved. For small defects, the lateral skin and mucosa can be mobilized and closed on the midline in two layers, with the orifice of the prepuce being extended cranially (Ader and Hobson, 1978). This may be ineffective for some defects (Pope and Swaim, 1986) and more aggressive reconstruction may be required. This requires both mucosal and skin reconstruction. For larger defects, a free autogenous, oral mucosal graft from the buccal area can be harvested and used to create a preputial lining, either as a staged procedure (Pope and Swaim, 1986) or at the time of the skin reconstruction (Smith and Gourley, 1990). Reconstruction of the prepuce has been described using local advancement flaps (Pope and Swaim, 1986) or axial pattern flaps based on the caudal superficial epigastric artery (Smith and Gourley, 1990). Staged procedures may be required.

Castration of puppies with hypospadias should be recommended and can be performed at the same time as reconstructive surgery.

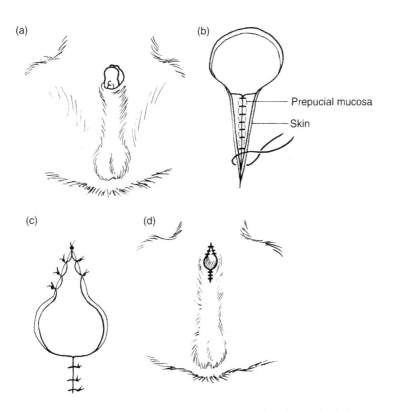

Figure 9.16 (a) Closure of glandular hypospadias. (b) The edges of the defect are trimmed and the defect is closed ventrodorsally in two layers (preputial mucosa and skin). (c, d) The cranial aspect of the orifice is then extended; a full-thickness incision is made and then the mucosa is apposed to the skin edge along each side.

For penile, scrotal and perineal hypospadias, urethrostomy is required. If the urethral opening is distal to the scrotum or at the level of the scrotum (penile or scrotal hypospadias), castration and scrotal urethrostomy can be performed. For perineal hypospadias, a perineal urethrostomy should be performed. Concurrent castration is also recommended. The urethral groove and remnants of the prepuce and penis are excised.

Scrotal urethrostomy

The scrotal urethrostomy is the site of choice for a urethral stoma because the urethra is most superficial at this point, has a large diameter and creates a stoma in a dependent site which prevents urine scalding.

The puppy is positioned in dorsal recumbency and prepared for aseptic surgery. A sterile urinary catheter should be passed intraoperatively if possible. If obstruction precludes passing a catheter it can be placed after the urethrotomy incision. An elliptical skin incision is made around the base of the scrotum and the skin is completely excised. Castration is performed. This will expose the penis. The retractor penis muscle is dissected from the ventral surface and sutured laterally to the subcutaneous tissue. This should expose the corpus spongiosum with the urethra directly dorsal (the catheter should be palpable; Fig. 9.17). A midline penile incision into the corpus spongiosum and urethra is made using a number 11 scalpel blade. The length of the incision should be a minimum of 10 mm and up to 20 mm, depending on the size of the puppy. The tunica albuginea (which covers the corpus cavernosum) can be sutured to the subcutaneous fascia to minimize haemorrhage from the penile tissue. Alterna-

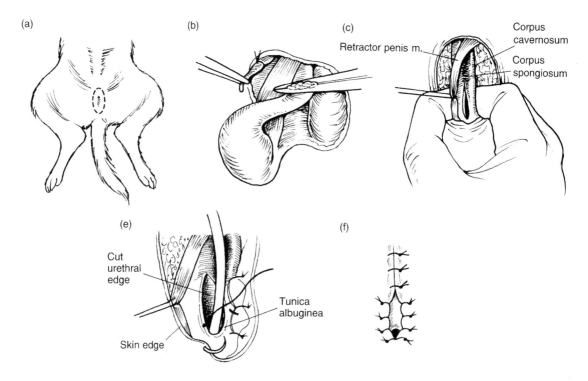

Figure 9.17 Scrotal urethrostomy. (a) An elliptical skin incision is made around the base of scrotum and the skin is completely excised. (b) The testicles are exposed and castration is performed. (c) The penis should be subsequently exposed and the retractor penis muscle is dissected from the ventral surface and sutured laterally to the subcutaneous tissue. The underlying corpus spongiosum with the urethra directly dorsal (the catheter should be palpable) and the lateral corpus cavernosum are exposed. A midline penile incision into the corpus spongiosum and urethra is made using a number 11 scalpel blade and extended with sharp scissors if necessary. (d) The tunica albuginea (which covers the corpus cavernosum) can be sutured to the subcutaneous fascia to minimize haemorrhage from the penile tissue. (e) The urethral mucosa is then sutured to the skin. The remainder of the skin incision is closed routinely.

tively, the tunica albuginea can be incorporated in the simple interrupted sutures (4-0 or 5-0 monofilament, absorbable) that approximate the urethral mucosa to the skin. The remainder of the skin incision is closed routinely.

Perineal urethrostomy

The perineal site is less desirable for a permanent stoma because the urethra is deep and urine extravasation into tissues may be a problem, in addition to urine scald. More penile tissue must be incised to reach the urethra and postoperative bleeding can be a problem.

For the perineal urethrostomy, the puppy is placed in sternal recumbency, or dorsal recumbency with the legs flexed forwards. A pursestring is placed in the anus to prevent intraoperative contamination. A sterile urinary catheter should be passed intraoperatively. A midline perineal skin incision is made midway between anus and scrotum. The subcutaneous tissue is dissected until the retractor penis muscle is identified. It is elevated and retracted laterally. The bulbospongiosum muscles are separated along their median raphe to expose corpus spongiosum penis. A midline penile incision is made into the corpus spongiosum and urethra. The tunica albuginea (which covers the corpus cavernosum) can be sutured to the subcutaneous fascia to minimize haemorrhage from the penile tissue and reduce tension on the urethra to skin suture line. The urethral mucosa is then sutured (4-0 or 5-0 monofilament, non-absorbable) in a simple interrupted pattern to the skin, starting with the most proximal sutures (2 and 10 o'clock), and finishing with the two most distal sutures (5 and 7 o'clock). The remainder of the skin incision is closed routinely.

Table 9.8 Postoperative considerations after penile or urethrostomy surgery

Consideration	Comment
Self-trauma	Protection of surgical site imperative
	Elizabethan collars recommended
Indwelling urethral catheters	Should not be used as they cause irritation of the stoma site and promote stricture
	Catheter predisposes animal to ascending urinary tract infection
Haemorrhage	Expected during urination or excessive excitement and can continue for 1–2 weeks
	Monitor haematocrit as decreases of up to 10% can be recorded
	Topical cold therapy can be applied
	Tranquilization (low-dose phenothiazine) may be indicated
	Attempts to remove clots from the stoma site should be avoided as later urine flow usually dislodges the clot
Urine scald	More likely after perineal urethrostomy
	Application of a water-repellent ointment (petroleum jelly) to the skin surrounding the stoma is beneficial in preventing urine scald
Urine extravasation	Extravasation into the tissues is the result of poor urethral mucosa-to-skin apposition
	Severe tissue inflammation and necrosis can occur
Suture removal	If non absorbable suture is used, sedation is recommended to allow atraumatic suture removal and careful examination of the urethrostomy site. Alternatively, absorbable suture can be used
Ascending urinary tract infection	May be more common in animals after urethrostomy due to loss of normal urethral defence mechanisms
	Attention to urination patterns and colour (increased frequency, blood-tinged urine) as early signs of urinary tract infection is important
	Regular long-term monitoring (urinalysis) may be indicated
Stricture	Long-term complication, generally as a result of poor technique
	Surgical revision may be necessary

Postoperative considerations and complications

Postoperative considerations after preputial reconstruction require prevention of self-mutilation. Suture line dehiscence or graft failure may occur and should be treated appropriately; however, if surgery is successful, normal urinary function is likely.

Postoperative considerations after urethrostomy are listed in Table 9.8.

Phimosis

Phimosis is the inability to protrude the penis beyond the preputial orifice. It may be congenital or secondary to scarring following trauma (Table 9.9).

Clinical signs

Congenital phimosis is usually associated with a distended prepuce full of urine and the inability to urinate normally. The preputial orifice appears abnormally small. Urine may pass in drops or a small stream. Retention of urine in the prepuce may induce balanoposthitis with varying degrees of ulceration and necrosis of the prepuce.

Diagnosis

Diagnosis is based on physical examination, clinical signs and the inability to extrude the penis. Sedation may be required for complete examination.

Table 9.9 Definition and characteristics of selected penile and preputial disorders of puppies and kittens

Disorder	Definition	Clinical signs and characteristic features
Persistent frenulum	Persistence of the immature connective tissue bands between the penis and the prepuce	Ventral deviation and presence of frenulum noticed during attempted extrusion of penis
		Pain during sexual excitement or when penis is extruded
Hypospadias	Anomaly of the male external genitalia resulting from failure of fusion of the urogenital folds with incomplete formation of the penis and penile urethra	External urethral orifice opens on the ventral surface of the penis, anywhere between the ischial arch and the normal opening
		Prepuce hypoplastic or incomplete. Classified as glandular, penile, scrotal and perineal based on location of urethral opening
		Urinary incontinence is not usually a clinical feature
Phimosis	Inability to protrude the penis beyond the preputial orifice	Distended prepuce with urine
		Urine dripping from prepuce
		Balanoposthitis
		Inability to extrude penis manually
Paraphimosis	Inability for the extruded penis to be replaced in the preputial sheath	Small preputial orifice or constricting hairs surrounding the preputial orifice. Occasionally, there is no preputial lesion but the tip of the penis is exposed
		The penis may be congested, discoloured or traumatized
		Severe damage and necrosis can occur after prolonged exposure
		Penis cannot be manually replaced in the prepuce
Priapism	Persistent erection of the penis not associated with sexual excitement	Penis can be manually retracted into the prepuce but will not stay in its normal position
		Penis may become congested, dry and necrotic
		There is no constricting preputial lesion and the penis can easily be reduced into the prepuce if secondary penile lesions have not developed

Treatment and surgical technique

Surgical reconstruction of the prepuce to enlarge the orifice is performed. With the animal in dorsal recumbency, the prepuce is prepared for aseptic surgery. A full-thickness wedge of preputial skin is taken from the dorsal or ventral aspect of the prepuce (Fig. 9.18). Dorsal meatotomy is less likely to expose the penis and is usually recommended. Ventral meatotomy sacrifices ventral support and subsequent coverage of the penis and may be more useful when there is redundant preputial skin. The size of the wedge depends on the degree of preputial stenosis, the size of the dog and the distance of the glans penis from the preputial orifice. As much tissue as possible is removed but the penis must remain covered. The cut edge of the skin is then sutured to the preputial mucosa using 4-0 or 5-0 monofilament, non-absorbable suture in a simple interrupted pattern.

An alternative technique to wedge resection is to resect the end of the prepuce. This technique is indicated if the constricting lesion does not extend beyond the tip of the prepuce. The preputial skin and mucosa are sutured using simple interrupted sutures of 4-0 or 5-0 monofilament non-absorbable suture.

Postoperative considerations and prognosis

Postoperative considerations include prevention of self-trauma. In general, the prognosis for normal urination is good.

Paraphimosis

Paraphimosis is the inability for the extruded penis to be replaced in the preputial sheath (Table 9.9). It is generally seen following coitus, trauma or masturbation and is often observed in young male dogs. A small preputial orifice or constricting hairs surrounding the preputial orifice may prevent complete penile retraction. Occasionally, there is no preputial lesion but the tip of the penis remains exposed.

Clinical signs

Clinical signs are variable, depending on the duration of paraphimosis. The exteriorized penis becomes congested and discoloured and may be traumatized by the dog licking the penis. Severe damage and penile necrosis can result from prolonged exposure.

Diagnosis

Diagnosis is based on physical examination. Sedation may be required for complete examination. The penis cannot be physically returned to the prepuce in its presenting state and as such the condition can be differentiated from priapism, thrombosis of the cavernosus tissue or veins and preputial or retractor penis muscle pathology. When the penis reduces easily, mechanical, vascular or neural causes should be suspected.

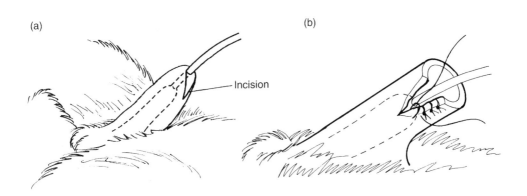

(a)   (b)   Incision

Figure 9.18 Surgical correction of phimosis. (a) A full-thickness wedge of prepuce is excised from the dorsal aspect and (b) the skin and preputial mucosa apposed with simple interrupted or simple continuous sutures.

Treatment and surgical technique

Immediate measures to return the penis to the prepuce may be attempted. After gentle cleansing of the penis, lubricants, hyperosmolar solutions and local cold therapy can be applied to the penis while attempts to push the penis caudally as the prepuce is drawn cranially are made. Any constricting hairs should be trimmed prior to these attempts.

If these attempts fail, temporary or permanent surgical enlargement of the preputial orifice (preputiotomy) is indicated. With the animal in dorsal recumbency, the prepuce and penis are carefully cleansed and prepared for aseptic surgery. A full-thickness incision through the preputial skin, subcutaneous tissue and dorsal preputial mucosa is made on the median raphe of the dorsal surface of the prepuce, beginning at the preputial orifice and extending caudally. The penis is returned to the prepuce and the incision closed carefully in three layers. The mucosa and subcutaneous tissue should be closed with 4-0 or 5-0 monofilament absorbable suture. The skin is closed routinely. Closure must be meticulous to prevent preputial orifice stricture. If a constricted preputial orifice was deemed as the cause of paraphimosis, then a full-thickness wedge of skin from the dorsal or ventral aspect of the prepuce can be excised (as for phimosis; Fig. 9.18). The specific cause of the paraphimosis should be addressed. Long-standing cases of paraphimosis may require partial penile amputation.

For those cases where there is no preputial lesion but the tip of the penis remains exposed, preputial advancement can be performed. A crescent-shaped incision is made in the skin cranial to the prepuce and the preputial muscles are imbricated or preferably partially resected (Fig. 9.19). The crescent-shaped defect is sutured in two layers (subcutaneous tissue and skin), thereby pulling the prepuce cranially. If there appears to be a ventrocaudal preputial orifice defect, the edges of the defect can be debrided and the preputial mucosa and skin closed as previously described. Care must be exercised in closing a preputial orifice so that phimosis does not occur.

Postoperative considerations and prognosis

Postoperative considerations include prevention of self-trauma. In general, the prognosis is fair since recurrence is not uncommon. Castration should be considered in recurrent cases. Paraphimosis with a deficient prepuce may require partial penile amputation.

Priapism

Priapism is persistent erection of the penis not associated with sexual excitement. It can be differentiated from paraphimosis in that the penis can be manually retracted into the prepuce but will not stay in its normal position. The penis often becomes congested, dry and eventually may become necrotic. Causes of priapism vary but include genitourinary infection, spinal cord trauma and constipation. It has been observed post general anaesthesia, after the use of phenothiazine tranquillizers (especially in the horse) and post-castration in the cat (Swalec and Smeak, 1989). Many cases are deemed idiopathic.

Priapism is classified as low-flow ischaemic or high-flow ischaemic, depending on whether the failure of detumescence is caused by haemostasis or disturbances in the neuroarterial reflex, or by increased arterial supply, respectively.

(a)   (b)   (c)

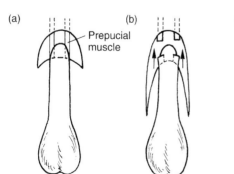
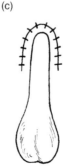

Prepucial muscle

Figure 9.19 Surgical advancement of the prepuce. (a) A crescent-shaped incision is made in the skin cranial to the prepuce. (b) The preputial muscles are partially resected. (c) The defect is sutured in two layers (subcutaneous tissue and skin), thereby pulling the prepuce cranially.

Clinical signs and diagnosis

Clinical signs are similar to paraphimosis except that there is no constricting preputial lesion and the penis can easily be reduced into the prepuce. However, note that if the penis has become severely congested or traumatized, it may not be able to be replaced in the prepuce.

Treatment and surgical technique

Treatment should be directed at remedying the primary cause, if this can be identified. In the case of phenothiazine-induced priapism in horses, administration of benztropine (an anticholinergic drug that is a combination of the active portions of atropine and diphenhydramine; Wilson *et al.*, 1983) could be tried but has not been shown successful for other causes of priapism in dogs and cats.

Topical therapy to reduce oedema and prevent desiccation can be attempted, as for paraphimosis. Surgical treatment to remove sequestered blood and establish venous drainage from the corpora cavernosa penis to the corpora spongiosa penis is used in humans. α-Adrenergic agents may be instilled into the corpora cavernosa penis in the early stages of priapism to recover cavernous and arterial smooth-muscle contractility.

Often, unless the cause can be identified, salvage procedures such as penile amputation and perineal urethrostomy are necessary (Swalec and Smeak, 1989).

Penile amputation

Indications for penile amputation include neoplasia, severe trauma to the penis or prepuce, persistent paraphimosis and unresponsive priapism. In the dog, penile amputation may be performed at varying levels and the requirement for urethrostomy depends on the length of penis remaining. In the cat, penile amputation with perineal urethrostomy is the only option.

The dog is placed in dorsal recumbency and the penis, prepuce and surrounding skin are cleaned and prepared for aseptic surgery. The penis is extruded if necessary and a sterile urinary catheter is placed. A tourniquet is placed caudal to the level of amputation (Fig. 9.20). If the penis cannot be extruded, a ventral midline incision in the prepuce can be made to expose the penis. Two lateral flaps in the penile tissue are created at the level of amputation. The os penis and the urethra must be preserved. The os penis is dissected and transected as far caudally as possible using bone cutters. The urethra, which must be dissected free from the groove in the os penis using a small periosteal elevator, is transected just distal to the level of amputation. Transection of the urethra can be performed without removal of the catheter but one or two stay sutures should be placed in the urethra prior to transection. The tourniquet is loosened and the dorsal artery of the penis is ligated using 4-0 monofilament, absorbable suture. The urethra is incised longitudinally on its ventral midline and the urethral mucosa is sutured to the tunica albuginea of the penis using 4-0 or 5-0

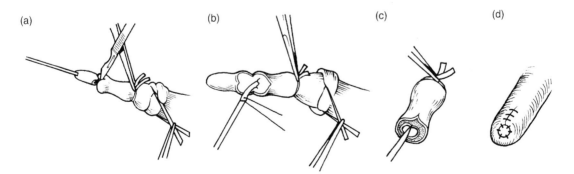

Figure 9.20 Partial penile amputation. (a) Two lateral flaps in the penile tissue are created at the level of amputation. (b) The urethra is dissected free from the groove in the os penis and transected distal to the level of penile amputation; the os penis is transected as far caudally as possible using bone cutters. The tourniquet is loosened and the dorsal artery of the penis is ligated. (c, d) The urethra is incised longitudinally on its ventral midline and the urethral mucosa is sutured to the tunica albuginea of the penis using simple interrupted sutures. The dorsal aspect of the penile flaps should be sutured together.

monofilament absorbable simple interrupted sutures. The sutures should pass through some of the cavernosus tissue to reduce postoperative haemorrhage. The dorsal aspect of the penile flaps should be sutured together. A simple interrupted or simple continuous pattern is suitable; a simple continuous pattern may be more effective in controlling haemorrhage from the penile tissue.

The prepuce may require shortening to prevent urine pooling in the prepuce. A full-thickness section of preputial skin and mucosa is resected (Fig. 9.21).

For penile amputation at the level caudal to the os penis, the skin incision extends from cranial to the prepuce to caudal to the scrotum. The penis is amputated as above, except that the cut end of the penis is ligated and the penile flaps are sutured together. A urethrostomy is created in the scrotal region as described previously.

Penile amputation and perineal urethrostomy in the cat

Penile amputation and perineal urethrostomy in the cat can be regarded as a salvage procedure for penile lesions but are also indicated to relieve obstruction of the penile urethra. Complications, particularly bacterial urinary tract infection, have led to investigation of the basic surgical procedure. The basic surgical procedure for perineal urethrostomy adopted by most veterinary surgeons was originally described by Wilson and Harrison (1971). The description below includes the author's interpretation of these modifications (Hosgood and Hedlund, 1992).

The cat is placed in sternal recumbency with the perineum elevated and the perineal area prepared for aseptic surgery. A pursestring suture (3-0 or 4-0) is placed in the anus to prevent faecal contamination. The penis is extruded and, if possible, the urethra is catheterized perioperatively to allow later identification of the urethra (Fig. 9.22). An elliptical incision is made to excise the scrotum and prepuce. Avoid excision of excessive perineal skin; additional skin can be removed prior to closure if necessary. The spermatic cords are exposed in the intact male cat and castration is performed. Scrotal vessels are ligated or electrocoagulated. The dorsal artery of the penis may be apparent and must be ligated. Attention to haemostasis is imperative to allow accurate visualization of structures during the procedure.

Allis tissue forceps are used to clamp the end of the prepuce to the catheter to aid in mobilization of the penis. The penis is reflected dorsolaterally first to one side, and then to the other, to allow sharp dissection of the loose tissue surrounding the penis. This dissection extends laterally and ventrally towards the penile attachments at the ischial arch. The dissection should be external to the crus of the penis to avoid damage to the covering ischiocavernosus muscle and subsequent haemorrhage. The penis is then elevated dorsally to allow sharp dissection and severance of the ventral penile ligament. The ischiocavernosus and ischiourethralis muscles are closely associated with each other and can be palpated ventrolaterally extending from the penis to the ischium. These should be sharply transected close to their insertion on the ischium to avoid damage to branches of the pudendal nerves. If possible, branches of the pudendal nerves should be identified and preserved during any further sharp dissection that is required to free the ventral penis from the pelvic floor.

The penis is then reflected ventrally to expose the dorsal surface. The bulbospongiosus muscle is evident on the dorsal surface. Minimal sharp dissection external to these muscles is required to expose the bulbourethral glands slightly proximal and dorsal to the bulbospongiosus muscle and cranial to the severed ischiocavernosus and ischiourethralis muscles. Although there appears to be no difference in the effect of

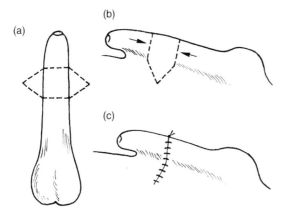

Figure 9.21 Preputial shortening. (a, b) A full-thickness section of prepuce is excised. (c) The prepuce is reconstructed by suturing the mucosa and skin in separate layers.

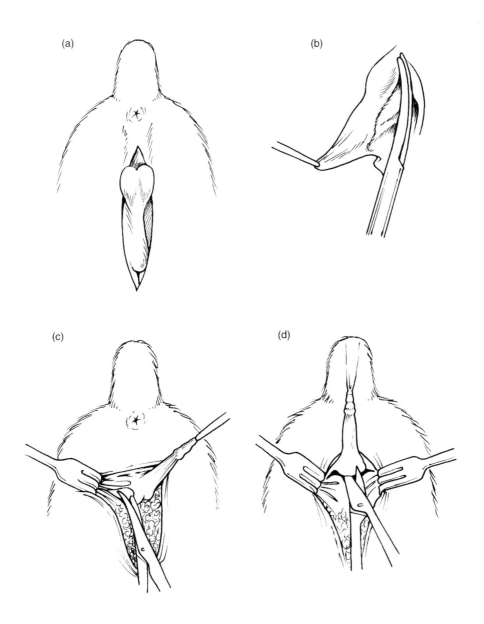

(a)

(b)

(c)

(d)

Figure 9.22 *continued on following page*

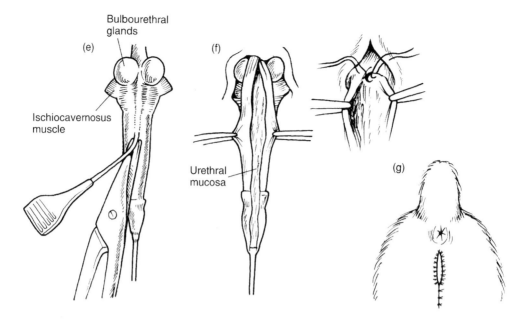

Figure 9.22 Perineal urethrostomy in the cat. (a) An elliptical incision is made around the base of the scrotum and penis. (b) The subcutaneous tissues are dissected to expose the spermatic cords and the intact cat is castrated. (c) Careful dissection is performed laterally and ventrally towards the penile attachments at the ischial arch. The ischiocavernosus and ischiourethralis muscles are elevated (using a periosteal elevator) from the ischium or alternatively, ligated and severed. (d) The penis is then elevated dorsally to allow sharp dissection and severance of the ventral penile ligament. (e) The retractor penis muscle is elevated and excised from the dorsal surface of the penis, exposing the urethra underneath. (f) After incising the dorsal aspect of urethra, the urethral incision is extended approximately 5 mm beyond the level of the bulbourethral glands. The most proximal sutures are placed first, with sutures placed at the apex of the urethral opening at approximately 45° to the skin. The remaining sutures are placed down the incised edges of the urethra, including approximately two-thirds of the penile urethra. The remainder of the penis is amputated prior to ligation. (g) Additional skin sutures may be required to close the skin incision.

blunt versus sharp dissection on urethralis muscle function after surgery (Sackman *et al.*, 1991), precise sharp dissection offers better control over the extent of tissue damage and is recommended. Dorsal dissection should be conservative, especially at the most dorsal aspect, to avoid damage to neurovascular structures necessary for urethralis muscle function (Sackman *et al.*, 1991).

The bulbourethral glands are approximately 0.5–0.7 cm in diameter in the intact male cat, but may be atrophied and barely visible in the castrated male cat. The bulbourethral glands should not be removed. The catheter should be palpable on the dorsal surface of the penis. The urethra is covered by the retractor penis muscle, which is carefully elevated and excised. The catheter should then be more evident. The urethra is incised longitudinally on the most

dorsal aspect at the level of the penile urethra using a number 11 blade. Incising on to the catheter, which is held firmly to avoid rolling, prevents incising through the entire urethra. Continuation of the urethral cut can be made using sharp, pointed iris scissors or sharp-sharp tenotomy scissors. The incision must be continued into the pelvic urethra, approximately 5 mm beyond the level of the bulbourethral glands. Some haemorrhage will occur as the bulbospongiosus muscle is incised at the level of the pelvic urethra. The diameter of the pelvic urethra should allow passage of a pair of closed Halstead mosquito haemostats to the level of the box-locks without resistance.

The urethral mucosa is sutured to the skin using 4-0 monofilament-absorbable suture on a taper-cut swaged-on needle. No subcuticular sutures are required. It is imperative that the edge of the urethral mucosa is identified and that periurethral tissue (which may have a mucosa-like appearance) is not sutured to the skin inadvertently. The most proximal sutures are placed first, with sutures placed at the apex of the urethral opening at approximately 45° to the skin. The remaining sutures are placed down the incised edges of the urethra, including approximately two-thirds of the penile urethra. Sutures must be tight enough to achieve apposition of the urethral mucosa and skin without strangulating the tissue. The remaining penis is amputated. An absorbable mattress suture can be placed through the body of the penis to control haemorrhage from the distal cavernosus body. The final two sutures are placed through the ventral end of the urethral flap, at 45°, to widen the ventral end of the urethral flap. Additional skin sutures may be required to close the skin incision.

Postoperative considerations and prognosis

Generally, unless response to medical management is seen early in the course of the condition, the prognosis for recovery is poor and salvage procedures are necessary.

Postoperative considerations are listed in Table 9.8. The prognosis for functional recovery after penile amputation and/or urethrostomy is good.

Special considerations for cats after penile amputation and perineal urethrostomy include the use of shredded paper in the litter tray to avoid litter particles adhering to the surgery site until suture removal. Short-term complications are rare. However, stomal stricture is probably the most common long-term complication, the result of incomplete mobilization and dissection of the penis and its pelvic attachments or failure to extend the urethral incision to the level of the pelvic urethra. Urine extravasation into the periurethral tissue with sloughing of the perineal skin occurs infrequently. Bacterial urinary tract infection after perineal urethrostomy is frequently reported in cats operated on for urethral obstruction. Urinary tract infection was reported in 23% of cats treated for urethral obstruction in one study (Gregory and Vasseur, 1983). Urinary tract infection is typically not a characteristic feature of cats with urethral obstruction, with reports of 1–3% incidence.

Balanoposthitis/preputial foreign bodies

Balanoposthitis occurs in young intact male dogs and presents as a copious yellow or sanguineous purulent preputial discharge. Occasionally it occurs secondary to foreign bodies such as plant material. The animals frequently lick the prepuce.

Clinical signs

Clinical signs include obvious preputial discharge with erythema of the preputial and penile mucosa. Occasionally, ulcerated and vesicular lesions on the mucosal surfaces may be observed.

Diagnosis

Diagnosis is made by clinical signs. Bacterial culture of the discharge reveal normal aerobic bacteria: *Escherichia coli*, *Proteus vulgaris*, *Staphylococcus* spp., haemolytic streptococci, *Pseudomonas aeruginosa* and *Mycoplasma* spp. Fungal balanoposthitis may occur occasionally. The significance of vesicular lesions is unknown but may be caused by a herpesvirus. Careful inspection of the prepuce for evidence of foreign bodies is essential and may require sedation. The penis should be completely extruded and the prepuce lavaged with warm, normal saline after specimens are taken for culture. Any suspicious lesions should be biopsied.

Treatment

Treatment requires 3–4 weeks of systemic antibiotic therapy based on bacterial culture and sensitivity testing and daily lavage of the prepuce with dilute antiseptic solution (0.1% iodine or 0.5% chlorhexidine) followed by infusion of a broad-spectrum antibiotic ointment. Preventing the animal licking the area is important.

Prognosis

Balanoposthitis, in the absence of foreign bodies or trauma, has a poor prognosis since recurrence is common. In some cases, castration resolves the problem.

Vaginal anomalies

Congenital anomalies of the vagina are caused by faulty embryogenesis of the urogenital sinus. Most lesions are located immediately cranial to the urethral orifice. The cranial vagina, uterus and urinary system are often normal as they are derived from the Müllerian and Wolffian ducts. Anomalies reported include vertical septum at the vaginovestibular junction, outpouching of the vagina, caudal vaginal agenesis, incomplete fusion of the Müllerian ducts resulting in partition of a portion of the length of the vagina and stenosis at the vaginovestibular junction (Fig. 9.23). A persistent hymen is the result of failure of the Müllerian ducts to unite with each other or cannulate with the urogenital sinus. It can be confused with hypoplasia of the vagina which has a lumen but lacks the fibrous ring seen with hymen remnants. Vulval stenosis is generally seen at the vestibulovulval junction, although it may occur within the vestibule.

Clinical signs

Some cause no clinical signs and are only found on fertility examinations, while others cause vaginal discharge, urine pooling or apparent urinary incontinence. Breeding or whelping difficulties may be observed. Vaginal abnormalities may be associated with ectopic ureter and ectopic ureter should be ruled out as a cause of urinary incontinence.

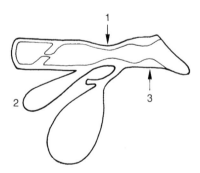

Figure 9.23 Sites of congenital lesions of the vagina: (1) vertical septum at the vaginovestibular junction or hypoplasia at the vaginovestibular junction; (2) outpouching of the vagina; (3) caudal vaginal agenesis or stenosis at the vaginovestibular junction.

Diagnosis

Diagnosis is based on clinical signs and digital vaginal examination. Vaginal examination may be facilitated by sedation of general anaesthesia. Vertical bands or central partitions can be palpated. Annular strictures of hypoplastic lesions may prevent digital examination. Vaginal examination using a speculum or endoscopic examination may be useful but can miss some lesions (as they slide past). Vaginograms, performed using water-soluble contrast material administered via a Foley catheter, may help to demonstrate the expandability of the vagina but may not differentiate between the types of lesions. These are important in determining the extent of the lesion should surgery be considered.

Treatment

Incidental findings in animals not intended for breeding require no treatment. Surgical correction may be necessary in animals with associated clinical signs. The ethics of surgical correction in animals intended for breeding is questionable.

Surgery is best performed via an episiotomy (Fig. 9.14). The urethra should be catheterized. The vertical band is identified and a curved instrument placed cranial to the band. The dorsal and ventral attachments of the band are incised. The vaginal mucosa may require closure for large bands. For hypoplastic or annular lesions, resection of the submucosal fibrous tissue or vaginoplasty is required. The episiotomy is extended through the dorsal wall of the vagina beyond the stenotic region. The vaginal wall is then closed in a T, using monofilament absorbable suture, in an attempt to increase the lumen size. The episiotomy is closed routinely in three layers.

For strictures more than 2 cm cranial to the vaginal opening, an abdominal approach with pubic symphysiotomy may be required. En bloc excision of the lesion with vaginal anastomosis may be attempted.

For animals with urine pooling after vaginal septum excision, vaginectomy via an abdominal approach is indicated at the time of ovariohysterectomy. The vagina is isolated from its peritoneal reflections followed by ligation of the vaginal branches of the urogenital artery and vein. The vagina is transfixed just cranial to the urethral opening, which should be identified with urinary catheter placed prior to surgery. Extreme care should be exercised to avoid compression of the urethral opening or damage to the ureters or neurovascular structures of the urinary bladder.

For animals with vestibulovulval stenosis, the ventral third of the episiotomy is closed with mucocutaneous apposition of each side, to enlarge the vulva permanently.

Postoperative considerations and prognosis

General considerations after surgery include preventing self-trauma and monitoring for normal urine function and any abnormal vaginal discharge. A serosanguineous discharge is expected for 1 or 2 days after surgery. The prognosis for normal function without reproductive expectations is generally good. Changes in the conformation of the vestibule may increase exposure to bacteria. These animals may be predisposed to urinary tract infection. The prognosis for normal breeding and whelping, particularly with hypoplastic lesions, is poor and the ethics of treating for this reason are questioned.

Vaginitis

Puppies often develop vaginitis before their first oestrus. Although juvenile vaginitis is not normal, it usually subsides following the first oestrus and does not require medical treatment. Puppies with atypical vaginal discharges, however, may require treatment. Atypical discharges include an offensive odour from the vaginal discharge or evidence of fresh blood in the vaginal discharge.

Puppies younger than 6 months harbour significantly more coagulase-positive staphylococci than older animals. Many types of bacteria can be cultured from the prepubertal posterior vagina of puppies. If puppy vaginitis does not respond to appropriate symptomatic therapy then a bacterial culture should be obtained. Once a potential pathogen is isolated, antimicrobial sensitivity testing should be performed in order to formulate proper antimicrobial therapy.

Treatment

Conservative medical therapy usually allows vaginal inflammation and discharge to resolve spontaneously at puberty. Conservative therapy may include cleaning the perivulvar area to prevent moist dermatitis. In puppies with atypical vaginal discharges, intravaginal infusion of a commercial human douching solution followed by copious infusion of normal saline solution is performed every 2 weeks until the vaginal discharge resolves. At the same time, systemic antimicrobial therapy is administered daily for 2–3 weeks.

Prevention

Although the means for dissemination of vaginal bacteria is unknown, puppies grouped together seem to harbour similar vaginal bacteria. In general, clipping hair in the perivulval area and keeping the puppies in clean surroundings will reduce the incidence of puppy vaginitis.

References

Ader, P.L. and Hobson, H.P. (1978) Hypospadias: a review of the veterinary literature and a report of three cases in the dog. *Journal of the American Animal Hospital Association*, **14**, 721–727.

Alexander, S.A. (1994) Characteristics of animals adopted from an animal control center whose owners complied with a spay/neutering program. *Journal of the American Veterinary Association*, **205**, 472–476.

Arohnson, M.G. and Fagella, A.M. (1993) Surgical techniques for neutering 6 to 14-week-old kittens. *Journal of the American Veterinary Association*, **202**, 53–55.

Autran de Morais, H.S., DiBartola, S.P. and Chew, D.J. (1996) Juvenile renal disease in golden retrievers: 12 cases (1984–1994). *Journal of the American Veterinary Medical Association*, **209**, 792–797.

Bloomberg, M.S. (1996) Surgical neutering and nonsurgical alternatives. *Journal of the American Veterinary Association*, **208**, 517–519.

Chastain, C.B. (1992) Pediatric cytogenetics. *Compendium of Continuing Education for the Practicing Veterinarian*, **14**, 333–341.

Edney, A.T.B. and Smith, P.M. (1986) Study of obesity in dogs visiting veterinary practices in the United Kingdom. *Veterinary Record*, **118**, 391–396.

Fagella, A.M. and Arohnson, M.G. (1993) Anesthesia techniques for neutering 6 to 14-week-old kittens. *Journal of the American Veterinary Association*, **202**, 56–62.

Grandy, J.L. and Dunclop, C.I. (1991) Anesthesia of pups and kittens. *Journal of the American Veterinary Association*, **198**, 1244–1249.

Gregory, C.R. and Vasseur, P.B. (1983) Long-term examination of cats with perineal urethrostomy. *Veterinary Surgery*, **12**, 210–212.

Hart, B.L. and Cooper, L. (1984) Factors relating to urine spraying and fighting in prepubertally gonadectomized cats. *Journal of the American Veterinary Association*, **184**, 1255–1258.

Hosgood, G. (1992) Anesthesia and surgical considerations of puppies and kittens. *Compendium of Continuing Education for the Practicing Veterinarian*, **14**, 345–359.

Hosgood, G. and Hedlund, C.S. (1992) Perineal urethrostomy in cats. *Compendium of Continuing Education for the Practicing Veterinarian*, **14**, 1195–1205.

Houpt, K.A., Coren, B., Hintz, H.F. and Hildebrandt, J.E. (1979) Effect of sex and reproductive status on sucrose preference, food intake, and body weight of dogs. *Journal of the American Veterinary Medical Association*, **174**, 1083–1085.

Johnston, S.D. (1991) Questions and answers on the effects of surgically neutering dogs and cats. *Journal of the American Veterinary Association*, **198**, 1206–1214.

Kelly, G.E. (1980) The effect of surgery on dogs on the response to concomitant distemper vaccination. *Australian Veterinary Journal*, **56**, 556–557.

Le Roux, P.H. and Van der Walt, L.A. (1977) Ovarian autograft as an alternative to ovariectomy in bitches. *Journal of the South African Veterinary Association*, **48**, 117–123.

Le Roux, P.H. (1983) Thyroid status, oestradiol level, work performance and body mass of ovariectomized bitches and bitches bearing ovarian transplants in the stomach wall. *Journal of the South African Veterinary Association*, **54**, 115–117.

Lieberman, L.L. (1987) A case for neutering pups and kittens at two months of age. *Journal of the American Veterinary Medical Association*, **191**, 518–521.

Marshall, L.S., Oehlert, M.L., Haskins, M.E., Selden, J.R. and Patterson, D.F. (1982) Persistent Müllerian duct syndrome in miniature schnauzers. *Journal of the American Veterinary Medical Association*, **181**, 798–801.

Meyers-Wallen, V.N. and Patterson, D.F. (1989) Sexual differentiation and inherited disorders of sexual development in the dog. *Journal of Reproduction and Fertility Supplement*, **39**, 57–64.

Meyers-Wallen, V.N., Wilson, J.D., Griffin, J.E. *et al.* (1989) Testicular feminization in a cat. *Journal of the American Veterinary Medical Association*, **195**, 631–634.

Millis, D.L., Hauptman, J.G. and Johnson, C.A. (1992) Cryptorchidism and monorchidism in cats: 25 cases (1980–1989). *Journal of the American Veterinary Medical Association*, **200**, 1128–1130.

Moulton, C. (1990) Early spay/neuter: risks and benefits for shelters. *American Humane Shoptalk*, **7**, 1–6.

Nemzek, J.A., Homco, L.D., Wheaton, L.G. and Grman, G.L. (1992) Cystic ovaries and hyperestrogenism in a canine female pseudohermaphrodite. *Journal of the American Animal Hospital Association*, **28**, 402–406.

O'Farrell, V. and Peachey, E. (1990) Behavioural effects of ovariohysterectomy on bitches. *Journal of Small Animal Practice*, **31**, 595–598.

Olson, P.N., Seim, H.B., Park, R.D., Grandy, J.L., Freshman, J.L. and Carlson, E.D. (1989) Female pseudo-

hermaphroditism in three greyhound siblings. *Journal of the American Veterinary Medical Association*, **194**, 1747–1749.

Pope, E.R. and Swaim, S.F. (1986) Surgical reconstruction of a hypoplastic prepuce. *Journal of the American Animal Hospital Association*, **22**, 73–77.

Richardson, E.F. and Mullen, H. (1993) Cryptorchidism in cats. *Compendium of Continuing Education for the Practicing Veterinarian*, **15**, 1342–1345.

Romagnoli, S.E. (1991) Canine cryptorchidism. *Veterinary Clinics of North America [Small Animal Practice]*, **21**, 533–544.

Root, M.V. and Johnston, S.D. (1995) The effect of early spay-neuter in the development of feline obesity. *Veterinary Forum*, **12**, 38–43.

Root, M.V., Johnston, S.D. and Olson, P.N. (1996) Effect of prepubertal and postpubertal gonadectomy on heat production measured by indirect calorimetry in male and female cats. *American Journal of Veterinary Research*, **57**, 371–374.

Sackman, J.E., Sims, M.H. and Krahwinkel, D.J. (1991) Urodynamic evaluation of lower urinary tract function in cats after perineal urethrostomy with minimal and extensive dissection. *Veterinary Surgery*, **20**, 55–60.

Salmeri, K.R., Bloomberg, M.S., Scruggs, S.L. and Shille, V. (1991a) Gonadectomy in immature dogs: effects on skeletal, physical and behavioral development. *Journal of the American Veterinary Association*, **198**, 1193–1203.

Salmeri, K.R., Olson, P.N. and Bloomberg, M.S. (1991b) Elective gonadectomy in dogs: a review. *Journal of the American Veterinary Medical Association*, **198**, 1183–1192.

Schneider, R., Dorn, C.R. and Taylor, D.O.N. (1969) Factors influencing canine mammary cancer development and postsurgical survival. *Journal of the National Cancer Institute*, **43**, 1249–1253.

Smith, M.M. and Gourley, I.M. (1990) Preputial reconstruction in a dog. *Journal of the American Veterinary Medical Association*, **196**, 1493–1496.

Sommer, M.M. and Meyers-Wallen, V.N. (1991) XX true hermaphroditism in a dog. *Journal of the American Veterinary Medical Association*, **198**, 435–438.

Stone, E.A. and Barsanti, J.A. (1992a) Diagnosis and medical therapy of congenital disorders. In: Stone, E.A. and Barsanti, J.A. (eds) *Urologic Surgery of the Dog and Cat*, pp. 201–204. Philadelphia: Lea & Febiger.

Stone, E.A. and Barsanti, J.A. (1992b) Postoperative management and surgical complications of congenital disorders. In: Stone, E.A. and Barsanti, J.A. (eds) *Urologic Surgery of the Dog and Cat*, pp. 210–211. Philadelphia: Lea & Febiger.

Stone, E.A. and Barsanti, J.A. (1992c) Surgical therapy for congenital disorders. In: Stone, E.A. and Barsanti, J.A. (eds) *Urologic Surgery of the Dog and Cat*, pp. 205–209. Philadelphia: Lea & Febiger.

Stone, E.A. and Mason, K.L. (1990) Surgery of ectopic ureters: types, method of correction and postoperative results. *Journal of the American Animal Hospital Association*, **26**, 81–88.

Swalec, K.M. and Smeak, D.D. (1989) Priapism after castration in a cat. *Journal of the American Veterinary Medical Association*, **195**, 964–964.

Wilson, G.P. and Harrison, J.W. (1971) Perineal urethrostomy in cats. *Journal of the American Veterinary Medical Association*, **159**, 1789–1793.

Wilson, D.V., Nickels, F.A. and Williams, M.A. (1983) Pharmacologic treatment of priapism in two horses. *Journal of the American Veterinary Medical Association*, **199**, 1183–1184.

Localization of neurologic lesion

Neurologic examination on puppies and kittens older than 8 weeks of age is the same as for adult animals. Prior to that age, development is not complete (see Chapter 1). Neurologic examination should allow the lesion to be localized to the brain, cervical spinal cord, brachial plexus, thoracolumbar spinal cord, lumbosacral plexus or sacrococcygeal region. The fore and hind limbs should be evaluated to determine whether they are normal or showing signs of an upper motor neuron (UMN) or a lower motor neuron (LMN) lesion (Table 10.1).

Once the status of the fore limbs, hind limbs and cranial nerves has been established, the lesion can be localized to one of six sites (Table 10.2). If LMN signs are present in both the hind and fore limbs a generalized peripheral neuropathy or myopathy is most likely. It could also indicate two separate lesions, one in the lumbosacral plexus and one in the brachial

Table 10.1 Clinical signs associated with upper and lower motor neuron spinal lesion

Lower motor neuron signs	Upper motor neuron signs
Paralysis (flaccid)	Paresis to paralysis
Hyporeflexia to areflexia	Normal to hyperreflexia
Neurogenic muscle atrophy (early onset and severe)	Disuse muscle atrophy (late onset and less severe)
Decreased muscle tone	Normal to increased muscle tone
Abnormal electromyogram 5–7 days after insult	Normal electromyogram
Anaesthesia of innervated region with paraesthesia or hyperaesthesia of adjacent regions	Decreased proprioception, diminished pain perception

Table 10.2 Localization of clinical signs of spinal disease to spinal cord segments

Site of spinal cord lesion	Clinical signs
S1–3	UMN signs to tail LMN signs to anal sphincter, urinary bladder Normal hind limbs Normal fore limbs Normal mental status and cranial nerves
L4–S2 (lumbosacral plexus)	UMN signs to tail UMN or LMN signs to sphincters, urinary bladder LMN signs to hind limbs Normal fore limbs Normal mental status and cranial nerves
T3–L3	UMN signs to hind limbs, urinary bladder, sphincter Normal fore limbs Normal mental status and cranial nerves
C6–T2 (brachial plexus)	Normal or UMN signs to hind limbs, urinary bladder LMN signs to fore limbs Normal mental status and cranial nerves
C1–6	Normal or UMN signs to hind limbs, urinary bladder UMN signs to fore limbs Normal mental status and cranial nerves
Brain	Normal or UMN signs to hind limbs, urinary bladder Normal or UMN signs to fore limbs Abnormal mental status, gait, postural reactions or cranial nerves; head tilt

C = Cervical; L = lumbar; T = thoracic; S = sacral; UMN = upper motor neuron; LMN = lower motor neuron.

plexus, but this would be very unlikely. Complete spinal cord destruction could also cause LMN signs in both the hind and fore limbs but death due to respiratory arrest would probably occur first. If LMN signs are present in the hind limbs and UMN signs are present in the fore limbs, it is either a diffuse disease or a multifocal disease with one lesion in the lumbosacral plexus and one lesion in the brain or C1–5 region. Monoparesis or monoparalysis is usually due to peripheral nerve lesions which usually occur secondary to limb trauma or neoplasia.

Thoracolumbar and lumbosacral spinal cord diseases

Paraparesis is weakness of the hind limbs, and paraplegia is paralysis of the hind limbs. Animals with hind limb paresis should be thoroughly evaluated to determine whether the problem is related to the musculoskeletal or neurological system. All bones, joints and muscles should be carefully evaluated for asymmetry or pain. Proprioception, pain perception and spinal reflexes should be evaluated in all four limbs. If hind limb paresis is present with normal cranial nerves and fore limbs, the lesion is caudal to spinal cord segment T2. The hind limb reflexes are evaluated to determine if the lesion is in the T3–L3 or L4–S2 spinal segments. If the hind limb reflexes are decreased or absent, the lesion is in the L4–S2 spinal segments. If the hind limb reflexes are normal or exaggerated, the L4–S2 segments are functioning and the lesion is between T3 and L3. A lesion in the T3–L3 region causes a loss of the UMN inhibitory influence on the LMNs, resulting in exaggerated reflexes. After the lesion has been localized to a particular segment of the spinal cord, the possible aetiologies should be considered (Tables 10.3 and 10.4).

Treatment of spinal cord trauma in the puppy and kitten is similar to that of an adult animal and is beyond the scope of this text. In addition, there are a large number of toxins which can affect an animal of any age. Anomalous

Table 10.3 Causes of thoracolumbar spinal cord diseases (modified from Oliver and Lorenz, 1993a)

Aetiology	Thoracolumbar spinal cord diseases (T3–L3)
Degenerative	Demyelinating diseases (Table 10.19)
	Neuronopathies (Table 10.8)
Anomalous	Spinal dysraphism
	Vertebral anomalies
Neoplastic	Multiple cartilaginous exostosis (Chapter 12)
Inflammatory	Viral (distemper, feline infectious peritonitis), bacterial, protozoal, mycotic myelitis (Table 10.20)
	Discospondylitis (Table 10.20)
	Granulomatous meningoencephalitis (Table 10.20)
Toxic	Various neuropathies
Traumatic	Vertebral fractures/luxations
	Traumatic disc rupture
	Haemorrhagic myelomalacia

T = Thoracic; L = Lumbar

conditions of the thoracic, lumbar and sacral spinal cord are discussed below. Degenerative disc disease is not included, because it is not a paediatric condition. Degenerative and inflammatory conditions which are not specific to the thoracolumbar or lumbosacral spinal cord are discussed later.

Table 10.4 Causes of lumbosacral spinal cord and cauda equina diseases (modified from Oliver and Lorenz, 1993a)

Aetiology	Lumbosacral and cauda equina diseases (L4–S3)
Degenerative	Neuronopathies (Table 10.8)
Anomalous	Spinal dysraphism
	Vertebral anomalies
Inflammatory	Viral (distemper, feline infectious peritonitis), bacterial, protozoal, mycotic myelitis (Table 10.20)
	Discospondylitis (Table 10.20)
	Post vaccinal rabies or distemper (Table 10.20)
	Granulomatous meningoencephalitis (Table 10.20)
Toxic	Various neuropathies
Traumatic	Vertebral fractures/luxations
	Traumatic disc rupture
	Haemorrhagic myelomalacia

L = Lumbar; S = Sacral

Vertebral anomalies

Vertebral anomalies are most common in the English and French Bulldog, Boston Terrier, Pug and Pekinese (Bailey, 1975). Block vertebrae occur with incomplete separation of the bodies, arches or entire vertebrae. They are usually stable and rarely clinically significant (Morgan, 1968). Hemivertebrae occur when half of the vertebral body fails to ossify, resulting in unilateral, dorsal or ventral hemivertebra. Unilateral hemivertebra causes scoliosis, dorsal hemivertebra causes kyphosis and ventral hemivertebra causes lordosis. A butterfly vertebra is a form of hemivertebra and is characterized by a sagittal cleft in the vertebral body. Transitional vertebrae have characteristics of two major divisions of the vertebral column and they can be seen in the cervicothoracic, thoracolumbar, lumbosacral and sacrocaudal junctions.

Clinical signs

Clinical signs of hemivertebrae are uncommon but can be caused by intermittent compression of the spinal cord due to instability. Instability may also cause secondary osseous changes which can further compress the cord. Paraparesis, urinary and faecal incontinence, vertebral pain and muscle atrophy of affected limbs may be observed.

Transitional vertebrae in the cervicofore and thoracolumbar region are generally clinically insignificant. Lumbosacral anomalies may be associated with clinical signs, although it has not been proven. In sacralization of the lumbar vertebra, the seventh lumbar vertebra may fuse with the first sacral segment. If the sacralization is unilateral the pelvis is deviated, resulting in abnormal conformation. It has been postulated that this may cause painful spinal nerve root compression, but the pain may be due to secondary arthritic changes. Lumbarization of the sacrum results in transverse processes on the first sacral segment. The union between the ilium and the lumbar transverse processes is stronger than the union which forms with a sacral transverse process. This less stable formation could cause arthritic changes as the animal ages (Oliver and Lorenz, 1993a).

Diagnosis

It is important to verify spinal cord compression by myelography before attempting surgery.

Treatment

In some animals, surgical decompression and fixation may help restore spinal cord function.

Spinal dysraphism

Failure of normal neural tube closure causes dysraphic conditions. Dysraphic conditions affecting the vertebral column or spinal cord include spinal dysraphism, syringomyelia, spina bifida with or without myelomeningocele and caudal vertebral hypoplasia. Spinal dysraphism has been reported as a genetic condition in the Weimaraner (McGrath, 1965). Syringomyelia is fluid-filled cavitations within the spinal cord, seen commonly in dysraphic spinal cords.

Clinical signs

Clinical signs are usually seen between 4 and 8 weeks of age and include a symmetrical hopping gait (bunny-hopping), a crouched posture and a wide-based stance. Proprioception of the hindlimbs is abnormal and postural reactions (hopping, hemiwalking, wheelbarrowing) are depressed. Spinal reflexes are normal. Other signs include abnormal hair whorls in the dorsal cervical region, tail kinking, scoliosis and depression of the sternum. The neurologic signs are non-progressive but become more apparent as the dog matures (Oliver and Lorenz, 1993a).

Treatment

There is no treatment but affected dogs can lead a normal life.

Spina bifida

Spina bifida is the incomplete fusion of the dorsal vertebral arches. It is most common in the English Bulldog and the Manx cat, but can occur in any breed (Wilson *et al.*, 1979; Fingeroth *et al.*, 1989). Spina bifida most com-monly affects the lumbar vertebrae and it may be associated with a meningocele (protrusion of the meninges) or a myelomeningocele (protrusion of the spinal cord and meninges). A meningocele or myelomeningocele may adhere to the skin producing a small dimple at the site of attachment. If the defect is open, spinal fluid may leak on to the skin and cause skin ulceration. Since the meninges are exposed, there is a risk of meningitis. Myeloschisis, tethered spinal cord and hydrocephalus may be associated with spina bifida.

Clinical signs

Signs vary with the severity of the involvement of the spinal cord or the cauda equina. Mild to moderate hindlimb ataxia and paresis can occur and faecal and urinary incontinence are usually present. The hindlimb may be fixed in extension if there is decreased innervation by the sciatic nerve. There may be diminished pain perception in the perineal region and hind limbs. In the absence of a myelomeningocele, spina bifida is not associated with neurological deficits (Oliver and Lorenz, 1993a).

Diagnosis

The diagnosis is confirmed with spinal radiographs and myelography (Oliver and Lorenz, 1993a).

Treatment

There is no specific treatment and loss of nerve supply to the urinary bladder and anus is not reversible. Meningoceles can be closed to prevent leakage of cerebrospinal fluid and to prevent meningeal infection. Euthanasia is recommended for animals with severe neurological deficits (Oliver and Lorenz, 1993a).

Prognosis

The prognosis is guarded to poor.

Caudal dysgenesis

Congenital malformations of the sacrococcygeal spinal cord and vertebrae have been reported in

Manx cats. Manx cats are bred for taillessness but other anomalies may occur as well, including sacral hypoplasia, spina bifida, spinal dysraphism, syringomyelia, meningocele and myelomeningocele (Leipold *et al.*, 1974). Abnormal development of nerves in the cauda equina can result in plantigrade posture, bunny-hopping, faecal and urinary incontinence and perineal analgesia. Severely affected cats have ataxia and paraparesis or paraplegia. Diagnosis is based on history, clinical signs and lumbosacral radiographs. There is no treatment and the prognosis is poor.

Cervical spinal cord diseases

Tetraparesis and tetraplegia are used to describe motor dysfunction of all four limbs, depending on the severity of the affliction. Hemiparesis describes a weakness of the two limbs on the same side of the body and occurs with a unilateral lesion. Paresis may be apparent as a gait abnormality or as abnormal postural reactions. Tetraparesis is usually secondary to neurologic disease, although it can be a result of diffuse muscle or skeletal disease. Generalized muscle weakness or depression associated with severe metabolic disease must also be ruled out.

Neurologic tetraparesis results from a lesion in the cerebral cortex, brainstem, cervical spinal cord or LMNs. Animals with diffuse cerebral cortex disease have abnormal postural reactions, and usually have a normal or slightly abnormal gait. Other signs of cerebral dysfunction include altered mental status, seizures or blindness. Lesions in the brainstem and cranial cervical spinal cord (C1–5) cause identical UMN signs in all four limbs, so these lesions must be differentiated by examination of the cranial nerves. Lesions in the brachial plexus can also cause tetraparesis but will cause LMN signs in the fore limbs and UMN signs in the hind limbs. There are many conditions which can cause signs preferable to the cervical spinal cord (Table 10.5). Atlantoaxial luxation, cervical spondylomyelopathy, and other cervical vertebral anomalies are discussed below. Some of the degenerative and inflammatory diseases which are less specific to the cervical region will be discussed later.

Table 10.5 Causes of cervical spinal cord diseases (modified from Oliver and Lorenz, 1993b)

Aetiology	Cervical diseases (C1–T2)
Degenerative	Cervical vertebral spondylopathy Demyelinating diseases (Table 10.19) Axonopathies and neuronopathies (Tables 10.8 and 10.9) Storage diseases (Table 10.18)
Anomalous	Atlantoaxial luxation Spinal dysraphism Vertebral anomalies
Nutritional	Hypervitaminosis A (Chapter 12)

Inflammatory	Viral (distemper myelitis, feline infectious
	    peritonitis), bacterial, protozoal,
	    fungal myelitis (Table 10.20)
	Discospondylitis (Table 10.20)
	Granulomatous meningoencephalitis
	    (Table 10.20)

Traumatic	Vertebral fractures/luxations Traumatic disc rupture Haemorrhagic myelomalacia

C = Cervical; T = Thoracic

Atlantoaxial luxation

Instability of the atlantoaxial joint can result in dorsal displacement of the axis into the vertebral canal with spinal cord compression (Oliver and Lewis, 1973; Fig. 10.1). Congenital joint instability can be a result of separation, absence or malformation of the dens. The dens (odontoid process) is the bony, cranial projection of the axis which is attached to the ventral arch of the atlas by the transverse ligament (Fig. 10.1). The dens is attached to the occipital bone by an apical and two lateral (alar) ligaments. These attachments prevent flexion between the atlas and axis. If the ligamentous support, especially the transverse ligament, is not properly developed the axis luxates dorsally and the spinal cord is pinched between the dens and the dorsal atlantal arch (Watson and DeLahunta, 1989). Agenesis or hypoplasia of the dens is also associated with atlantoaxial instability. Neurological signs are less severe if there is also congenital malformation of the dens because there is less compression of the spinal cord.

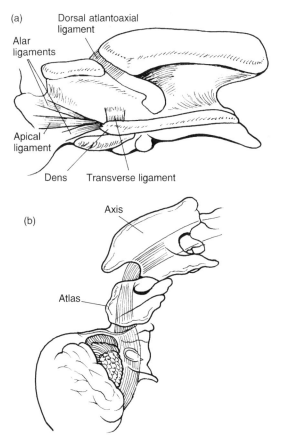

(a) Alar ligaments, Dorsal atlantoaxial ligament, Apical ligament, Dens, Transverse ligament

(b) Axis, Atlas

Figure 10.1 (a) Anatomy of the atlantoaxial region. (b) Dorsal displacement of the axis with compression of the spinal cord.

Clinical signs

Congenital atlantoaxial luxations are most common in toy or miniature breeds. Neurological signs are usually seen within the first year of life. Onset of signs may be insidious or acute. Signs range from cervical pain to severe paresis or paralysis (Geary *et al.*, 1967). Motor deficits may affect the hind limbs only or all four limbs. Severely affected animals may be non-ambulatory and tetraparetic. Flexing the neck may cause severe pain and neurological injury. If atlantoaxial luxation is suspected, the neck should not be flexed. Displacement of an intact dens into the spinal canal may precipitate respiratory paralysis and death. If the animal is under anaesthesia the neck should be carefully supported and maintained in extension at all times.

Diagnosis

Atlantoaxial luxation should be suspected in any toy or miniature breed with cervical pain, paresis or paralysis. Lateral and ventrodorsal radiographic views usually reveal displacement of the axis. On the lateral view, an increased space is seen between the arch of the atlas and the spinous process of the axis. There is also angulation of the atlas relative to the axis. A hypoplastic or aplastic dens may also be apparent, although oblique views may be needed to visualize it. Flexed radiographic views are usually not needed and flexion of the neck can cause severe spinal cord compression.

Treatment and surgical technique

Conservative management can be attempted in animals with minimal clinical signs. Strict cage rest is enforced and the head and neck are splinted in extension. A fibreglass splint is maintained for 6 weeks to allow fibrous tissue to stabilize the joint. Initial short-term corticosteroids (dexamethasone 0.2–1.1 mg/kg IM b.i.d. for 2 days) or analgesics may be used. If the animal has moderate to severe neurologic deficits or recurrent episodes of neck pain which are unresponsive to medical management, surgical stabilization is indicated. Various techniques have been described which allow reduction and stabilization through a dorsal or ventral approach (Oliver and Lewis 1973; Chambers *et al.*, 1977; Cook and Oliver, 1981; Sorjonen and Shires, 1981).

Dorsal stabilization may be accomplished by using stainless-steel wire, non-absorbable suture material or the nuchal ligament to attach the spinous process of the axis to the dorsal arch of the atlas (Fig. 10.2). Heavy suture is passed under the dorsal lamina of the atlas and through holes placed in the dorsal spine of the axis. Spinal cord trauma and respiratory arrest may result from the surgical manipulation.

A ventral approach allows arthrodesis of the atlantoaxial joint (Fig. 10.3). This is especially indicated for animals in which the dorsal bony structures will not support fixation devices or if the dens is angulated and needs to be removed (Swaim and Greene, 1975). A cancellous bone graft is placed in the joint and pins or screws are placed across the joints (Sorjonen and

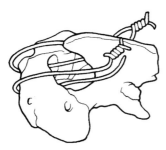

Figure 10.2 Dorsal stabilization of atlantoaxial luxation using wire or suture.

Shires, 1981; Denny *et al.*, 1988). Methylmethacrylate may be used on the pin ends to prevent migration.

Postoperative considerations and prognosis

A neck brace is recommended for 4–6 weeks postoperatively. When using a dorsal approach the suture may break, or tear through the dorsal arch of the atlas before adequate fibrous tissue has formed (Renegar and Stoll, 1979; Cook and Oliver, 1981). Complications associated with the ventral approach include improper pin placement and pin migration. Prognosis is fair for animals with moderate neurologic deficits and guarded for animals with tetraplegia (Oliver and Lorenz, 1993b).

Cervical spondylomyelopathy

Cervical spondylomyelopathy is also termed cervical spondylopathy, caudal cervical vertebral malformation–malarticulation, cervical vertebral instability, wobbler syndrome and cervical vertebral stenosis. The exact aetiology is unknown but neurologic signs develop because of spinal cord compression from surrounding soft-tissue or bony vertebral structures. The disease occurs most commonly in Dobermanns and Great Danes as well as other large-breed dogs. Although the disease is similar in all dogs, certain changes are more characteristic of each breed (Table 10.6; Fig. 10.4). One or more of these abnormalities may occur in one dog. Static spinal cord compression is constant pressure on the spinal cord regardless of neck position. Dynamic spinal cord compression can result from intervertebral instability or ligamentous hypertrophy that buckles against the spinal cord with neck movement.

Clinical signs

Clinical signs are related to the amount of spinal cord compression and are usually much more pronounced in the hindlimbs. There is usually an insidious onset of hindlimb ataxia and hypermetria. Dogs usually have proprioceptive deficits and may knuckle the digits when walking.

(a)   (b)

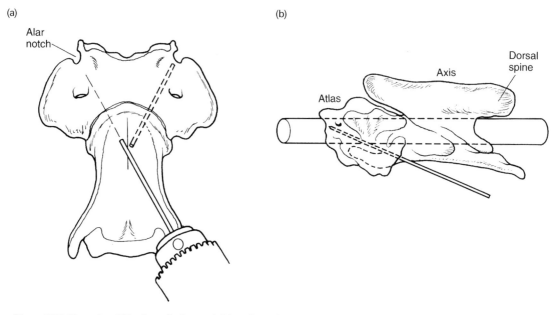

Figure 10.3 Ventral stabilization of atlantoaxial luxation using pins. (a) Ventral and (b) lateral views of pin placement.

Table 10.6 Characteristics of cervical vertebral lesions associated with spondylomyelopathy

Common site	Type of lesion	Location of compression	Static or dynamic	Surgical treatment
	Dobermann; onset of clinical signs at 5–7 years			
C5–6 and C6–7 disc spaces	Type II disc protrusion with hypertrophy or hyperplasia of the annulus fibrosis	Ventral	Static	Ventral slot
C6 or C7	Tipping of craniodorsal surface of vertebral body into spinal canal	Ventral	Dynamic	Distraction and stabilization
	Great Dane; onset of clinical signs at 3–18 months			
Any level of the cervical spine	Hourglass compression: hypertrophy or hyperplasia of annulus fibrosus or dorsal longitudinal ligament (ventral), hypertrophy of the ligamentum flavum (dorsal), degenerative joint disease or malformation or malarticulation of articular facets (lateral)	Ventral, dorsal and lateral	Static or dynamic	Dorsal laminectomy if static Distraction and stabilization if dynamic
C4–7	Ligamentum flavum hypertrophy and vertebral arch malformation	Dorsal	Dynamic and static	Dorsal laminectomy if static Distraction and stabilization if dynamic
	Congenital bony malformation: stenosis of cranial vertebral canal orifice, articular facet deformities, malformation of the vertebral pedicles or malformation of the vertebral arches	Ventral, lateral and dorsal	Static	Dorsal laminectomy

C = Cervical vertebrae

The hind limbs may abduct widely and cross each other when turning. Ataxia and paresis or hypermetria may be present in the forelimbs, but abnormalities are usually subtle. Affected dogs may have ambulatory or non-ambulatory tetraparesis. Neck pain is usually not present. Urinary incontinence may develop with progression of the disease.

Diagnosis

Diagnosis is confirmed by cervical radiographs and myelogram. Changes on survey radiographs include changes in the shape and density of the articular facets, stenosis of the vertebral canal, malformed or misshapen vertebral bodies and misshapen dorsal spinous processes (Van-Gundy, 1989a). Myelographic evaluation may demonstrate bony or soft-tissue compression of the spinal cord and there may be more than one site of compression. Radiographic views taken with the neck in traction may reduce protrusion by soft tissues, thus demonstrating a dynamic lesion. Dynamic lesions may also be demonstrated by taking radiographic views with the neck in extension or flexion, but caution

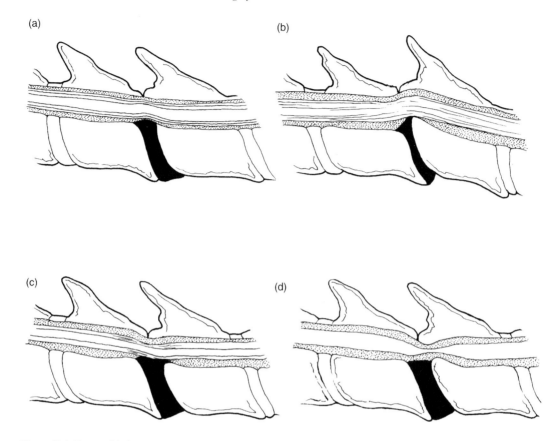

Figure 10.4 Types of lesions seen with cervical spondylomyelopathy. (a) Type II disc protrusion. (b) Tipping of the vertebra. (c) Ligamentum flavum hypertrophy. (d) Bony malformation causing stenosis of the vertebral canal.

must be used to avoid excessive spinal cord compression. Before considering surgical options, a myelographic examination is essential to determine the exact location and extent of the lesion or lesions and whether the lesions are dynamic or static.

Treatment and surgical technique

Mild neurological signs may improve with medical management which includes restricting movement of any dynamic lesions and systemic treatment of spinal cord inflammation. Medical management involves cage rest, a neck brace, a harness rather than a neck collar and anti-inflammatory medication. If the neurologic status improves within 3–4 weeks, the dog may gradually return to normal activity. Some dogs may be maintained for months to years with medical management.

If there is unsatisfactory response to medical management or if the condition deteriorates, surgery may be considered. However, if abnormal vertebrae occur at multiple levels, it may not be surgically correctable (Ellison *et al.*, 1988; Bruecker *et al.*, 1989a; 1989b; VanGundy, 1989b; McKee *et al.*, 1990; Lyman and Seim, 1991). Surgical techniques are directed at decompression, stabilization or both. Decompression may be done through a ventral or dorsal approach, depending on the location of the compressive lesion. A ventral slot is used to decompress ventral compressive lesions, caused by intervertebral disc protrusion. A dorsal laminectomy is used to decompress dorsal compressive lesions, including bony malformations and hypertrophy of the ligamentum flavum.

Vertebral stabilization is usually not indicated unless gross instability can be demonstrated during myelography. The choice of stabilization procedure depends on the type of pathology and the experience of the surgeon. It is difficult to stabilize the cervical region through a dorsal approach but it can be performed by placing screws through the articular facets or placing bone plates to the dorsal spines. Stabilization is usually performed through a ventral approach with the goal of fusing the vertebrae. If a dynamic lesion is present, the vertebrae are maintained in distraction while they are stabilized. Ventral stabilization techniques include screws placed through the vertebral bodies, plates applied to the ventral vertebral bodies, Harrington rods, pins applied to the vertebral bodies and stabilized with methylmethacrylate and placement of bone grafts or methylmethacrylate into a ventral slot defect (Ellison *et al.*, 1988; Bruecker *et al.*, 1989a; 1989b; Walker, 1990).

Postoperative considerations and prognosis

The prognosis is guarded to poor regardless of treatment since the disease is progressive. Prognosis for disc-associated lesions is better than that for malformation or instability. Prognosis is poor if there are multiple sites of compression or if the dog is tetraplegic. Factors which contribute to the poor prognosis include irreversible spinal cord damage, failure to stabilize the vertebrae adequately and complications associated with rehabilitation of a recumbent large-breed dog. Many dogs that benefit from the surgery initially develop neurological signs later in life due to destabilization at an adjacent site (Oliver and Lorenz, 1993b).

Other vertebral anomalies

Occipitoatlantoaxial malformations

Occipitoatlantoaxial malformations have been reported in dogs and cats. Dogs may have dorsal angulation of the dens and in cats the atlas may be fused to the occipital bone (Parker *et al.*, 1973; Jaggy *et al.*, 1991; Oliver and Lorenz, 1993b). Signs are related to a compressive lesion of the cervical spinal cord.

Anomaly of the third cervical vertebra

A deformity of C3 resulting in spinal cord compression has been reported in young male Basset Hounds (Palmer and Wallace, 1967). The deformed veterbral body results in pressure necrosis of overlying cord. This causes signs of a compressive cervical lesion in dogs from birth to 6 months of age.

Diseases with diffuse lower motor neuron signs

Tetraparesis associated with diffuse LMN signs can be due to lesions in the motor neurons of the spinal cord (neuronopathy), the axonal processes (axonopathy or peripheral neuropathy) or the neuromuscular end-plate (motor end-plate disorder; Table 10.7). Polyradiculoneuritis, tick paralysis, botulism, aminoglycoside paralysis, chronic polymyositis and metabolic disorders are less likely to occur in puppies

Table 10.7 Diseases with diffuse lower motor neuron signs. Diseases more likely to occur in young animals are printed in *italics*

Acute progressive disorders	*Chronic progressive disorders*	*Episodic progressive disorders*
Polyradiculoneuritis	*Motor neuronopathies* (Table 10.8)	*Myasthenia gravis* (Chapter 12)
Tick paralysis	*Polyneuropathies* (Table 10.9)	Metabolic disorders: *hypoglycaemia* hyperkalaemia hypercalcaemia hypocalcaemia hypothyroidism hyperadrenocorticism
Botulism	*Polymyopathies* (Tables 10.10 and 10.11; Chapter 12)	Chronic relapsing polymyositis
Aminoglycoside paralysis		

and kittens, and dicussion is beyond the scope of this text. Motor neuronopathies, polyneuropathies and polymyopathies are discussed below.

Motor neuronopathies

Motor neuronopathies are characterized by progressive denervation of muscle fibres resulting in paresis, paralysis and severe muscle atrophy. Few neuronopathies have been reported in dogs and cats (Table 10.8).

Polyneuropathies

Polyneuropathies are chronic progressive diseases with an insidious onset. They generally progress slowly over several months but may have periods of spontaneous improvement. The hereditary neuropathies are rare (Table 10.9). Storage diseases (Table 10.18) and demyelinating diseases (Table 10.19) can also cause peripheral neuropathies.

Polymyopathies

The signs of diffuse muscle disease are similar to those of diffuse polyneuropathies. Diseased muscles are usually weak, and may exhibit myalgia, myotonia or cramping. Myopathies result from inflammation or degeneration. Polymyositis is diffuse muscle inflammation of infectious or non-infectious origin. Infectious polymyositis is rare. Polymyopathies which are seen in puppies and kittens are listed in Tables 10.10 and 10.11 and further described in Table 12.25.

Ataxia

Ataxia is characterized by uncoordinated movements of the head, trunk or limbs which may

Table 10.8 Motor neuronopathies reported in the dog

Motor neuronopathies	Signalment (breed, age)	Clinical signs
Spinal muscle atrophy of Brittany spaniels (spinal abiotrophy; Lorenz *et al.*, 1979)	Brittany Spaniel < 4 months of age hereditary	Atrophy of paraspinal and pelvic muscles. Crouched, waddling gait. Cranial nerves V, VII and XII may be involved. Early-onset form has signs by 1 month and tetraparesis by 3–4 months of age. Intermediate onset form has weakness at 4 6 months and tetraparesis at 2–3 years of age. Dogs with late-onset form may live several years. No treatment
Hereditary neuronal abiotrophy of the Swedish Lapland Dog (Sandefeldt *et al.*, 1973)	Swedish Lapland Dog 5–7 weeks of age Hereditary	Paresis of fore or hindlimbs, become tetraparetic within 2 weeks. Does not progress after 2 weeks. No treatment
Stockard's paralysis (Stockard, 1936)	Great Dane, Bloodhound, or Great Dane–St Bernard mix	Hindlimb paralysis, atrophy of the distal limb muscles. Non-progressive after a few days
Spinal muscle atrophy of Pointers (Inada *et al.*, 1978)	Pointers 5 months of age	Similar to Brittany Spaniel disease. May be a storage disease
Spinal muscle atrophy of German Shepherd Dogs (Cummings *et al.*, 1989)	German Shepherd Dog	Weakness and atrophy of thoracic muscles
Spinal muscle atrophy of Rottweiler dogs (Shell *et al.*, 1987)	Rottweiler 8 weeks of age	Similar to Brittany Spaniel disease. May also have megaoesophagus
Multisystem neuronal degenerations	Cairn Terriers, Cocker Spaniels 4–7 months of age	Hindlimb paresis progresses to tetraplegia in weeks to months (Cummings *et al.*, 1988; Palmer and Blackmore, 1989) Cocker Spaniels had behavioural changes, ataxia, and dysmetria (Jaggy and Vandevelde, 1988)

Table 10.9 Characteristics of congenital or hereditary peripheral neuropathies

Disease	Signalment (breed, age)	Comment
Progressive axonopathy in Boxer dogs (Griffiths *et al.*, 1980)	Boxer 2–3 months of age	Hind limb ataxia which progresses to fore limbs. Good muscle strength, no atrophy, bilateral patellar areflexia. Signs may stabilize after 1–2 years and dog can live a relatively normal life
Giant axonal neuropathy in German Shepherd Dogs (Duncan, 1991)	German Shepherd Dog 14–16 months of age Hereditary	Paraparesis and ataxia. Proprioceptive deficits, areflexia, distal muscle atrophy, diminished pain sensation in hindlimbs. Megaoesophagus develops at 18 months
Neurofibrillary accumulation (deLahunta and Shively, 1975; Vandevelde *et al.*, 1976)	Dog: Collie Cat: domestic cat	Generalized weakness that progresses to tetraplegia
Hypertrophic neuropathy (Cummings and deLahunta, 1974; Cooper *et al.*, 1984)	Tibetan Mastiff Dogs 7–12 weeks of age	Generalized weakness and decreased reflexes. Become tetraplegic within 3 weeks
Sensory neuropathy (Cummings *et al.*, 1983; Nes, 1986; Wouda *et al.*, 1983)	Longhaired Dachshunds (8 weeks), Pointers (3–9 months), Golden Retrievers, Dobermann, Siberian Husky, Whippet, Scottish Terrier	Dachshund: urinary incontinence, hindlimb ataxia, loss of proprioception, depressed patellar reflexes, diminished pain sensation over entire body. No treatment Pointer: self-mutilation of the extremities, anaesthesia of the hind limb digits and diminished sensation in fore limbs and trunk
Laryngeal paralysis	Siberian Husky, Bouvier des Flandres 4–6 months of age Hereditary	Stridor, pharyngitis, exercise intolerance. Treat as for acquired laryngeal paralysis

occur without spasticity, paresis or involuntary movements. Clinically, ataxia can be classified as sensory, vestibular or cerebellar. Sensory ataxia is evidenced by loss of proprioception in the limbs. Sensory ataxia is frequently associated with motor dysfunction (paresis) and the lesion is located as for motor dysfunctions (Table 10.2). Diseases which cause sensory ataxia have already been discussed.

Table 10.10 Causes of inflammatory polymyopathies of puppies and kittens

Infectious
  Toxoplasma gondii
  Neospora caninum
  Leptospira ictorohaemmorrhagiae
  Clostridium spp.
  Hepatozoon *Canis*
  Dirofilariaimmitis

Non-infectious
  Dermatomyositis of Collie and Border Collies

Table 10.11 Degenerative polymyopathies of puppies and kittens

Inherited

Muscular dystrophies
Dog: Labrador Retriever, Golden Retriever, Bouvier des Flandres, Samoyed, Rottweiler, Irish Terrier
Cat: domestic cats

Mitochondrial myopathy
Dog: Sussex Spaniel, Clumber Spaniel, German Shepherd Dog

Myotonic myopathy
Dog: Chow Chow, Staffordshire Terrier, Great Dane, Rhodesian Ridgeback, Cavalier King Charles Spaniel, Golden Retriever

Phosphofructokinase deficiency
Dog: Springer Spaniel

Nutritional

Vitamin E/selenium deficiency

Vestibular ataxia

The vestibular system uses sensory input to modify and coordinate movement. The vestibular system controls the muscles which maintain equilibrium, position the head and regulate eye movements. A head tilt usually indicates vestibular system disease. Head tilt is not seen with cerebellar or sensory ataxia. Asymmetrical ataxia and nystagmus may be seen with vestibular ataxia. Neurological examination can be used to localize vestibular ataxia to a peripheral vestibular lesion or a central vestibular lesion (brainstem). If nystagmus changes direction with altered head position, proprioceptive deficits are present, or paresis is present, the lesion is in the central vestibular region rather than peripheral.

If neurological examination indicates peripheral vestibular disease, diagnostic evaluation should include otoscopic examination, bulla radiographs and possibly computed tomography or magnetic resonance imaging (Table 10.12).

Table 10.12 Differential diagnosis for peripheral vestibular diseases

Congenital vestibular disease
Otitis media or interna
Idiopathic vestibular disease (older dogs, any-age cat)
Ototoxic drugs (aminoglycosides)
Head trauma

Congenital vestibular syndromes occur sporadically in pure-bred dogs and cats. Animals with congenital vestibular syndrome have signs from birth until several weeks of age. Unilateral or bilateral deafness may also be present. The pathogenesis is unknown. Some animals gradually improve while others have persistent head tilt and deafness. There is no treatment.

Central vestibular disorders may be caused by diseases which produce multifocal neurological signs or systemic signs (Table 10.13).

Cerebellar ataxia

The cerebellum coordinates motor activity. It controls muscle movements, helps maintain equilibrium and controls posture. Characteristic signs of cerebellar disease include a hypermetric

Table 10.13 Central vestibular diseases

Storage diseases (Table 10.18)
Degenerative diseases (Table 10.19)
Hydrocephalus
Hypoglycaemia
Thiamine deficiency of cats
Encephalitis: viral (canine distemper, feline infectious peritonitis), bacterial, fungal (Table 10.20)
Toxicities: metronidazole, lead, others
Head trauma

wide-based gait, truncal ataxia, head tremor and intention tremors. Tremor-like nystagmus may be seen, but head tilt is rare. There may be slight proprioceptive deficits, but cerebellar disease does not cause paresis. Acute cerebellar dysfunction is characterized by opisthotonus, tonic extension of the fore limbs and clonic movement of the hind limbs. Possible causes of cerebellar ataxia are listed in Table 10.14. Dysmyelinogenesis and congenital cerebral disorders are discussed below. The other cerebellar diseases seen in puppies and kittens are addressed in the section on systemic and multifocal neurologic diseases.

Dysmyelinogenesis

Dysmyelinogenesis is not a degenerative disease but a condition with abnormal myelin forma-

Table 10.14 Differential diagnoses for cerebellar diseases

Aetiology	Cerebellar diseases
Degenerative	Cerebellar abiotrophies (Table 10.15) Storage diseases (Table 10.18) Demyelinating diseases (Table 10.19) Neuroaxonal dystrophies (Table 10.15 and 10.19) Spongiform degeneration (Table 10.19)
Anomalous	Malformations: hypoplasia and dysplasia Dysmyelinogenesis Occipital dysplasia (see hydrocephalus)
Nutritional	Thiamine deficiency (early)
Inflammatory	Viral (distemper, feline infectious peritonitis), toxoplasmosis, fungi, bacteria, parasites (Table 10.20)
Toxic	Lead, hexachloraphene, organophosphates, plants, others
Traumatic	Head trauma

tion. It has been reported in Chow Chows, Springer Spaniels, Lurchers, Weimaraners and a Dalmatian (Kornegay, 1986). Signs include ataxia, involuntary limb movement and head tremor at 4–6 weeks of age. Signs in Chow Chows and Weimaraners usually gradually improve and are absent by 6–12 months (Vande-velde *et al.*, 1981). Cerebrospinal hypomyelino-genesis was also reported in a 5-week-old Dalmatian with body tremors and inability to walk (Greene *et al.*, 1977). Spontaneous remis-sion of dysmyelinogenesis differentiates it from the storage diseases which are progressive and from cerebellar hypoplasia which is static. There is no treatment.

Congenital cerebellar disorders

Congenital cerebellar disorders can be classified as viral infections, malformations or abiotro-phies (Table 10.15). Neonatal syndromes are present at birth or prior to normal ambulation.

These syndromes have symmetrical clinical signs and a non-progressive course. Postnatal syndromes are due to abiotrophies which are considered to be degenerative diseases because there is premature neuron death. There is a variable period of normal function followed by onset of cerebellar signs (ataxia, dysmetria, tremors). Diagnosis of cerebellar abiotrophy is confirmed by cerebellar biopsy or necropsy.

Altered mentation

Altered mental status is always related to abnor-mal brain function. Causes are varied (Table 10.16). A depressed animal is lethargic but will react to its environment normally. A disoriented animal responds inappropriately to its environ-ment. A stuporous animal appears to be asleep but can be roused. A comatose animal is uncon-scious and has no behavioural reaction to any stimulus.

Table 10.15 Congenital cerebellar diseases

Aetiology and disease	Signalment (breed, age)	Clinical signs
Neonatal syndromes		
Viral infections		
Canine herpesvirus	Dog 3–4 weeks of age	Cerebellar ataxia. Diarrhoea, crying, dyspnoea up to 2 weeks. Usually die within 1–3 days. Surviving puppies may have cerebellar deficits when walking
Feline panleukopenia	Cat 3–4 weeks of age	*In utero* infection causes cerebellar hypoplasia with ataxia, head tremors, hypermetria
Malformation		
Cerebellar hypoplasia and lissencephaly	Dog: Wire-haired Fox Terriers, Irish Setters 3–4 weeks of age	Non-progressive cebellar dysfunction
Cerebellar hypoplasia	Dog: Chow Chows, Miniature Poodle, others 6 weeks of age	Tremor and dysmetria. Signs are not progressive and may improve with compensation
Abiotrophies		
Abiotrophies	Dog: Beagle, Labrador, Retriever, Samoyed, Irish Setter, Bull Mastiff, Australian Kelpie 3–4 weeks of age	Non-progressive cerebellar dysfunction
Olivopontocerebellar atrophy	Cat: domestic cat	May be secondary Panleucopenia virus

Table 10.15 (continued)

Aetiology and disease	Signalment (breed, age)	Clinical signs
Postnatal syndromes		
	Abiotrophies	
Abiotrophies	Dog: Akita, Airedale, Beagle, Bern Running Dogs; Bernese Mountain Dog; Brittany Spaniels; Border Collie; Cairn Terrier, Clumber Spaniel; Cocker Spaniel, Finnish Harriers, Fox Terrier, Golden Retriever; Gordon Setters (6–30 months), Great Dane, Kerry Blue Terriers (2–4 months), Labrador Retriever, Miniature Poodle, Miniature Schnauzer × Beagle, Rough Coated Collies (1–2 months) hereditary	Hindlimb stiffness and incoordination, dysmetria to hypermetria, broad-based stance. Bunny-hopping and forelimb stiffness has been reported. Some dogs have head tremors or nystagmus
Neuroaxonal dystrophy	Cat 5–6 weeks of age Hereditary Dog 2–4 months of age Hereditary	Cat: Head tremors and shaking, incoordinated gait and hypermetria Dog: Slowly progressive cerebellar ataxia with incoordination, hypermetria, wide-based stance

Table 10.16 Diseases causing stupor and coma

Aetiology	Stupor and coma
Degenerative	Storage diseases (10.18)
Anomalous	Hydrocephalus Brain malformation: lissencephaly, hydranencephaly, otocephaly Narcolepsy
Metabolic	Hypoglycaemia Hepatic encephalopathy Congenital defects with associated metabolic disorders (renal insufficiency, diabetes, hypothyroid) Heat stroke Hypoxia
Nutritional	Thiamine deficiency (late stages)
Inflammatory	Severe bacterial, viral, protozoal, fungal or rickettsial infections (Table 10.20)
Toxic	Heavy metals, barbiturates and other drugs, carbon monoxide, various plants, many others
Traumatic	Head trauma with cerebral haemorrhage or oedema

Hydrocephaly

Hydrocephalus is a condition in which the cerebral ventricular system is enlarged secondary to increased volume of cerebrospinal fluid (CSF). An abnormality of CSF flow or absorption is responsible for the increased fluid. Hydrocephalus can be an acquired disease in puppies as young as 6 weeks old or it can be congenital. Hydrocephalus can occur sporadically in cats or in any breed of dog. Congenital hydrocephalus is commonly seen in small-breed dogs such as the Chihuahua, Cocker Spaniel, English Bulldog, Maltese, Yorkshire Terrier, Lhasa Apso, Pomeranian, Toy Poodle, Cairn Terrier, Boston Terrier, Pug and Pekinese.

Clinical signs

Puppies or kittens with acquired hydrocephalus secondary to infection have an acute onset of neurologic signs at 6–8 weeks of age. They suddenly become irritable and hyperexcitable. They may circle and seem blind. The skull may rapidly enlarge. Clinical signs in animals with congenital hydrocephalus are often recognized between 2 and 3 months of age. The head is dome-shaped and there is ventrolateral strabismus. Open fontanelles or sutures may be palpable. The animal is often smaller than its littermates. Some animals have minimal or no clinical signs. Other animals may demonstrate depression, behavioural changes or seizures. They may be difficult to house-train, and have visual or auditory deficits. Motor function can range from a normal gait to severe tetraparesis. Some puppies have also been reported to have occipital dysplasia, which is an abnormally large foramen magnum (Parker and Park, 1974). Neurologic signs are usually attributed to the hydrocephalus.

Diagnosis

The diagnosis is usually based on clinical signs. Electroencephalogram traces have a characteristic pattern and can be used to support a diagnosis of hydrocephalus. A ventricular tap may also be performed. A 22-gauge spinal needle is inserted through an open suture line approximately midway between the lateral canthus of the eye and the external occipital protuberance, and 5–10 mm from midline (Savell, 1974). Needles should be placed bilaterally and fluid may be allowed to escape through the spinal needle. Negative pressure should not be used. Two millilitres (mlh) or less can be removed from normal animals and 5–10 ml may be removed from each ventricle in animals with hydrocephalus. The CSF may be submitted for analysis to determine whether an infection is present. Congenital hydrocephalus will have a normal CSF analysis and normal pressures. Skull radiographs can be made to identify open suture lines and fontanelles, thinning of the calvarium and a homogeneous or 'ground-glass' appearance to the cranial vault. Pneumoventriculography may be performed by replacing the CSF that was removed with the same volume of air. Radiographs are made using a horizontal beam. Less invasive diagnostic procedures include the use of ultrasound through an open fontanelle. Computed tomography and magnetic resonance imaging can also be used to demonstrate dilated ventricles.

Treatment and surgical technique

The recommended treatment depends on the status of the animal. If an animal has stable neurological signs over several months and its behaviour is acceptable, no treatment is required. Anticonvulsant therapy may be necessary if seizure activity is frequent. If neurologic signs are progressive, medical treatment is attempted in an effort to reduce CSF production (Simpson, 1989). Dexamethasone, 0.25 mg/kg PO t.i.d. or q.i.d., or prednisolone 0.25–0.5 mg/kg PO b.i.d., has been effective in some animals. The dose should be tapered over 2–4 weeks. Many animals will stabilize and require chronic alternate-day therapy or intermittent steroids for exacerbation of signs.

Surgery is recommended for cases which cannot be stabilized medically. A drainage tube is placed from the lateral ventricle to the right atrium or peritoneal cavity (Few, 1966; Gage, 1968).

Postoperative considerations and prognosis

Hydrocephalics tend to be frail and have poor tolerance to many drugs commonly used to treat non-specific illnesses such as diarrhoea and vomiting. Prognosis for progressive hydrocephalus is poor because of the irreversible brain damage. It has not been determined whether surgical management is any more effective than medical management. Although the shunts may be very effective, problems include occlusion by fibrous tissue or clots, infection and shifting of the catheter. Some animals may require tube replacement with a larger tube as the animal grows. Severely affected animals may not improve after shunting. Prognosis is poor.

Other cerebral malformations

Lissencephaly is the reduction or absence of cerebral gyri and has been reported in the Lhasa Apso and a cat (Greene *et al.*, 1976). It has also been reported with concomitant cerebellar hypoplasia in Wire-haired Fox Terriers and Irish Setters. It can cause erratic behaviour and visual deficits by 3 months of age and generalized seizures by 1 year. Diagnosis may be confirmed by asynchronous wave patterns on electroencephalogram or absence of gyri on magnetic resonance imaging. Treatment is symptomatic but the animals are often not acceptable pets.

Hydranencephaly is the absence of cerebral hemispheres and results in blind ataxic animals that are unable to suckle. It is thought to be associated with feline panleukopenia virus in the cat. Hydranencephaly is usually not compatible with life.

Seizures

Seizures are paroxysmal stereotyped behavioural changes and can include loss of consciousness, change of muscle tone or movement, altered sensation (e.g. hallucinations), disturbances of the autonomic nervous system (e.g. salivation, urination, defaecation) and behavioural changes (e.g. rage, fear). Seizures always indicate abnormal brain function and can be caused by any process that alters neuronal function (Table 10.17). If an animal has more than one seizure a minimum data base is recommended to help determine the cause.

A minimum data base includes the physical and neurologic examination, as well as CBC, urinalysis and serum chemistry. Blood lead levels may also be indicated. The minimum data base should be used to determine whether the seizures are due to a primary neurologic disease or a systemic disorder. Computed tomography, MRI, skull radiographs, CSF analysis and EEG may be required for a definitive diag-

nosis or to rule out true epilepsy. Recurrent or intense seizures should be treated, but their management is beyond the scope of the text.

Systemic or multifocal neurological diseases

Systemic or multifocal diseases should be suspected if the neurological examination indicates involvement of two or more regions of the nervous system which are not closely related anatomically. Diseases which are likely to cause systemic or multifocal signs in puppies and kittens include storage diseases and abiotrophies.

Storage diseases

The storage diseases are rare, inherited (usually recessive) enzyme deficiencies which result in the accumulation of various metabolic products within cells (Table 10.18). The two categories of storage diseases are neuronal storage diseases and leukodystrophies. Neuronal storage diseases are characterized by product accumulation within the neurons and leukodystrophies are characterized by progressive myelin destruction. Clinical signs of the neuronal storage diseases include attitude changes, seizures, tetraparesis, intention tremor and blindness. Euthanasia is usually required as the disease progresses. The behaviour of the storage diseases is similar. Affected animals are usually normal at birth but may have stunted growth and develop neurologic signs within a few months of age. In general, these are slowly progressive, fatal, and there is no treatment.

Degenerative diseases

Most degenerative diseases are hereditary and are characterized by premature ageing of neurons. Abiotrophy is a term used for the process of degeneration which implies inherent lack of a trophic or nutritive factor. The degeneration can be primarily motor neuronal, peripheral, cerebellar or multisystemic (Table 10.19). An example of a primary motor neuronal abiotrophy is that of the Swedish Lapland Dog (Table 10.8). The sensory neuropathy of Dachshunds and Pointers (Table 10.9) are examples of peripheral degenerative diseases. Examples

Table 10.17 Disorders causing seizures in young dogs and cats

Hydrocephalus
Lissencephaly
Storage diseases (Table 10.18)
Hypoglycaemia
Hepatic encephalopathy due to portosystemic shunt
Thiamine deficiency
Canine distemper, feline infectious peritonitis, other
   infectious diseases (Table 10.20)
Lead, organophosphates, other toxins
Acute head trauma
True epilepsy (pure-bred dog or cat)

Table 10.18 Storage diseases

Storage disease	Signalment (breed, age)	Signs
Gangliosidosis GM1	Dog: Beagle mix (3 months), Portuguese Water Dog (5 months) Cat: Siamese, Korat and domestic cats (2–3 months)	Tremor, incoordination, spastic paraplegia, impaired vision
Gangliosidosis GM2	Dog: German Shorthaired Pointer (6–9 months), Japanese Spaniel (18 months), mixed-breed dog (1.5 years) Cat: domestic cats (2 months)	Pointer: (amaurotic idiocy): incoordination, nervousness and decreased training ability, progressive ataxia and impaired vision by 9–12 months, dementia. Mixed-breed: ataxia, incoordination, tremor, hypermetria Cat: same as GM1
Mannosidosis	Cat: domestic cat (7 months), Persian cat (8 weeks)	Ataxia, incoordination, tremor
Glycogenosis	Dog: Lapland Dogs (1.5 years); English Springer Spaniel (11 years) Cat: domestic and Norwegian Forest cats (5 months)	Incoordination, exercise intolerance
Glucocerebrosidosis	Dog: Australian Silky Terrier (6–8 months)	Ataxia, incoordination, hypermetria
Sphingomyelinosis	Dog: Poodles (2–4 months) Cat: Siamese, Balinese, domestic cats (2–4 months)	Ataxia, incoordination, hypermetria, polyneuropathy
Ceroid lipofuscinosis	Dog: English Setter (1 year); Dachshund (3.5–7 years); Cocker Spaniel (1.5 years); Chihuahua, Saluki (2 years); Tibetian Terrier (3 years); Australian Cattle Dog (14 months); Border Collie (18–22 months); Blue Heeler (12 months); mixed breed (4 months) Cat: Siamese, domestic cat (2–7 years)	Personality change, visual impairment, ataxia, incoordination, jaw champing, seizures
Fucosidosis	Dog: Springer Spaniel (2 years)	Incoordination, behavioural changes, dysphonia, dysphagia, seizures
Glycoproteinosis	Dog: Beagle, Basset Hound, Poodle (5 months–9 years)	Depression, progressive seizures
Mucopolysaccharidosis	Dog: Plott Hound (3–6 months); mixed dog (4–6 months) Cat: Siamese, domestic cat (4–7 months)	Progressive paraparesis (Chapter 12)
Globoid cell leukodystrophy	Dog: Cairn Terrier, West Highland White Terrier (2–3 months); Beagle, Blue Tick Hound (4 months); Miniature Poodle (2 years), Basset Hound (1.5–2 years), Pomeranian (1.5 years), possibly Dalmatian Cat: domestic cat (5–6 weeks)	(Krabbe's disease): ataxia, incoordination, hypermetria, tremor, blindness, paraparesis progressing to tetraplegia
Metachromatic leukodystrophy	Cat: domestic cat (2 weeks)	Progressive motor dysfunction, seizures, opisthotonos

Table 10.19 Degenerative neurological diseases

Degenerative diseases	Signalment (breed, age)	Clinical signs
Cerebellar ataxia	Dog: Cocker Spaniel (1 year); Cairn Terrier (2.5–5 months); Bull Mastiff (6–9 weeks)	Cerebellar ataxia, spastic paresis Mastiff: cerebellar ataxia, head tremor, abnormal nystagmus, behaviour change, visual abnormality, hydrocephalus
Ataxia of Fox Terriers	Smooth Fox Terrier, Jack Russell Terrier (2–6 months) Hereditary	Weakness, hindlimb incoordination, dysmetria, spasticity
Degenerative myelopathy	Dog: German Shepherd Dog, Siberian Huskies, others (4–5 years)	Progressive hindlimb ataxia and paresis
Dalmatian leukodystrophy	Dalmatian (3–6 months) May be hereditary	Progressive visual deficit and ataxia and weakness of all limbs
Leukoencephalomyelopathy of Rottweilers	Rottweiler (1.5–3.5 years) Hereditary	Ataxia, dysmetria, tetraparesis
Myelin degeneration	Dog: Labrador Retriever (4–6 months), Saluki (3 months), Afghan Hound (3–13 months) Hereditary	Labrador: extensor rigidity, opisthotonos, progressive cerebellar ataxia Saluki: seizures, behaviour change Afghan: hindlimb ataxia and paresis, progresses to paraplegia in 7–10 days. Forelimbs become weak within 1–2 weeks. Death is due to respiratory failure within 2 to 6 weeks (Cockrell, 1973)
Neuronaxonal dystrophy	Dog: Collie (2–4 months), Rottweiler (1–2 years), Chihuahua (7 weeks), German Shepherd Dog (15 months); Boxer (1–7 months) Cat: Siamese (5 weeks)	Collie: progressive cerebellar ataxia, tremor Shepherd: progressive hindlimb paresis and ataxia Boxer: spastic hindlimb paresis, late tetraparesis Cat: progressive cerebellar ataxia
Neurofilament degeneration	Dog: Collie Cat: domestic cats (3 weeks)	Paresis
Demyelinating myelopathy	Dog: Miniature Poodles (2–4 months) May be hereditary	Paraparesis progressing to spastic paraplegia and tetraplegia
Spongiform degeneration	Dog: Samoyed (12 days), Australian Silky Terrier, Labrador Retrievers (4–5 months) Cat: Egyptian Mau cat (7 weeks) May be hereditary	Ataxia and dysmetria, hyporeflexia and extensor rigidity. Samoyed: hindlimb tremor progressing to body tremors over 5 days Australian Silky Terrier: uncontrolled intermittent contractures of paravertebral muscles Labrador: episodes of extensor rigidity and opisthotonus Cat: hindlimb ataxia and hypermetria. Intermittent depression and hindlimb flicking
Fibrinoid leukodystrophy	Dog: Labrador Retrievers, Scottish Terrier (6 months)	Paraparesis, ataxia, generalized weakness, personality change
Hereditary quadriplegia and amblyopia	Dog: Irish Setter (affected at birth) Hereditary	Look like swimmer puppies at 3 days. Visual impairment, head tremors, seizures. No pathology (Palmer *et al.*, 1973)

of cerebellar abiotrophies are listed in Table 10.15. Most of these degenerative diseases are hereditary, occur in young animals, are slowly progressive and result in death. The degenerative process can affect various parts of the neuron including the cell body, cell process, myelin or neurofilaments. Diagnosis of degenerative diseases is based on ruling out the acquired diseases.

Hypoglycaemia

Hypoglycaemia in puppies and kittens may be due to malnutrition, severe parasitism, stress or gastrointestinal abnormality. Glycogen storage diseases have also been reported, but are rare. Clinical signs usually include severe depression or coma, and seizures may be present. Blood glucose levels are very low. Treatment is administration of intravenous glucose. Diazepam may be given for seizures if the animal does not respond to glucose. If mental status does not improve, corticosteroids and mannitol may be given for brain swelling.

Infectious and inflammatory diseases

There are a number of infectious agents that cause clinical signs of central nervous system disease (Table 10.20).

Aural disorders

Congenital deafness

Congenital deafness has been reported in several dog breeds (Table 10.21) and appears to occur more often in blue-eyed white cats. Dalmatians appear to be at highest risk (30% of all dogs), with 22% affected unilaterally and 8% bilaterally. A 1% incidence of deafness is estimated in blue-eyed white cats (Strain, 1991) and several characteristic features of the incidence in affected cats have been noted. Either sex is affected, unilaterally or bilaterally, that is, not correlated with the side of blue eye colour. Longhaired cats appear to be affected more often than shorthaired cats. Shorthaired cats are more likely to have unilateral hearing loss (Mair, 1973).

Congenital deafness has been shown to be hereditary, transmitted by autosomal dominant, recessive or sex-linked modes. Autosomal dominant appears to be most consistent in canine and feline deafness, although recessive transmission has been documented in Bull Terriers. Sex-linked modes of transmission have not been established.

The correlation of deafness and coat colour is apparent and is frequently associated with the merle gene (Collie, Shetland Sheepdog, Harlequin Great Dane, Dappled Dachshund, American Foxhound, Norwegian Dunkerhound) and the piebald or extreme piebald gene (Bull Terrier, Samoyed, Great Pyrenees, Sealyham

Table 10.20 Infectious agents causing central nervous system infection or inflammation

Infectious agent	Age of onset of clinical signs	Clinical signs
	Viral	
Feline panleukopenia	2–3 weeks	Ataxia, incoordination, tremor. Signs rarely progress, and usually improve due to compensation
Feline infectious peritonitis (coronavirus)	Usually less than 2 years	Infected *in utero* or postnatal ingestion. Signs of meningitis (fever, hyperaesthesia, cranial nerve abnormalities), seizures, paraparesis, tetraparesis, ataxia, behavioural changes. If there are neurologic signs, there are not usually signs of pleural or peritoneal involvement
Canine herpesvirus	Less than 1 week	Depressed, persistent crying, diarrhoea, do not suckle, rhinitis, opisthotonus, seizures. Surviving puppies may be blind or ataxic
Canine parvovirus	Within first few weeks of life	Cerebellar degeneration. May also have systemic signs

Table 10.20 (continued)

Infectious agent	Age of onset of clinical signs	Clinical signs
Canine distemper	Any age	May have neurologic signs 1–3 weeks after systemic illness. Post vaccinal distemper has been reported 1–2 weeks after vaccination with a modified live virus. Non-specific neurologic signs: seizures, cerebellar and vestibular signs, sensory ataxia, myoclonus
Adenovirus (infectious canine hepatitis)		Has predilection for vascular endothelium, but can cause encephalitis in rare cases. Rapidly progressive tetraparesis, coma, seizures, death. Also vomiting, abdominal pain, fever, jaundice may occur
Pseudorabies (Aujeszky's disease)		Exposure is usually by consumption of contaminated tissues. Intense pruritus on face and limbs, fever, emesis, excessive salivation, dyspnoea followed by incoordination, vocalization, ptosis, anisocoria, facial tremors, convulsions, coma and death within 1–2 days
Rabies	Any age	Signs after exposure to rabid animal or after vaccination (modified live vaccine). Behavioural changes or progressive lower motor neuron paralysis
Rickettsia and spirochaetes Lyme disease	Any age	Signs after tick exposure. Fever, anorexia, oculonasal discharges, lymphadenopathy, lethargy, stupor, seizures, coma, paraparesis, ataxia
Bacteria		
Canine brucellosis (many others)	Any age	Occurs especially after history of breeding. Behavioural changes, anisocoria, ataxia, hyperaesthesia, head tilt, circling
Discospondylitis	Any age	Infection of intervertebral disc and vertebral end-plates. Usually young, male, large-breed dogs.
Staphylococcus is most common. Also *Brucella, Nocardia, Streptococcus* and fungi		Signs range from hyperaesthesia to paresis or paralysis. May be anorexic and pyrexic. Diagnosis by clinical, laboratory data and radiographs. Blood or urine cultures may identify the agent
Fungi		
Cryptococcosis more common than blastomycosis, histoplasmosis or coccidiomycosis	Any age	Signs after inhaling the saprophyte. Ataxia, paresis, cranial nerve involvement, seizures
Parasites		
Many		Related to abberrant migration

Table 10.20 (continued)

Infectious agent	Age of onset of clinical signs	Clinical signs
Algae		
Prototbecosis	Any age	Signs after exposure to water or organic matter. Persistent bloody diarrhoea, blindness, ataxia, circling, paresis or paralysis
Protozoa		
Neospora caninum *Toxoplasma gondii*	Prenatal infection: puppies less than 10 days old Postnatal infection: dogs and cats of any age	Inflammation of the peripheral nerves, muscles or central nervous system. Prenatal infection: diarrhoea, respiratory compromise, ataxia. Postnatal infection: seizures, paraparesis, ataxia, polymyositis. It may be difficult to distinguish the two organisms. Early treatment may be beneficial (Chapter 12)
Idiopathic		
Granulomatous meningoencephalomyelitis (reticulosis)	Usually adult animals	May have signs similar to a space-occupying mass or have multifocal signs with diffuse form of disease
Pug encephalitis	9 months to 4 years	Seizures, circling, and visual deficits. Death in 1–6 months is preceded by coma or status epilepticus
Feline polioencephalomyelitis	Any age	Possibly viral aetiology. Incoordination, paresis, hypermetria. Intention tremors of the head. Guarded prognosis. No known treatment

Table 10.21 Dog breeds reported with congenital deafness (Strain, 1991)

Affected breeds	
Akita	Fox Terrier
American Staffordshire Terrier	Great Dane (harlequin)
Australian Cattle Dog	Great Pyrenees
Australian Shepherd	Maltese Terrier
Beagle	Mixed-breed
Border Collie	Norwegian Dunkerhound
Boston Terrier	Old English Sheepdog
Bull Terrier	Papillon
Catahoula	Pointer
Cocker Spaniel	Poodle (miniature)
Collie	Rhodesian Ridgeback
Dachshund (dappled)	Scottish Terrier
Dalmatian	Sealyham Terrier
Dobermann	Shetland Sheepdog
Argentine Mastiff	Shropshire Terrier
English Bulldog	Walker American Foxhound
English Setter	West Highland White Terrier
Foxhound	

Terrier, Greyhound, Bulldog, Dalmatian, Beagle). However, deafness has not been reported in all these breeds. The syndrome of hereditary deafness associated with pigmentation abnormalities may show variable features such as piebaldism, partial albinism, heterochromia iridis (blue iris due to lack of pigment), absence of retinal pigment, absence of cochlea stria vascularis pigment and various facial defects (Strain, 1991; Greibrokk, 1994). The absence of cochlea stria vascularis pigment, required for normal function, appears to be the critical factor in determining deafness (Strain, 1991). The syndrome appears to be inherited as an autosomal dominant trait. Selective breeding excluding blue-eyed animals will control the incidence of the syndrome and deafness (Greibrokk, 1994).

The pathophysiology of congenital deafness is variable, although most hereditary deafness results from cochleosaccular degeneration, the result of a vascular disorder beginning in the stria vascularis.

Table 10.22 Acquired causes of deafness

Causes of acquired deafness	Comment
Meningitis	
Viral infection	Distemper can cause demyelination changes in the auditory pathway to the brainstem and cerebrum and typically causes partial rather than complete hearing loss
Anoxia	
Otitis	Conduction interference due to external canal obstruction and tympanic membrane damage
	Progressive disease due to otitis media and interna may cause irreversible damage to vestibular, cochlear and auditory structures
Ototoxicity	Prolonged systemic aminoglycoside administration most commonly implicated and mostly affect auditory system but may affect vestibular system. Animals can be deaf with or without vestibular signs. Immediate discontinuation of administration may result in improvement of vestibular signs but deafness is usually irreversible
	Topical antiseptics also cause ototoxicity, particularly if instilled into the middle ear through a damaged tympanic membrane. Chlorhexidine, iodophors and quaternary ammonium compounds are implicated (Mansfield, 1990); however, toxicity appears to be concentration-dependent and some dilute solutions, 0.2% chlorhexidine (Merchant *et al.*, 1993) or 0.1% iodine solution (Morizono and Sikora, 1982) appear safe
Noise	
Malformation of external ear canal	
Hydrocephalus	
Unknown	

Other causes of deafness in young puppies and kittens may be acquired and are usually because of problems in sound conduction or nerve impulse transmission (Table 10.22).

Diagnosis

Diagnosis may require several procedures to rule out causes, particularly in animals that are not typically affected by hereditary deafness (Table 10.23; Neer, 1995).

Definitive diagnosis of deafness requires brainstem auditory-evoked potential testing, although lateral testing can usually be detected by orifice testing. These test procedures, while they require specialized equipment, can usually be performed without chemical restraint. Brainstem auditory-evoked potential testing can be performed once the ear canals are open, as early as 30–40 days of age in dogs and by 3–4 weeks of age in cats, although waiting until 5 weeks of age, when cochlear degeneration has occurred to a sufficient degree, may be more accurate (Strain, 1991).

Pinna lacerations

Pinna lacerations are not uncommon and may be the result of the dam picking up the puppy or of rough play between puppies. In older puppies, traumatic lacerations tend to occur more often in pendulous-eared dogs. Lacerations may be incomplete, through one skin layer or the cartilage, or complete, through both skin

Table 10.23 Characteristics of congenital and acquired hearing loss

Procedure	Diagnostic evaluation for congenital hearing loss	Diagnostic evaluation for acquired hearing loss
History	Known predisposed breed. Evidence of hearing loss since birth, no previous ear problems	Current or previous otitis externa, media or interna. Clinical signs related to involvement of other body systems (e.g. canine distemper, aminoglycoside administration)
Physical and neurologic findings	Normal except for hearing loss. Associated bilateral congenital vestibular deficits may occur	Altered ear canal and/or tympanic membrane. Focal or multifocal neurological defects. Symptoms of vestibular disease
Ancillary diagnostic procedures	None required	Cytological study of ear discharge. Culture and sensitivity testing of discharge. Skull radiographs to evaluate tympanic bullae and petrous temporal bone structure. Cerebrospinal fluid analysis and cerebrospinal fluid distemper titre
Electrodiagnostic procedures	Electroencephalogram (EEG) arousal response test. Brainstem auditory-evoked potential testing	EEG arousal response test. Brainstem auditory-evoked potential testing. Impedance audiometry test

layers and cartilage. They are associated with a considerable amount of bleeding.

Treatment and surgical technique

Treatment involves basic wound management and, typically, surgical repair of the laceration for first-intention healing. The owners should be directed to apply pressure to the area with a clean cloth until they can present the animal. Attention as soon as possible reduces the chance of infection and possible abscessation, and will allow surgical repair.

Small lacerations may be repaired under sedation and local anaesthesia; however, large or highly traumatized and contaminated lacerations will require general anaesthesia. The wound should be clipped free of hair and the surrounding skin prepared for aseptic surgery. The edges of the laceration should be debrided if traumatized or contaminated. Any torn cartilage should be excised. The wound should be lavaged with normal saline.

Although a very small skin laceration will heal by second intention (contraction and epithelialization), primary closure of most lacerations is preferred to potentiate a cosmetic outcome. Single-surface skin wounds can be closed with simple interrupted sutures of 4-0 or 5-0 monofilament, non-absorbable suture material, making sure the sutures penetrate the skin only, and skin apposition is complete. No cartilage should be exposed as it does not support a granulation tissue bed and will delay skin healing over its surface.

Single-surface wounds which penetrate the skin and cartilage should not be left to heal by second intention and require suturing. Vertical mattress sutures can be used to help stabilize the cartilage if necessary; the deep bite of the suture aligns cartilage while the superficial bite aligns the skin (Fig. 10.5). Again, skin apposition over the cartilage is imperative.

Closure of full-thickness lacerations is difficult, especially if they involve the helical border. They can be treated as a combination of a single-surface laceration and a incomplete laceration involving the cartilage; that is, one side is closed in simple interrupted sutures through the skin and the other by vertical mattress sutures through the skin and cartilage.

Occasionally, severe trauma may require amputation of a portion of the pinna. For this procedure, non-traumatic forceps such as a Doyen, Pean or Carmalt are placed across the pinna to crush tissue slightly. The pinna is trimmed along the edge of the clamp with a scalpel or, in cats or small-eared dogs, through the middle of the crushed tissue with scissors after removal of the clamp. Alternatively, scissors can be used to resect the pinna without using clamps. The scissors will have a crushing effect on the trimmed edge which will help to control bleeding without sufficiently traumatizing the

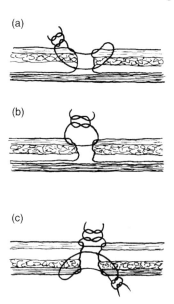

Figure 10.5 Suture closure of (a, b) incomplete and (c) complete pinna laceration using a combination of simple and vertical mattress sutures.

tissue to delay healing. In some cases, it may be advantageous to cut and suture as the pinna is amputated, in order to control bleeding.

The pinna margin is sutured in a simple continuous pattern with 4-0 or 5-0 monofilament, non-absorbable suture, including only the skin in the suture bites. This ensures that the skin edges roll over the end of the cartilage and are apposed to allow healing. Again, it is important that no cartilage is exposed as this interferes with skin healing and may result in a poor cosmetic outcome.

Postoperative considerations and prognosis

If lacerations are sutured, it is unnecessary to attempt to bandage the pinna. Once sutured, bleeding is usually minimal. An Elizabethan collar should be placed on the animal to prevent self-trauma of the pinna. Wounds left to heal by second intention are usually difficult to bandage and it is often best to leave them covered and protect with an Elizabethan collar. Animals with lacerations that are presented as acute injuries do not require antimicrobial therapy. Animals with infected lacerations or abscessed wounds should be treated with systemic broad-spectrum antimicrobial therapy for 7–10 days.

Most pinna lacerations heal quickly and cosmesis with primary closure is very good. Laceration causing considerable cartilage damage may result in a less cosmetic outcome.

Aural haematoma

Aural haematomas are a common condition of the dog's ear and in puppies, often secondary to parasitic otitis externa. Aural haematomas do occur in cats but much less frequently. The cause of the haematomas is not completely understood but in most animals is thought to result from excessive head-shaking (secondary to ear irritation from otitis externa, otic foreign bodies, flies) causing capillary disruption. Some animals with no apparent underlying disease develop aural haematomas. Coagulation disorders should be ruled out in these animals.

Clinical signs and diagnosis

An aural haematoma characteristically appears as a fluctuant swelling on the concave side of the ear. Both external ear canals should be examined thoroughly to determine any coexisting otic disease. Typically diagnosis is based on clinical signs alone. Aspiration of the swelling will reveal a sterile serosanguineous fluid that can confirm the diagnosis but is usually unnecessary. Aspiration of the haematoma risks introduction of bacteria and development of an aural abscess.

Treatment and surgical technique

Apart from addressing the haematoma, treatment should always be directed at the underlying or concurrent aural problem. Aseptic needle aspiration and bandaging of the ear to prevent redevelopment of the haematoma have been used as a treatment since it is inexpensive and easily performed in the conscious animal. Unfortunately, it is rarely successful and risks the development of an aural abscess. The authors do not recommend performing this.

Teat tube

Surgical options include the use of an indwelling catheter (bovine teat tube) or a closed-suction drain, or surgical incision and drainage (Table 10.24). Both these techniques require general

Table 10.24 Advantages and disadvantages of surgical options for aural haematoma

Technique	Advantages	Disadvantages
Teat tube	Very good cosmetic outcome Tube is inexpensive Minimal surgery time	Requires high degree of owner compliance for a prolonged period of time (21 days or more) Messy May require sedation for removal May be inadvertently dislodged Resolves condition in only 83% of cases (Wilson, 1983)
Closed-suction drainage	Drainage system is inexpensive Minimal surgery time Removal can be performed without chemical restraint Materials are inexpensive Very good cosmetic outcome	Requires high degree of owner compliance and possible repeated bandage maintenance Drainage system complications can occur (dislodgement, breakage) Resolves condition in less than 80% of cases (Swaim and Bradley, 1996)
Incisional drainage	Requires little owner compliance Reliable outcome Materials are inexpensive Suture removal can be performed without chemical restraint	Can be messy Technique takes longer to perform than alternatives Fair to good cosmetic outcome

anaesthesia. The ear is clipped and prepared for aseptic surgery. The bovine teat tube is a tapered, singly fenestrated nylon tube with two flexible retaining barbs that is modified slightly (the screw cap is discarded and the round collar on top of the teat tube is trimmed to lie flat against pinna) before use (Fig. 10.6; Wilson, 1983). A stab incision is made at the distal end of the haematoma on the concave side of the pinna and a sterile haemostat is inserted into the haematoma to break down any fibrinous adhesions. The haematoma is evacuated and the cavity flushed with normal saline. The tube is placed in the incision so that the self-retaining barbs help to anchor it in place. A suture (3/0 or 4/0 monofilament non-absorbable) is placed around the collar of the tube and passed full-thickness through the ear tip.

Postoperatively, the ear is not bandaged but the owners are instructed to 'milk' fluid out of the haematoma through the tube daily and keep the pinna clean. The tube is typically left in place for at least 21 days, depending on the amount of fluid present. Some animals may require the tube to be left in longer than this. As with any ear surgery, placement of an Eliza-bethan collar on the animal until the condition is resolved is essential.

Tube removal may require sedation since the barbs make quick extraction difficult. The procedure is associated with a good cosmetic outcome with minimal scarring. Up to 85% of 47 animals in one study had successful resolution with minimal ear deformity (Wilson, 1983). Removal before 21 days appears likely to result in recurrence of the haematoma.

Closed-suction drainage

Use of closed-suction drain (see Chapter 7) is an alternative to the teat tube. The fenestrated drain is placed through a stab incision at the proximal region of the haematoma and secured at this point and at the distal end of the haematoma (Swaim and Bradley, 1996). The drain is connected to the collection tube to establish closed-suction drainage.

Postoperatively, the ear must be bandaged to allow the collection tube to be secured. The collection tube should be changed twice daily for 7 days and this requires client compliance. The bandage must be maintained during this time and may require changing several times during

(a)   (b)   (c)

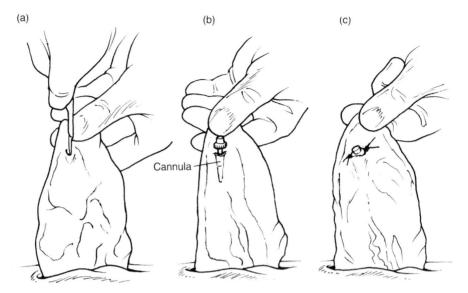

Cannula

Figure 10.6 Teat tube placement for aural haematoma. (a) A stab incision is made at the distal end of the haematoma on the concave side of the pinna and a sterile haemostat is inserted into the haematoma to break down any fibrinous adhesions. (b) After flushing the cavity, the tube is placed in the incision such that the self-retaining barbs help to anchor it in place. (c) A suture (3/0 or 4/0 monofilament absorbable) is placed around the collar of the tube and passed full-thickness through the ear tip.

this period. After 7 days, the drain is removed and the ear bandaged for a further 7 days. Placement of an Elizabethan collar on the animal until the condition is resolved is essential.

Following this regime, 7 of 9 dogs had resolution of the problem with a good cosmetic outcome (Swaim and Bradley, 1996). Breaking of the needle of the butterfly catheter occurred and the authors have recognized this to be a common problem associated with use of this drainage system, particularly when repeated collection tubes are required over a prolonged period of time. The authors have no experience with this technique but would suggest using as large a gauge of butterfly catheter as available (at least 19-gauge) and possibly leaving the drain in place longer than 7 days.

Incisional drainage

Incisional drainage and suture apposition of the skin to the auricular cartilage require a full-thickness longitudinal skin incision made over the haematoma on the concave side of the ear. The cartilage should not be incised. The contents of the haematoma are removed and the cavity is lavaged with normal saline. A thin margin (1 mm) of skin can be removed from the incision line so that when suturing, the edges of the incision stay apart approximately 1 mm. Mattress sutures (4/0 monofilament non-absorbable suture) are placed from the convex side, full-thickness through the ear, oriented longitudinally (Fig. 10.7) to avoid occluding the blood supply to the pinna, which traverses the ear longitudinally. The sutures can be stented (buttons, X-ray film, plastic, plastic tubing) if necessary but sutures should not be tight enough to cut through tissue and are placed to appose the skin to cartilage.

Postoperatively, the ear is left uncovered and the sutures are removed at 14 days. Some drainage may continue postoperatively and the owners should keep the pinna clean. Placement of an Elizabethan collar on the animal until suture removal is essential. Resolution of the problem with this technique is reliable (close to 100% in the authors' experience); however, the cosmetic appearance is only fair to good as some fibrosis and pinna thickening are usually observed. Complications of focal pinna necrosis have been reported. The advantage of the technique is, however, that it reliably resolves the problem and relies on very little owner compliance.

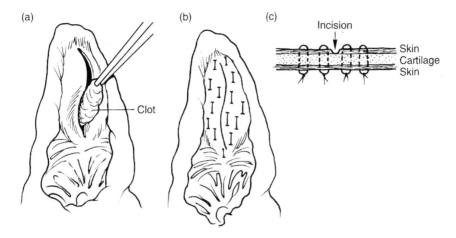

Figure 10.7 Suture placement after incisional drainage of an aural haematoma. (a) A full-thickness longitudinal skin incision is made over the haematoma on the concave side of the ear; the contents of the haematoma are removed and the cavity is lavaged with normal saline. (b) A thin margin (1 mm) of skin can be removed from the incision line so that, when suturing, the edges of the incision stay apart approximately 1 mm. (c) Mattress sutures are placed from the convex side full-thickness through the ear, oriented longitudinally. The sutures can be stented if necessary.

Otitis externa

Otitis externa is not uncommon in puppies and kittens and is most often caused by bacterial or parasitic infections.

Bacterial otitis externa

Bacterial otitis externa is the most common ear problem encountered in puppies and kittens. Their external ear canals are inhabited by various bacteria and yeasts. The type of bacteria and their frequency of isolation vary. Pathogenic bacteria that frequently colonize the healthy external ear canals of puppies and kittens in low numbers are *Staphylococcus intermedius*, β-haemolytic *Streptococcus* spp., *Proteus* spp., *Pasteurella multocida*, *Escherichia coli* and, in rare instances, *Pseudomonas* spp. The yeasts, *Malassezia* spp., may also be found in low numbers in the healthy ear canals of puppies and kittens. When conditions in the external ear canal are favourable, these pathogenic bacteria and yeasts are readily available to infect the ear canal secondarily and cause otitis externa.

Clinical signs

The physical findings associated with bacterial otitis externa are ear pruritus, increased exudation and a foul-smelling odour. Typically there is an obvious exudate in the vertical portion of the ear canal; however, in some cases it may be limited to the horizontal portion of the canal. The colour and odour of the exudate often provide insight into the underlying cause of the otitis. Infections with *Malassezia* spp. usually produce a dark-brown, sweet-smelling discharge. In contrast, the discharges seen with staphylococcal and streptococcal infections are more often dark-yellow or light-brown and creamy.

Diagnosis

Diagnosis of otitis externa is based on physical and laboratory examination via otoscopy, and cytological examination and culture and sensitivity of ear canal contents. Puppies and kittens are born with closed external ear canals. The ear canals open between 6 and 14 days of age (average 9 days), and are completely open by 17 days. The healthy ear canal is lined by stratified squamous epithelium at birth with an abundance of associated sebaceous and apocrine glands and some hair follicles. Once the external ear canal of the puppy or kitten opens, the epithelial lining cells desquamate readily during the first week. Cytologic examination at this time shows an abundance of desquamating epithelial cells. This does not represent a disease state but the normal adjustment of the ear canal lining to the external environment after the canal opens.

Both external ear canals are always examined, since ear problems are more often bilateral than unilateral, with one ear canal being more severely affected than the other. Examination of the least affected ear canal should precede that of the more affected one. Cytologic smears and, when deemed necessary, bacterial, yeast or fungal cultures of discharges from external ear canals should be taken before otoscopy. Cytologic smears are best taken directly from the horizontal portion of the ear canal. For collection, a dry cotton swab (3 mm diameter) is passed into the external ear canal and turned gently several times. Smears are then made by rolling the cotton swab on to a clean glass slide, which is immediately fixed in alcohol or air-dried and stained with either a cytologic or a haematologic stain. Smears are examined microscopically under high-power magnification for number and morphology of bacteria and yeasts, fungal hyphae, leukocytes and debris.

A thorough otoscopic examination can usually be made in a 3-weeks and older puppy or kitten. The tip of the otoscope cone should reach to within 0.5–1 cm of the tympanic membrane. Excessive manipulation of an otoscope cone often traumatizes the external ear canal and pushes debris and discharges from the vertical portion of the external ear canal into the horizontal canal. This can readily happen in puppies and kittens, as most commercial otoscope cones are too large for their small ear canals. Visualization of the tympanic membrane should be attempted before any vigorous cleaning of an external ear canal occurs.

Treatment

General guidelines for treatment of bacterial otitis externa are presented in Table 10.25.

Parasitic otitis externa

Parasites commonly infest the external ear canals and pinnae of puppies and kittens. They include mites (i.e. *Otodectes cynotis, Sarcoptes scabiei, Notoedres cati* and *Demodex* spp.), ticks, fleas and chiggers. The whole body, as well as the infested ears, should be treated with an effective parasiticide.

Table 10.25 General guidelines for the treatment of bacterial otitis externa

A thorough otic examination should be performed before initiating therapy for bacterial otitis externa, including cytologic examination, ear mite examination, bacterial culture and sensitivity testing, and otoscopy

The external ear canals should be thoroughly cleaned and dried before applying topical medication. Normal saline solution is the preferred cleaning solution for the ear canals of puppies and kittens

Most commercially available otic preparations are combination drugs. They usually contain one or more of the following: ceruminolytic, antibacterial, anti-inflammatory, antiparasitic and antifungal agents. Combination drug selection should be restricted to puppies and kittens older than 12 weeks of age. In puppies and kittens younger than 12 weeks of age use only an antibacterial product for topical treatment of a bacterial otitis externa. Systemic use of antimicrobial agents is indicated in ulcerative otitis, as shown by the cytologic examination, and in animals with a febrile response

When medicating ears, the entire ear canal is treated. This is accomplished by massaging the ears after instillation of the otic preparation. Owner education should focus on instillation of the otic preparation and periodic superficial cleaning of the ear canals with normal saline solution by the owner. Periodic re-examinations of the ear canals by the veterinarian are warranted until complete resolution of the otitis externa occurs

Otodectes cynotis infestation

The psoroptid ear mites, *Otodectes cynotis*, are highly contagious and infest many animal species. They do not burrow but live on the surface of the epidermis where they feed on epidermal debris and tissue fluids. The mite is easily seen on otoscopic and ear swab examinations. The mite generally prefers the external ear canals but may be found on other parts of the body, especially the neck, rump and tail.

Treatment of otodectic otitis externa is accomplished by using a variety of commercial parasiticidal otic preparations. There are several points to remember when treating for *O. cynotis* infestation. First, the treatment should extend throughout the life cycle of the mite, which is approximately 3 weeks. Second, all other animals in the household should be treated at the same time, even if asymptomatic, to prevent reinfestation and cyclic spread of the mites. Last, if recurrent infestations occur with consistent otic treatment, an insecticide spray, foam or sponge-on treatment applied weekly for 3 weeks reduces the likelihood of self-reinfestation from mites that have migrated to other parts of the body.

Sarcoptes scabiei and *Notoedres cati* infestations

Sarcoptes scabiei and *Notoedres cati* are similar mites whose life cycles last 17–21 days and are completed only on their respective hosts. Because these mites prefer skin with sparse hair, the external ear canals and pinnae are affected and may be the only areas initially involved. Infested lesions are reddish, papulo-crustous eruptions that are usually pruritic. Alopecia, thick yellow crusts and excoriations are seen secondary to the intense pruritus. The diagnosis is made by the demonstration of mites, eggs and/or faecal pellets in superficial skin scrapings. The entire animal should be treated with a topical acaricidal product. The pinnae and external ear canals should always be thoroughly soaked.

Demodex infestation

Demodex spp. may infest the pinnae and external ear canals as part of a generalized skin problem. They may cause an erythematous, ceruminous otitis externa. Ear swab examination of cerumen may reveal numerous demodectic mites at varying stages of development. Treatment with most of the parasiticidal otic preparations or with mineral oil is curative.

Tick infestation

Ixodid (hard) ticks frequently infest the pinnae and external ear canals of young dogs and cats. The argasid (soft) tick, *Otobius megnini*, may be found in the external ear canals of young dogs and cats, but its range is limited to certain regions of the world. The larvae and nymphs of this tick infest the ear canals of their host and produce an otitis externa. The ear canals may be packed with the immature ticks, but in some cases only a few ticks are found on otoscopic examination. Both ixodid and argasid ticks may cause severe head-shaking without appreciable inflammatory disease. Parasiticidal dip, sponge-on or powder are effective treatments for dogs and cats older than 3 months of age. Manual removal of ticks is preferred in younger puppies and kittens. Treatment of otitis externa may be needed after effective tick removal.

Ophthalmological disorders

Ocular abnormalities account for up to 15% of all congenital defects in the dog and 9% of cats (Priester, 1972). Familial and inherited disorders are reported. Careful ocular examination (Table 10.26) of the young puppy or kitten should be performed, not only in animals with obvious abnormalities, but also in apparently normal individuals, particularly of predisposed breeds, to monitor for their presence (Tables 10.27–10.35).

Table 10.26 Normal features of the eye of the newborn puppy and kitten (Glaze and Carter, 1995)

Eye component	Characteristics
Globe position	Kittens demonstrate a divergent strabismus until the second postnatal month
Cornea	Mild corneal cloudiness resolves in 2–4 weeks as the level of hydration approximates that of the normal adult cornea
Iris	The newborn iris is blue-grey and changes to adult coloration within a few weeks of birth
Lens	A remnant of the hyaloid artery may be seen attached to the posterior lens capsule for a few days after the eyelids open
Fundus	The tapetum is blue-grey, gradually assuming the adult coloration by 4 months of age. The optic disc may appear slightly smaller due to incomplete myelination, but the calibre and the distribution of the retinal vessels are like those of adults

Table 10.27 Selected congenital and acquired abnormalities of the eyelids of puppies and kittens

Abnormality	Affected breeds	Comment
Congenital		
Agenesis		Unilateral or bilateral Affects the cat more than the dog Temporal or upper eyelid affected most often Defects of more than one-third require reconstructive surgery
Distichiasis	English Bulldog, Toy and Miniature Poodle, Cocker Spaniel, Golden Retriever, Pekinese	Extra row of eyelashes exiting from the orifices of the meibomian glands along the eyelid margins causing keratitis and conjunctivitis Cryoepilation required in dogs with clinical signs
Trichiasis		Misdirected eyelashes causing keratitis May be secondary to entropion or facial folds Electroepilation or cryoepilation indicated to remove cilia
Ectopic cilia		Cilium that has erupted through the palpebral conjunctiva of the eyelid causing keratitis and possibly corneal ulceration En bloc resection of the palpebral conjunctiva and affected meibomian gland is indicated
Entropion	Multiple breeds	Eyelid deviates inwards Lower eyelid more often affected May be result of presence of other conformation abnormalities; narrow palpebral fissure (Chow Chow), redundant facial fold (Chinese Shar-Pei) or deeply set globes (Golden Retriever) A temporary tacking procedure may be indicated in severely affected animals (Chinese Shar-Pei) at 3–4 weeks of age followed by permanent surgical correction at a later age
Ectropion	Observed in breeds with lax lower eyelids; Bloodhound, Cocker Spaniel, Basset Hound, St Bernard	Eversion of the eyelid exposing the bulbar conjunctiva Surgical correction is indicated if lubrication of the exposed conjunctiva is unsuccessful or for cosmetic reasons
Acquired		
Premature opening of the eyelids in neonates		Eyelids normally open at 7–10 days Premature opening results in corneal desiccation, keratitis, ulceration and conjunctivitis since tear production is inadequate Temporary intermarginal tarsorrhaphy indicated with bactericidal and lubricating ointments applied through a gap left at the medial canthus Sutures are removed after 7–10 days
Lacerations		Not uncommon. May be parallel or perpendicular to lid margin Require immediate attention with careful debridement and meticulous sutured apposition to avoid functional defects Laceration through the lid margin must be closed in two layers – the conjunctival margin and then the skin
Parasitic infections		Clinical signs of alopecia, erythema, pruritus of eyelids Most commonly *Demodex canis, Notoedres cati, Otodectes cynotis, Sarcoptes scabiei* Diagnosis is by serial skin scrapings
Bacterial infections		Commonly staphylococcal folliculitis may involve the eyelids causing swelling and postural dermatitis of the eyelids, face and muzzle Diagnosis is confirmed by culture and sensitivity testing of tarsal secretion Topical and systemic antimicrobial therapy is indicated in addition to systemic corticosteroid administration Local compress therapy may facilitate drainage of pustules

Table 10.28 Selected congenital and acquired abnormalities of the conjunctiva of puppies and kittens

Abnormality	Affected breeds	Comment
Congenital Dermoid		Congenital masses of tissue in the conjunctiva containing varying components of normal skin: epidermis, dermis, fat hair follicles, sebaceous glands Most often observed at the lateral limbus Infrequently involves the third eyelid Dermoid and associated hair growth causes ocular irritation Surgical excision indicated
Aberrant canthal dermis	Dogs: Shih Tzu, Pekinese, Lhasa Apso, Poodles and Chinese Pugs Cat: Persian	Canthal trichiasis Long hairs extend from the medial canthal caruncle on to the corneal surface Moisture wicks along the hair causing facial staining Corneal pigment may develop because of corneal irritation Cryotherapy of hair follicles in caruncle or surgical excision of caruncle indicated
Acquired Conjunctivitis		Inflammation of the conjunctiva causing hyperaemia, chemosis (swelling) and discharge May be due to bacteria, viral, *Mycoplasma* or feline *Chlamydia* infection Conjunctival scrapings and cytology are indicated in the diagnosis Treatment varies with cause but usually includes daily cleansing and topical broad-spectrum antimicrobial therapy (tetracycline for *Mycoplasma* infections). Topical corticosteroids are occasionally used for non-infectious causes

Table 10.29 Characteristic cytological findings for conjunctivitis in puppies and kittens (Lavach *et al.*, 1977)

Conjunctivitis	Cytological findings
Acute bacterial	Predominantly neutrophils, few mononuclear cells, many bacteria, degenerating epithelial cells
Chronic bacterial	Predominantly neutrophils, many mononuclear cells, bacteria may or may not be present; degenerate or keratinized epithelial cells, goblet cells, mucus and fibrin
Feline herpesviral	Pseudomembrane formation, giant cells, red blood cells, varying numbers of neutrophils and mononuclear cells
Feline mycoplasmal	Predominantly neutrophils, few mononuclear cells, basophilic coccoid or pleomorphic organisms on cell membrane
Feline chlamydial	Predominantly neutrophils, many mononuclear cells in subacute disease, plasma cells, giant cells, basophilic cytoplasmic inclusion early in disease
Keratoconjunctivitis sicca	Keratinized epithelial cells, goblet cells, mucus, marked neutrophilic response and bacteria if there is severe infection; bacteria
Canine distemper	Variable findings depending on stage of disease, early disease shows giant cells and mononuclear cells, late disease shows neutrophils, goblet cells, mucus and occasional intracellular inclusion
Allergic conjunctivitis	Eosinophils, high number of neutrophils, possible basophils

Table 10.30 Selected congenital and acquired abnormalities of the nictitating membrane and lacrimal system of puppies and kittens

Abnormality	Affected breeds	Comment
Congenital Cartilage eversion	Dog: Great Dane, St Bernard, German Shepherd Dog, Weimaraner, German Shorthaired Pointer, English Bulldog, Golden Retriever Cat: Burmese	Characteristic scroll-like eversion of the membrane's leading edge Requires surgical excision of the affected portion of the cartilage through the bulbar conjunctiva
Prolapse of the gland	Dog: Beagle, Boston Terrier, Cocker Spaniel, Lhasa Apso, English Bulldog Cat: Burmese	Result of poorly developed soft-tissue attachments at base of gland Surgical replacement is indicated Excision of gland should not be performed since it contributes to 30–57% of tear production
Congenital atresia, ectopia or imperforate puncta		Imperforate puncta most common Characterized by epiphora and inability to cannulate puncta Most often obstructed by layer of conjunctiva over puncta Overlying conjunctiva is excised Kittens may develop cicatrix of the puncta secondary to herpesvirus infection

Table 10.31 Selected congenital and acquired disorders of the globe and orbit of puppies and kittens

Abnormality	Affected breeds	Comment
Congenital Microphthalmos	Australian Shepherd Dog – autosomal recessive, associated with multiple colobomas, linked to hair coat colour Miniature Schnauzer, Old English Sheepdog, Akita, Cavalier King Charles Spaniel – associated with inherited congenital cataracts Bedlington Terrier, Sealyham Terrier, Labrador, Dobermann – associated with retinal dysplasia	Smaller than normal globe Characterized by varying degrees of enophthalmos and may be associated with other ocular defects Griseofulvin administration to pregnant cats has produced offspring with microphthalmos
Abnormal eye position	Brachycephalic dog and cat breeds, particularly Boston Terrier	Strabismus (outwards or inwards deviation) Divergent strabismus normal for kittens less than 2 months of age Convergent (inwards) strabismus inherited in Siamese cat (autosomal recessive) Wandering ocular movement (ocular nystagmus) generally characteristic of congenital blindness
Acquired Proptosis	Brachycephalic dog breeds	Displacement of the globe from the orbit Should be treated immediately Requires replacement under general anaesthesia with intermarginal tarsorrhaphy and systemic and topical antimicrobial administration with decreasing levels of oral corticosteroid administration Sequelae include strabismus, blindness, reduced tear production and phthisis bulbi

Table 10.32 Selected congenital and acquired conditions of the corena of puppies and kittens

Abnormality	Affected breeds	Comment
Congenital Opacity		Normal neonatal corneal opacity should clear by 2–4 weeks of age Animals with premature eyelid-opening may develop opacity due to corneal oedema Lysosomal storage disease in cats causes fine granular opacities of cornea as early as 8 weeks of age Persistent pupillary membrane adheres to inner corneal surface and causes deep corneal opacity which may eventually diminish over several weeks to months. Condition is inherited in the Basenji. No treatment indicated
Dermoids	Dog: Dachshund, St Bernard, German Shepherd Dog, Dalmatian Cat: Burman, Burmese	Similar to conjunctival dermoids Require surgical excision (keratectomy)
Acquired Dystrophy	Dog: Siberian Husky, Airedale Terrier, Shetland Sheepdog Cat: Manx	Familial, bilaterally symmetrical opacities affecting any layer of the cornea Stromal dystrophies of dogs characterized by deposition of triglycerides, phospholipids and fat in the cornea. The cat shows corneal oedema and ulceration more often Typically changes are observed after 1 year of age but have been reported as early as 5–6 months of age Siberian Husky lipid dystrophy – characteristic greyish central round or horizontally oval opacity. Inherited as recessive trait. Breeding discouraged; no treatment Airedale triglyceride and fat dystrophy – progressive axial dystrophy Shetland Sheepdog – multifocal opacities at 6 months of age described that progressed to epithelial erosions at 3–4 years of age Manx cat – progressive dystrophy characterized by outer stromal oedema with development of stromal vesicles and corneal stroma and epithelial breakdown. Possibly autosomal recessive inheritance
Melanosis	Brachycephalic dog breeds:Pug, Shih Tzu, Lhasa Apso, Pekinese	Superficial corneal pigment associated with mild chronic keratitis from exposure of prominent globes May also result from keratitis due to distichiasis, trichiasis or subclinical keratoconjunctivitis sicca
Sequestra	Cat: any breed, most commonly Persian, Siamese	Characteristic corneal degeneration of cat resulting in brown to black plaque on cornea Exact cause unknown Differentiated from melanosis since peripheral cornea spared Requires excision (superficial keratectomy)
Keratoconjunctivitis sicca	Dog: any breed, predisposed breeds include Shih Tzu, Lhasa Apso, Pekinese, Cocker Spaniel, Miniature Poodle, English Bulldog, West Highland White Terrier, Miniature Schnauzer	Causes in the young puppy and kitten vary – congenital lacrimal anomalies resulting in delayed separation of the lids and signs of corneal disease, canine distemper, feline upper respiratory disease, surgical removal of the gland of the third eyelid and certain drugs (sulphadiazine) Characterized by signs of keratitis. Blepharospasm (early sign), mucoid or mucopurulent discharge, corneal vascularization and pigmentation, dry, lustreless cornea, corneal ulceration and dry ispilateral nostril Diagnosis by clinical signs and Schirmer tear test Treatment may include topical administration of 2% cyclosporine, broad-spectrum antimicrobial agent, corticosteroids (in the non-ulcerated eye), mucolytic agent (5% acetylcysteine) and artificial tear ointment. Parotid duct transposition indicated for cases non-responsive to medical management

Table 10.33 Selected congenital conditions of the anterior uvea, lens and vitreous of puppies and kittens

Abnormality	Affected breeds	Comment
Congenital uveal abnormalities		
Iris cysts		Floating, fluid-filled vesicles in the anterior chamber
		Originate from the posterior iris epithelium
Pupil anomalies		Coloboma (notched defect) affects ventronasal border most often, causing keyhole-shaped pupil
		Eccentric pupil (corectopia) may occur with other ocular anomalies. Reported in the Australian Shepherd Dog
Heterochromia	Multiple breeds with coat colour albinism	Variation in iris colour, either within one iris or differently coloured irises
		Associated with lack of pigment, linked to coat colour (and deafness)
Congenital lens abnormalities		
Alterations in size and shape	St Bernard	Aphakia or congenital absence is rare, reported in St Bernard and a domestic shorthaired cat
		Microphakia reported in St Bernard, Beagle and cat. Luxation of the microphakic lens may lead to glaucoma
Congenital cataracts	Dog: Beagle, Cocker Spaniel, Old English Sheepdog, Australian Shepherd Dog, Bedlington Terrier, Sealyham Terrier, Labrador, Samoyed Cat: Persian	Lens opacity present at birth but often not noticed until 6–8 weeks of age. May be associated with persistent pupillary membranes or persistent hyaloid artery
Juvenile cataracts	Dog: Many breeds Cat: British Shorthair Himalayan	Develop any time between birth and 6 years of age. Hereditary (Table 10.34). Opacity is progressive with complete opacification in less than 1 year after diagnosis.
		Spontaneous resorption may occur. Surgical extraction may be indicated but the effect of lens opacity on visual pathway development must be considered
Congenital vitreous abnormalities Hyaloid remnants		Bloodless, white vermiform structures extending into the vitreous from the optic disc or the posterior lens capsule
Persistent hyperplastic primary vitreous	Dog: Dobermann, Staffordshire Bull Terrier, Bouvier des Flandres	Fibrovascular membrane on the posterior lens capsule manifested by congenital pupillary opacity, a fibrovascular sheath on the posterior aspect of the lens, elongated ciliary processes and secondary cataract formation

Table 10.34 Inherited cataracts in puppies and kittens (Glaze, 1995)

Breed	Inheritance
Afghan	Autosomal recessive
American Cocker Spaniel	Autosomal recessive (presumed)
Beagle	Autosomal recessive
Bedlington Terrier	Autosomal recessive
Boston Terrier	Autosomal recessive
Bouvier des Flandres	Unknown
British Shorthair cat	Autosomal recessive
Chesapeake Bay Retriever	Dominant with incomplete penetrance
English Sheepdog	Dominant with incomplete penetrance
English Toy Spaniel	Unknown
French Bulldog	Unknown
German Shepherd Dog	Autosomal recessive
German Shorthaired Pointer	Unknown
Golden Retriever	Dominant with incomplete penetrance
Himalayan	Autosomal recessive
Irish Setter	Unknown
Keeshond	Unknown
Labrador Retriever	Dominant
Norwich Terrier	Autosomal recessive
Pembroke Welsh Corgi	Unknown
Poodle (standard)	Autosomal recessive (presumed)
Samoyed	Autosomal recessive
Schnauzer (miniature)	Autosomal recessive
Siberian Husky	Autosomal recessive (presumed)
Staffordshire Terrier	Autosomal recessive
Welsh Springer Spaniel	Autosomal recessive
Welsh Terrier	Unknown
West Highland White Terrier	Autosomal recessive

Table 10.35 Selected congenital and acquired conditions of the retina and optic nerve of puppies and kittens

Abnormality	Breeds	Comment
Congenital		
Collie eye anomaly	Dog: Collie, Shetland Sheepdog, Border Collie, Australian Shepherd Dog	Autosomal recessive inheritance Non-progressive. Easily diagnosed at 6–8 weeks of age Varying abnormalities may be present and affected eyes usually have dissimilar lesions. Choroidal hypoplasia, optic nerve and scleral colobomas (defects) and retinal detachment (5–10% of affected animals) can be present Breeding of affected animals should be discouraged
Retinal dysplasia	Dog: Springer Spaniel (autosomal recessive), Labrador, Cocker Spaniel (recessive inheritance likely), Beagle Also reported in other breeds in association with other ocular defects Cat: Rare	Abnormal embryogenesis characterized by folds in the outer retinal layers and by retinal rosettes consisting of variably differentiated retinal cells around a central lumen. More severe cases may have retinal detachment May be associated with other ocular defects Non-progressive. Easily diagnosed at 6–8 weeks of age Severe retinal dysplasia with retinal detachment reported in Labrador in association with short-limbed dwarfism
Feline retinal degeneration	Cat: Persian cat (possible autosomal recessive) Domestic cat (possible dominant pattern)	Outer-segment retinal atrophy reported in a blind 15-week-old Persian kitten Photoreceptor degeneration in domestic mixed-breed cats with similar signs also reported

Table 10.35 (continued)

Abnormality	Breeds	Comment
Hemeralopia	Dog: Alaskan Malamute, Miniature Poodle	Day blindness observed in Alaskan Malamutes by 8 weeks of age
		Dogs visually impaired in daylight but function well at night
		Fundus appears grossly normal
		Electroretinography required for definitive diagnosis indicating abnormal cone response
Stationary night blindness	Dog: Tibetan Terrier, Briard (possible autosomal recessive)	Night blindness evident by 6 weeks of age
		Fundus appears grossly normal
		Diagnosis confirmed by electroretinogram
		In the Tibetan terrier, condition may not be a separate entity but represents a different stage of progressive retinal atrophy
Optic nerve hypoplasia	Dog or cat: Any breed	May be uni- or bilateral
		Bilateral lesions characterized by poor vision. May be incidental finding in unilaterally affected dogs as compensation by other eye masks clinical signs
		Affected optic disc appears small, often half normal size, centre is depressed and periphery pigments. Retinal vasculature is normal
		Note: the optic disc in a cat is relatively smaller than that of a dog and should not be misclassified as hypoplastic
Acquired Progressive retinal atrophy	Dog: Early onset – Collie, Norwegian Elkhound, Irish Setter	Typically a disease of adults, early onset reported in certain affected breeds. Also reported in young Miniature Schnauzers, Cardigan Corgis, Miniature Longhaired Dachshunds
		Visual loss noticed first in dim lighting. Progressive day vision loss to total blindness
		Characterized by attenuation of retinal vessels (peripheral arterioles followed by retinal veins) which progresses to complete absence of vessels, an increasingly granular and hyperreflective appearance of tapetum and a pale optic disc (lack of blood vessels)
Non-heritable retinal dysplasia	Dog or cat: Any breed	Normal maturation of retina continues until 6–8 weeks of age. Infectious agents (canine herpesvirus, canine parvovirus-2, canine adenovirus-1) may cause interference in this process. *In utero* or postnatal infection with feline panleukopenia infection will also cause changes. Retinal dysplasia has been reported with experimental infection with feline leukaemia virus but not with natural disease

References

Bailey, C.S. (1975) An embryological approach to the clinical significance of congenital vertebral and spinal cord abnormalities. *Journal of American Animal Hospital Association*, **11**, 426–434.

Bruecker, K.A., Seim, H.B.I. and Blass, C.E. (1989a) Caudal cervical spondylomyelopathy: decompression by linear traction and stabilization with Steinmann pins and polymethylmethacrylate. *Journal of American Animal Hospital Association*, **25**, 677–683.

Bruecker, K.A., Seim, H.B.I. and Withrow, S.J. (1989b) Clinical evaluation of three surgical methods for treatment of caudal cervical spondylomyelopathy of dogs. *Veterinary Surgery*, **18**, 197–203.

Chambers, J.N., Betts, C.W. and Oliver, J.E. (1977) The use of nonmetallic suture for stabilization of atlantoaxial subluxation. *Journal of American Animal Hospital Association*, **13**, 602–604.

Cockrell, B.Y., Herigstad, R.R., Flo, G.L. and Legendre, A.M. (1973) Myelomalacia in Afghan hounds. *Journal of American Veterinary Medical Association*, **162**, 362–365.

Cook, J.R. and Oliver, J.E. (1981) Atlantoaxial luxation in the dog. *Compendium of Continuing Education for the Practicing Veterinarian*, **3**, 242–252.

Cooper, B.J., deLahunta, A., Cummings, J.F., Lewis, D.H. and Karrema, G. (1984) Canine inherited hypertrophic neuropathy: Clinical and electrodiagnostic studies. *American Journal of Veterinary Research*, **45**, 1172–1177.

Cummings, J. and deLahunta, A. (1974) Hypertrophic neuropathy in a dog. *Acta Neuropathology*, **20**, 325–326.

Cummings, J.F., deLahunta, A., Braud, K.G. and Mitchell Jr., W.J. (1983) Animal model of human disease: heriditary sensory neuropathy. Nocioceptive loss and acral mutilation in pointer dogs: canine heriditary sensory neuropathy. *American Journal Pathology*, **112**, 36–138.

Cummings, J.F., deLahunta, A. and Moore, J.J. (1988) Multisystemic chromolytic neuronal degeneration in a cairn terrier. *Cornell Veterinarian*, **78**, 301–314.

Cummings, J.F., George, C., deLahunta, A., Valentine, B.A. and Bookbinder, P.F. (1989) Focal spinal muscular atrophy in two German shepherd pups. *Acta Neuropathologica*, **79**, 113–116.

deLahunta, A. and Shively, G.N. (1975) Neurofibrillary accumulation in a puppy. *Cornell Veterinarian*, **65**, 240–247.

Denny, H.R., Gibbs, C. and Waterman, A. (1988) Atlantoaxial subluxation in the dog: a review of thirty cases and an evaluation of treatment by lag screw fixation. *Journal of Small Animal Practice*, **29**, 37–47.

Duncan, I.D. (1991) Peripheral neuropathy in the dog and cat. *Progress in Veterinary Neurology*, **2**, 111–128.

Ellison, G.W., Seim, H.B. and Clemmons, R.M. (1988) Distracted spinal fusion for the management of caudal cervical spondylomyelopathy in large-breed dogs. *Journal of the American Veterinary Medical Association*, **193**, 447–453.

Few, A.B. (1966) The diagnosis and surgical treatment of canine hydrocephalus. *Journal of the American Veterinary Medical Association*, **149**, 286–293.

Fingeroth, J.M., Johnson, G.C., Burt, J.K., Fenner, W.R. and Cain, L.S. (1989) Neuroradiographic diagnosis and surgical repair of tethered cord syndrome in an English bulldog with spina bifida and myeloschisis. *Journal of the American Veterinary Medical Association*, **194**, 1300–1302.

Gage, D. (1968) Surgical treatment of canine hydrocephalus by ventriculoatrial shunting. *Journal of the American Veterinary Medical Association*, **153**, 1418–1431.

Geary, J.C., Oliver, J.E. and Hoerlein, B.F. (1967) Atlantoaxial subluxation in the canine. *Journal of Small Animal Practice*, **8**, 577–582.

Glaze, M.B. (1995) The lens and vitreous. In: Hoskins, J.H. (ed.) *Veterinary Pediatrics*, pp. 320–324. Philadelphia: WB Saunders.

Glaze, M.B. and Carter, J.D. (1995) The eye. In: Hoskins, J.D. (ed.) *Veterinary Pediatrics*, pp. 297–336. Philadelphia: WB Saunders.

Greene, C.E., Vandervelde, M. and Braud, K. (1976) Lissencephaly in two lhasa apso dogs. *Journal of the American Veterinary Medical Association*, **169**, 404–410.

Greene, C.E., Vandervelde, M. and Hoff, E.J. (1977) Congenital cerebrospinal hypomyelinogenesis in a pup. *Journal of the American Veterinary Medical Association*, **171**, 534–536.

Greibrokk, T. (1994) Heriditary deafness in the dalmatian: relationship to eye and coat color. *Journal of the American Animal Hospital Association*, **30**, 170–176.

Griffiths, I.R., Duncan, I.D. and Barker, J. (1980) A progressive axonopathy of boxer dogs affecting the central and peripheral nervous system. *Journal of Small Animal Practice*, **21**, 29–43.

Inada, S., Yamauchi, C., Igata, A. *et al.* (1978) Canine storage disease characterized by heriditary progressive neurogenic muscular atrophy in pointer dogs. *Japan Journal of Veterinary Science*, **40**, 539–547.

Jaggy, A. and Vandevelde, M. (1988) Multisystem neuronal degeneration in cocker spaniels. *Journal of Veterinary Internal Medicine*, **2**, 117–120.

Jaggy, A., Hutto, V.L., Roberts, R.E. and Oliver, J.E. (1991) Occipitoatlantoaxial malformation with atlantoaxial subluxation in a cat. *Journal of Small Animal Practice*, **32**, 366–372.

Kornegay, J.N. (1986) Congenital and degenerative diseases of the central nervous system. In: Kornegay, J.N. (ed.) *Neurologic Disorders*, pp. 109–129. New York: Churchill Livingstone.

Lavach, J.D., Thrall, M.A., Benjamin, M.M. and Severin, G.A. (1977) Cytology of normal and inflamed conjuctivitis in dogs and cats. *Journal of the American Veterinary Medical Association*, **170**, 722–727.

Keipold, H.W., Huston, K., Blauch, B. and Guffy, M.M. (1974) Congenital defects of the caudal vertebral column and spinal cord in the Manx cat. *Journal of the American Veterinary Medical Association*, **164**, 520–523.

Lewis, D.G. (1989) Cervical spondylomyelopathy ('wobbler syndrome') in the dog: a study based on 224 cases. *Journal of Small Animal Practice*, **30**, 657–665.

Lorenz, M.D., Cork, L.C., Griffin, J.W., Adams, R.J. and Price, D.L. (1979) Hereditary muscular atrophy in Brittany spaniels: clinical manifestations. *Journal of the American Veterinary Medical Association*, **175**, 833–839.

Lyman, R.L. and Seim, H.B. (1991) View point: wobbler syndrome. *Progress in Veterinary Neurology*, **2**, 143–150.

McGrath, J.T. (1965) Spinal dysraphism in the dog. *Pathology Veterinary Supplement*, **2**, 1–36.

McKee, W.M., Lavelle, R.B., Richardson, J.L. and Mason, T.A. (1990) Vertebral distraction–fusion for cervical spondylomyelopathy using a screw and double washer technique. *Journal of Small Animal Practice*, **31**, 21–26.

Mair, I.W.S. (1973) Hereditary deafness in the white cat. *Acta Otolaryngology [Supplement]*, **314**, 1–48.

Mansfield, P.D. (1990) Ototoxity in dogs and cats. *Compendium of Continuing Education for the Practicing Veterinarian*, **12**, 331–337.

Merchant, S.R., Neer, T.M., Tedford, B.L., Twedt, A.C., Cheramie, P.M. and Strain, G.M. (1993) Ototoxity assessment of a chlorhexidine otic preparation in dogs. *Progress in Veterinary Neurology*, **4**, 72–75.

Morgan, J.P. (1968) Congenital anomalies of the vertebral column of the dog: a study of the incidence and significance based on a radiographic and morphologic study. *Journal of the American Veterinary Radiology Society*, **9**, 21–29.

Morizono, T. and Sikora, M.A. (1982) The ototoxicity of topically applied povidone-iodine preparations. *Archives of Otolaryngology*, **108**, 210–213.

Neer, T.M. (1995) The ears. In: Hoskins, J.D. (ed.) *Veterinary Pediatrics*, pp. 283–296. Philadelphia: WB Saunders.

Nes, J. (1986) Electrophysiological evidence of sensory nerve dysfunction in 10 dogs with acral lick dermatitis. *Journal of the American Animal Hospital Association*, **22**, 157–160.

Oliver, J.E. and Lewis, R.E. (1973) Lesions of the atlas and axis in dogs. *Journal of the American Animal Hospital Association*, **9**, 304–313.

Oliver, J.E. and Lorenz, M.D. (1993a) Pelvic limb paresis, paralysis or ataxis. In: Oliver, J.E. and Lorenz, M.D. (eds) *Handbook of Veterinary Neurology*, pp. 128–169. Philadelphia: WB Saunders.

Oliver, J.E. and Lorenz, M.D. (1993b) Tetraparesis, hemiparesis, and ataxia. In: Oliver, J.E. and Lorenz, M.D. (eds) *Handbook of Veterinary Neurology*, pp. 170–127. Philadelphia: WB Saunders.

Palmer, A.C. and Blackmore, W.F. (1989) A progressive neuronopathy in the young cairn terrier. *Journal of Small Animal Practice*, **30**, 101–106.

Palmer, A.C. and Wallace, M.E. (1967) Deformation of the cervical vertebrae in basset hounds. *Veterinary Record*, **80**, 430–433.

Palmer, A.C., Payne, J.E. and Wallace, M.E. (1973) Hereditary quadriplegia and amblyopia in the Irish setter. *Journal of Small Animal Practice*, **14**, 343–352.

Parker, A.J. and Park, R.D. (1974) Occipital dysplasia in the dog. *Journal of the American Animal Hospital Association*, **10**, 520–525.

Parker, A.J., Park, R.D. and Cusick, P.K. (1973) Abnormal odontoid process angulation in a dog. *Veterinary Record*, **93**, 559–561.

Priester, W.A. (1972) Congenital ocular defects in cattle, horses, cats and dogs. *Journal of the American Veterinary Medical Association*, **160**, 1504–1510.

Renegar, W.R. and Stoll, S.G. (1979) The use of methylmethacrylate bone cement in the repair of atlantoaxial subluxation stabilization failures – case report and discussion. *Journal of the American Animal Hospital Association*, **15**, 313–318.

Sandefeldt, E., Cummings, J.F., deLahunta, A., Bjorck, G. and Krook, L. (1973) Hereditary neuronal abiotrophy in the Swedish Lapland dog. *Cornell Veterinarian*, **63**, 1–71.

Savell, C.M. (1974) Cerebral ventricular tap: an aid to diagnosis and treatment of hydrocephalus in the dog. *Journal of the American Animal Hospital Association*, **10**, 500–502.

Shell, L., Jortner, B. and Leib, M. (1987) Spinal muscle atrophy in two Rottweiler littermates. *Journal of the American Veterinary Medical Association*, **190**, 878–880.

Simpson, S.T. (1989) Hydrocephalus. In: Kirk, R.W. (ed.) *Current Veterinary Therapy*, pp. 842–846. Philadelphia: WB Saunders.

Sorjonen, D.C. and Shires, P.K. (1981) Atlantoaxial instability: a ventral surgical technique for decompression, fixation and fusion. *Veterinary Surgery*, **10**, 22–29.

Stockard, C. (1936) A hereditary lethal factor for localized motor and preganglionic neurons. *American Journal of Anatomy*, **59**, 1–53.

Strain, G.M. (1991) Congenital deafness in dogs and cats. *Compendium of Continuing Education for the Practicing Veterinarian*, **13**, 245–253.

Swaim, S.F. and Bradley, D.M. (1996) Evaluation of closed-suction drainage for treating auricular hematomas. *Journal of the American Animal Hospital Association*, **32**, 36–43.

Swaim, S.F. and Greene, C.E. (1975) Odontoidectomy in a dog. *Journal of the American Animal Hospital Association*, **11**, 663–667.

Vandevelde, M., Greene, C. and Hoff, E. (1976) Lower motor neuron disease with accumulation of neurofilaments in a cat. *Veterinary Pathology*, **13**, 428–435.

Vandevelde, M., Bruad, K.G., Luttgen, P.J. and Higgins, R.J. (1981) Dysmyelination in chow chow dogs: further studies in older dogs. *Acta Neuropathology*, **55**, 81–87.

VanGundy, T. (1989a) Canine wobbler syndrome: Part I. Pathophysiology and diagnosis. *Compendium of Continuing Education for the Practicing Veterinarian*, **11**, 144–158.

VanGundy, T. (1989b) Canine wobbler syndrome: Part II. Treatment. *Compendium of Continuing Education for the Practicing Veterinarian*, **11**, 269–284.

Walker, T.L. (1990) Use of Harrington rods in caudal cervical spondylomyelopathy. In: Bojrab, M.J. (ed.) *Current Techniques in Small Animal Surgery*, pp. 584–586. Philadelphia: Lea & Febiger.

Watson, A.C. and deLahunta, A. (1989) Atlantoaxial subluxation and absence of the transverse ligament of the atlas in a dog. *Journal of the American Veterinary Medical Association*, **195**, 235–237.

Wilson, J.W. (1983) Treatment of auricular hematomas, using a teat tube. *Journal of the American Veterinary Medical Association*, **182**, 1081–1083.

Wilson, J.W., Kurtz, H.J., Leipold, H.W. and Lees, G.E. (1979) Spina bifida in the dog. *Veterinary Pathology*, **16**, 165–179.

Wouda, W., Vandervelde, M., Oettli, P., van Ness, J.J. and Hoerlein, B.F. (1983) Sensory neuronopathy in dogs: a study of four cases. *Journal of Comparative Pathology*, **93**, 437–450.

Skin fold disorders

Skin fold dermatitis (intertriginous dermatitis) is not uncommon and may occur in many types of dogs with varying conformational changes that predispose them to a problem (Table 11.1). It is rarely a recognized problem in cats. These conditions often result in severe dermatitis associated with a foul odour. Ulceration of the affected tissue often occurs and the conditions are often quite painful.

Treatment and surgical technique

Medical management of any of these conditions using systemic antimicrobial medication and cleansers is rarely successful and surgical excision of the folds is indicated. It is particularly important for facial folds where there is a risk of serious ocular damage. Perioperative antimicrobials are indicated owing to the contaminated nature of the surgery and postoperative antimicrobials may be indicated in animals with severe infection. For surgery near the perineum (tail and vulval folds), a pursestring suture should be placed in the anus to prevent faecal contamination of the surgical site.

Cheiloplasty

Correction of lip fold dermatitis requires excision of the affected tissue within the fold. The animal is placed in dorsal recumbency to facilitate access to both sides of the mandible. The surgical sites are clipped and prepared for aseptic surgery. The fold is opened up and an elliptical incision made around the affected tissue, including a 2–3 mm margin of normal skin (Fig. 11.1). The skin is elevated and dissected free. Haemorrhage may be brisk due to the inflammation and should be controlled with pressure, electrocoagulation or ligation if necessary. The edges of the tissue are apposed using a subcutaneous and skin closure.

A second procedure has been described in order to elevate lower lips that are excessively droopy (Smeak, 1989). The mucocutaneous edge of the lower lip is incised in the area of droop and the edges undermined (Fig. 11.2). The lower lip is then elevated to a position so that the droop is eliminated but which does not interfere with mouth-opening. At this position, a horizontal incision is made in the mucosa of the upper lip along a line drawn from the commissure of the lip to the medial canthus of the eye. The mucosa is elevated and the mucosal edges of the upper and lower lip are apposed using stay sutures at the rostral

Table 11.1 Characteristics of intertriginous dermatitis

Skin fold dermatitis	Typical breeds	Characteristics
Lip	Dogs with drooping lips, particularly Cocker Spaniel, St Bernard	Food and saliva accumulate on a skin fold in the lower lip, caudal to the canine tooth, resulting in pyodermatitis
Facial	Typically brachycephalic breeds, particularly Pug, Pekinese, English Bulldog, Boston Terrier	Hairs from the folded skin may cause corneal irritation and possibly ulceration. Tears and ocular discharge can accumulate in the fold, causing dermatitis
Tail	Short-tailed dogs (and cats), particularly English Bulldog, Boston Terrier, Schipperke, Pug and Manx cat	Ventral deviation and corkscrewing of the tail result in deep skin folds lateral and ventral to tail which accumulate secretions, and sometimes faecal material resulting in moist pyodermatitis
Perivulval	Any breed; females with juvenile vulvas, typically animals ovariohysterectomized before maturity or animals that are obese	Vulval folds dorsal and lateral to the vulva allow accumulation of urine and moisture, resulting in urine scalding and pyodermatitis

and caudal ends of the wounds. The mucosal edges are then sutured together using monofilament absorbable suture.

Facial fold excision

Partial, or preferably complete excision of the facial fold is recommended. Partial excision may be adequate in animals with corneal irritation without fold dermatitis. A postoperative change in the animal's appearance should be discussed with the owner prior to surgery.

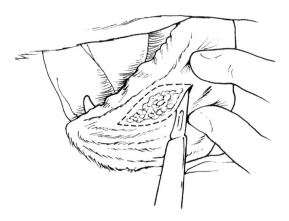

Figure 11.1 An elliptical incision is made around the skin fold with a margin of healthy tissue. The skin is excised and the defect closed.

The surgical site is prepared for aseptic surgery. Care is required to avoid antiseptic solutions, particularly alcohol, draining onto the eye. The fold is simply elevated and excised with scissors (Fig. 11.3). Although the use of scissors is more traumatic to the tissue than a scalpel, it does facilitate haemorrhage control by slightly crushing the tissue edges and facilitates a more accurate and uniform excision. Depending on the size of the fold, a subcutaneous closure may or may not be required. Care should be taken to ensure skin suture tags do not touch the cornea.

Tail fold excision

Tail fold excision requires tail amputation (caudectomy) and the client should be aware of this preoperatively. The animal is placed in ventral recumbency and the surgical site prepared for aseptic surgery. An eccentric elliptical incision is made around the tail including the skin folds (Fig. 11.4) and the skin dissected to expose the tail. Grasping the end of the tail with bone-holding forceps can aid in manipulation of the tail and facilitate identification of the caudal vertebral spaces. The coccygeal and levator ani muscles are severed close to their attachment on the caudal vertebrae. Care must be exercised in elevating the tail from the dorsal fascial attachments of the rectum. The caudal vertebra

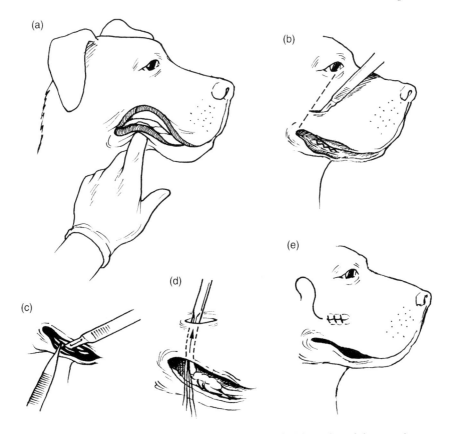

Figure 11.2 Cheiloplasty with elevation of the lower lip. (a, b) The region of the most droop is established and elevated to determine the site of the full-thickness horizontal cheek incision. (c) The mucocutaneous edge of the lower lip is incised in the area of droop and the edges undermined. (d) Stay sutures are placed in the lower-lip incision and pulled through the cheek incision. The mucosal edges of the upper- and lower-lip incisions are then sutured together using monofilament absorbable suture. (e) The cheek skin incision is then closed.

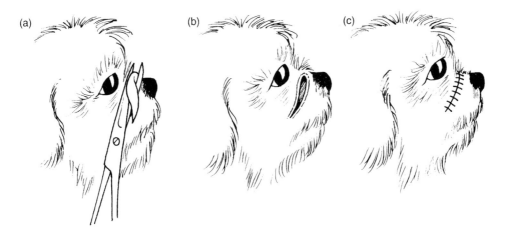

Figure 11.3 Excision of the facial fold. (a) The entire fold is excised with scissors, beginning laterally. (b) The defect is sutured. (c) Care is taken to place the knots anteriorly, away from the eye to avoid corneal abrasion. Alternatively, only partial excision (the top part of the fold) is carried out to maintain some facial fold for cosmetic purposes.

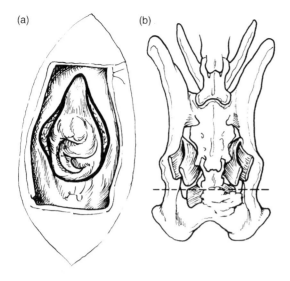

Figure 11.4 Caudectomy and excision of the tail folds. A pursestring suture is placed in the anus. (a) An eccentric elliptical incision (teardrop) is made around the tail base. (b) The coccygeal and levator ani muscles are severed close to their attachment on the caudal vertebrae and the bone is transected (dashed line).

is severed just cranial to the point of deviation. Ideally, transection between vertebrae is performed if possible using a scalpel blade, although it is often very difficult to determine the vertebral spaces accurately. Alternatively, the vertebrae are severed using bone cutters or Gigli wire. Caudal vessels are ligated and the severed muscles are sutured over the dorsal rectum. Subcutaneous and skin closure is routine.

Perivulval fold excision

The animal is placed in dorsal recumbency and the surgical site prepared for aseptic surgery. The vulval skin fold and underlying fatty tissue are excised from the dorsolateral aspect of the vulva (Fig. 11.5) using a horseshoe-shaped incision. Enough tissue must be excised to eliminate the fold but must not put undue tension on the closure. Subcutaneous closure is imperative to relieve tension on the skin closure.

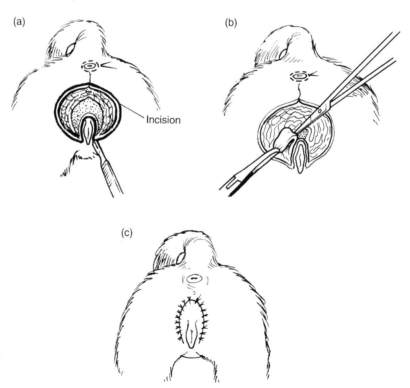

Figure 11.5 Excision of perivulval skin fold can be performed with the animal in dorsal or ventral recumbency. A purse string suture is placed in the anus. (a) Two horseshoe-shaped incisions are made around the vulva and (b) the skin between the incisions is excised. (c) The resultant defect is then closed in two layers.

Postoperative considerations and prognosis

An Elizabethan collar is required in all animals to prevent self-mutilation of the surgical site, regardless of location. Suture removal is performed in 7–10 days. The prognosis for all cases is generally excellent. The results of cheiloplasty for elevating lower lips have been reported as good (Smeak, 1989).

Pilonidal sinus

Pilonidal or dermoid sinus is an inherited anomaly (possibly simple recessive) reported most commonly in the Rhodesian Ridgeback but also reported in the Shih Tzu and Boxer. The authors have also observed it in Rottweiler and German Shepherd Dog breeds.

A pilonidal sinus is typically located cranial to or occasionally caudal to the ridge in the Rhodesian ridgeback and is the result of failure of the neural tube to separate completely from the skin during embryogenesis. This results in a tube of skin that may extend as far as the dura mater. Histologic examination shows that the sinus consists of squamous epithelium with secretory adnexal structures.

Clinical signs

Physical examination findings and clinical signs vary. A thin cord of tissue in the dorsal aspect of the neck may be palpated and hair projecting from a small hole in the skin surface may be observed. Infected sinuses or those associated with a lot of secretion may present as a swollen, draining abscess. Communication of the sinus with the dura mater may result in signs of meningitis if infection is present.

Diagnosis

Diagnosis is based on clinical signs and palpation of the sinus and can usually be made at a young age, before infection has developed. Radiography of the spine in the affected area is indicated to rule out vertebral malformation or spina bifida-type lesions that may be associated with the lesion. Metrizamide or iohexol fistulography may be indicated to determine the depth of the sinus.

Treatment and surgical technique

Surgical excision of the sinus is necessary and it is imperative that the entire sinus is removed. This can involve considerable dissection in some cases. Perioperative antimicrobials should be considered due to the risk of contamination of the surgical site from contents of the sinus and the possibility of having to incise the dura mater.

The dorsal aspect of the neck is clipped and prepared. An elliptical incision is made around the opening of the sinus and the sinus is carefully dissected using blunt dissection. Care must be taken not to tear or open the sinus for risk of contamination of the surgical site. The sinus may penetrate the nuchal ligament. In this case, the nuchal ligament is split around the sinus and repaired using tendon apposition sutures of non-absorbable monofilament suture. If the sinus ends at the vertebral spine, the proximal part of the vertebral spine is removed with the sinus. If the sinus extends through the vertebrae, a dorsal laminectomy must be performed and the dura mater is excised at the point of communication with the sinus. After excision, a piece of sinus tissue (preferably deep tissue) should be submitted for bacterial culture and sensitivity testing and the excised tissue submitted for histologic examination.

If there has been contamination of the surgical site, copious lavage with normal saline is indicated. A closed-suction wound drain may be required (passive drains such as Penrose drains will be ineffective as they will not be gravity-assisted in this location) if there has been contamination or excessive dissection. The wound is closed in several layers, apposing muscle, subcutaneous tissue and skin.

Postoperative considerations and prognosis

The wound does not require bandaging unless a drain has been placed. Maintenance of the drainage system may be needed for 2 or 3 days. Postoperative antimicrobial therapy should continue based on culture and sensitivity testing of the excised tissue.

The prognosis for complete recovery is good as long as the entire sinus has been excised and neurological signs were not present preoperatively. Any remnant is likely to result in recurrence of clinical signs, although the time for recurrence may be several months. Breeding of affected animals should be discouraged and neutering is recommended.

Dewclaw removal

The dewclaw is defined as the first digit of the rear leg, although the term is often used to refer to the first digit of the forelimb also. Rear dewclaws are absent in most dogs, although single and double dewclaws are a breed standard for some breeds (Great Pyrenees and Briard). Rear dewclaws often have no first or second phalanx (P1, P2) and are attached by skin only. Because of this flaccid attachment, they are predisposed to trauma. Front dewclaws usually have three phalanges and are firmly attached to the leg. Dewclaws are typically removed in the very young puppy at the owner's request, in dogs that require frequent grooming (Poodles, Schnauzers, Fox Terriers) or in hunting dogs to prevent trauma (Table 11.2). Occasionally, dewclaws may require amputation in older dogs after traumatic injury.

Surgical technique

Dewclaws are best amputated at 3–5 days of age. In animals presented at 1 week of age, local anaesthesia should be used. Surgery on animals older than 1 week should be postponed and performed under general anaesthesia at 12–16 weeks of age.

For puppies less than 1 week of age, the dewclaws are amputated using scissors. The dewclaw is not clipped. The dewclaw and the web of skin between the dewclaw and the metatarsus (or metacarpus) cleansed with antiseptic is to allow abduction of the digit. If there is skin attachment only, the dewclaw is simply cut off. If P1 and P2 are present, the digit is abducted so that the scissors can be slid up to the P1/P2 joint. All of P2 should be amputated. Cutting through the diaphysis of P2 or inadvertently cutting through P1 may expose the medullary cavity to contamination and may result in osteomyelitis.

Haemostasis is rarely a problem in young puppies, especially those with only skin attach-

Table 11.2 Dewclaw removal guidelines

Dog breeds in which dewclaw removal is acceptable (USA)

Alaskan Malamute
Belgian Malinois
Belgian Sheepdog
Belgian Tervueran
Bernese Mountain Dog
Boxer
Chesapeake Bay Retriever
Dalmatian
Dandie Dinmont Terrier
Kerry Blue Terrier
Komondor
Lakeland Terrier
Large Munsterlander
Norwegian Elkhound
Papillon
Pointer (front only)
Shetland Sheepdog
Siberian Husky
St Bernard
Vizsla
Weimaraner
Welsh Corgi-Cardigan Corgi

Dog breeds in which dewclaw removal may be acceptable

Basset Hound
Puli

Dog breeds in which dewclaw removal is unacceptable

Briard
Great Pyrenees

ments. Any bleeding can be controlled by pressure or topical application of styptics or silver nitrate sticks. Skin sutures are rarely required but may facilitate haemostasis. A single cruciate suture of monofilament non-absorbable suture can be placed (it requires removal) or the authors prefer to use chromic catgut, which will fall out on its own.

For older animals, general anaesthesia is required. The limbs are clipped and prepared for aseptic surgery. Use of a tourniquet may facilitate surgery. An elliptical incision is made around the dewclaw. Dissection is performed to expose the P1/P2 joint (Fig. 11.6). Disarticulation of the joint is performed using a scalpel. The tourniquet can be loosened so that the dorsal common and axial palmar digital arteries can be identified and ligated. The subcutaneous tissue and skin are closed.

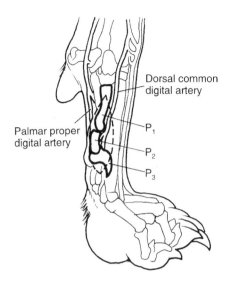

Figure 11.6 Removal of the first digit (dewclaw) with the first phalanx (P1) and second phalanx (P2) present. An elliptical incision is made around the base of the digit and it is amputated at the P1/P2 joint. The dorsal common digital artery (1) and palmar proper digital artery (2) are ligated.

Postoperative considerations

Bandages are not required for young puppies; however, a soft bandage is usually placed on the limbs of older dogs, left in place for 2–3 days postoperative. Suture removal, if necessary, is performed at 7–10 days.

Onychectomy

Onychectomy is the surgical amputation of the third phalanx and claw. It is typically an elective procedure performed on cats and is usually carried out at 12 weeks of age. Haemorrhage tends to be less when performed on cats of this age as opposed to adult cats. The assessment of the ethics of this procedure varies from clinician to clinician and from country to country. The authors present information on onychectomy and deep digital flexor tendonectomy neutral to their opinion of the procedures and include it for completeness of the text. However, the authors would comment that careful consideration of the animal's activity and environment (indoor/outdoor cat) should be made before the procedure is performed and particularly before both forelimb and hindlimb onychect-omy is performed. Rarely is onychectomy of all four limbs indicated.

Surgical technique

A complete understanding of the anatomy of the digit is imperative to surgical technique (Fig. 11.7). The ungual crest surrounds the nail bed with the ungual process extending into the claw. In the authors' opinion, techniques used to perform onychectomy are only acceptable if they result in complete excision of P3.

Onychectomy can be performed with nail clippers or with a scalpel blade. A tourniquet is placed on the leg above the elbow to avoid pressure on the median nerve and ulnar nerves. The feet are not clipped but cleansed with an antiseptic. The clipper is placed over the claw and over the top of the extensor process. The blade of the clippers is partially closed so it engages on the tissue. The claw is then extended using a forceps attached to the nail or fingers so that the clippers can be slid over the bottom of the flexor process, taking care to push the pad back with the clipper while doing this. The clipper is then completely closed and P3 severed. This manoeuvre is imperative to excise the flexor process of P3. Failure to extend the claw will result in a significant portion of P3 remaining with potential for regrowth, osteomyelitis or postoperative pain (Fig. 11.7). Alternatively, the entire procedure can be performed using a scalpel blade, again starting at the back of the extensor process.

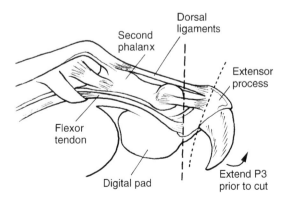

Figure 11.7 Normal anatomy of the digit of a cat. Dashed line marks the acceptable line of amputation. Cutting along the dotted line leaves a substantial amount of the third phalange, which may result in regrowth of the nail and expose the medullary cavity to contamination.

The wound is examined for remnants of P3. Any remnants should be excised with a scalpel blade. Overzealous use of the clippers can result in amputating a portion of P2. This should be avoided since exposure of the medullary canal of P2 will increase the risk of osteomyelitis and postoperative complications.

The author prefers to close the wound, regardless of the age of the cat, using absorbable sutures (3-0 or 4-0 chromic catgut) in a cruciate pattern. The sutures are placed so that wound closure is side to side. Although not used by the authors, tissue adhesives are preferred by some surgeons. These must be applied sparingly on the outer skin edge rather than within the wound since wound healing can only occur around the adhesive. The surgical field must be completely dry for them to be effective.

Postoperative considerations

A firm bandage is placed on the limb before release of the tourniquet. The bandage is checked after surgery to make sure it is in place. This must be left on no longer than 24 hours. If bleeding occurs at bandage removal, a second bandage can be placed and removed 12 hours later. While a bandage is in place, the animal must be hospitalized. At bandage removal, the toes can be inspected. Avoid cleansing the feet as this may only stimulate bleeding. Postoperative antimicrobials are unnecessary. Shredded paper should be used in the litter tray for a week. Suture removal is unnecessary.

Complications reported after onychectomy include persistent pain and reluctance to walk, osteomyelitis, infection and granuloma formation that is often associated with use of tissue adhesives, nail regrowth associated with inadequate amputation of P3, ischaemic necrosis of the feet that is associated with poor bandage maintenance, palmagrade stance and protrusion of P2 (Tobias, 1994). Regrowth and abscess formation require surgical exploration, debridement and excision of any remnants of P3 and appropriate antimicrobial therapy.

Deep digital flexor tendonectomy

Deep digital flexor tendonectomy has been reported as an alternative to onychectomy in

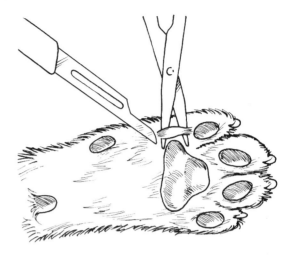

Figure 11.8 The deep digital flexor tendon is exposed via a ventral skin incision proximal to the digital pad. The tendon is dissected free and a 5-mm section is resected.

the cat (Rife, 1988). This procedure, by excising a portion of the deep digital flexor tendon, renders the cat unable to flex this tendon and expose the claw, which is held retracted by the dorsal elastic ligaments (Fig. 11.8). The claw must be kept trimmed or the cat will still be able to scratch and the untrimmed nail may grow into the digital pad.

Surgical technique

The foot is prepared as for onychectomy. A skin incision is made on the ventral aspect of the digit, just proximal to the digital pad. The deep digital flexor tendon will be exposed underneath the skin. The tendon is undermined using small, curved scissors and the tendon elevated and exteriorized from the wound by the scissors or haemostats. A 5-mm section of tendon is resected. The skin incision is closed using absorbable sutures or tissue adhesive. Tissue adhesive appears to reduce postoperative haemorrhage more effectively and obviates the need for postoperative bandages (Rife, 1988).

Postoperative considerations and prognosis

Postoperative considerations are as for onychectomy. It is imperative that the owner is aware of the need for regularly trimming the nails. An anecdotal report of cats suffering from reduced motion of the P2/P3 joint and increasing pain associated with manipulation of the joint has been reported (Kusba, 1988). This change appeared to make trimming the nails more difficult and these animals later required onychectomy.

Tail docking

The amputation of tails for cosmetic purposes and compliance with breed standards is referred to as tail docking. Length requirements vary for different breeds and also owners (Table 11.3). The veterinarian is advised to consult very closely with the client or reputable breeders

before amputating the tail. The authors include this information for completeness and express no opinion as to its endorsement. The procedure should be performed within the first few days of life to reduce morbidity. Surgery of animals older than 5 days requires general anaesthesia and may be associated with some morbidity, including postoperative pain, bleeding and dehiscence.

Surgical technique

The tail can be removed without anaesthesia in puppies less than 5 days of age. The tail is cleansed with antiseptic and the puppy is restrained. A piece of gauze or umbilical tape

Table 11.3 AKC breed standards for tail docking

Breed	Length for puppies < 1 week of age
Affenpinscher	Dock close to body. Leave $\frac{1}{3}$ in (8–9 mm)
Airedale	Leave two-thirds to three-quarters tail. The tip of the dock should be even with the top of the skull when the puppy is in show position
American Cocker Spaniel	Leave one-third tail; approx. $\frac{3}{4}$ in (19 mm)
Australian Silky Terrier	Leave one-third tail; approx. $\frac{1}{2}$ in (12–13 mm)
Australian Terrier	Leave two-thirds tail; cut $\frac{1}{16}$ in (1–2 mm) beyond tan hair on ventral surface of tail
Boston Terrier*	Naturally docked. If tail is too long, dock to natural length
Bouvier des Flandres	Leave $\frac{1}{2}$–$\frac{3}{4}$ in (12–19 mm)
Boxer	Leave $\frac{3}{4}$ in (19 mm)
Brittany Spaniel*	Leave $\frac{3}{4}$–1 in (19–25 mm)
Brussels Griffon	Leave one-quarter to one-third tail
Cavalier King Charles Spaniel	Optional. Leave at least two-thirds tail. Always leave white tip in broken-coloured puppies
Clumber Spaniel	Leave one-quarter to one-third tail. Dock at point of natural tail taper. Tail should be 4 in long in adult
Dobermann	Leave one-half to three-quarters tail or two vertebrae
English Bulldog*	
English Cocker Spaniel	Leave one-third tail or four to five vertebrae
English Toy Spaniel	Leave one-third tail
Field Spaniel	Leave one-third tail
Fox (Smooth and Wire-haired) Terrier	Leave two-thirds to three-quarters tail. The tip of the dock should be even with the top of the skull when the puppy is in show position
French Bulldog*	
German Short-haired Pointer	Leave two-thirds tail
German Wire-haired Pointer	Leave two-thirds tail

Table 11.3 (continued)

Breed	Length for puppies < 1 week of age
Irish Terrier	Leave two-thirds to three-quarters tail. The tip of the dock should be even with the top of the skull when the puppy is in show position
Kerry Blue Terrier	Leave one-half to two-thirds tail. The tip of the dock should be even with the top of the skull when the puppy is in show position
Lakeland Terrier	Leave two-thirds tail. The tip of the dock should be even with the top of the skull when the puppy is in show position
Miniature Pinscher	Leave $\frac{1}{2}$ in (12–13 mm) or two vertebrae. Tail must cover anus
Norwich Terrier	Leave one-quarter to one-third tail. Tail should be long enough to grasp and pull dog from fox hole
Old English Sheepdog*	Naturally docked. If necessary, dock as close to body as possible or leave one vertebra
Poodle – Miniature	Leave one-half to two-thirds tail; approx. $1\frac{1}{8}$ in (28–29 mm)
Poodle – Standard	Leave one-half to two-thirds tail; approx. $1\frac{1}{2}$ in (38 mm)
Poodle – Toy	Leave one-half to two-thirds tail; approx. 1 in (25 mm)
Rottweiler	Naturally docked. If necessary, dock as close to body as possible or leave one vertebra
Schipperke*	Dock close to body such that there is no tail left
Schnauzer – Giant	Leave $1\frac{1}{4}$ in (32 mm) or two or three vertebrae
Schnauzer – Miniature	Leave approx. $\frac{3}{4}$ in (19 mm). Tail should be less than 1 in (25 mm). Tail is docked at demarcation of white and grey hair on ventral tail. Tail must cover anus
Schnauzer – Standard	Leave 1 in (25 mm)or two vertebrae. Dock just beyond light markings on ventral tail surface
Sealyham Terrier	Leave one-third to one-half tail
Soft-coated Wheaten Terrier	Leave one-half to three-quarters tail
Spino Italiani	Leave three-fifths tail
Springer Spaniel – English	Leave one-third tail
Springer Spaniel – Welsh	Leave one-third to one-half tail
Sussex Spaniel	Leave one-third tail
Vizsla	Leave two-thirds tail
Weimaraner	Leave three-fifths tail; approx. $1\frac{1}{2}$ in (38 mm). Tail tucked between legs must cover genitalia
Welsh Pembroke Corgi*	Naturally docked. If necessary dock as close to body as possible or leave one vertebra
Welsh Terrier	Leave two-thirds to three-quarters tail. The tip of the dock should be even with the top of the skull when the puppy is in show position
Yorkshire Terrier	

*May be naturally docked.

is wrapped firmly at the base of the tail to act as a tourniquet. The amputation site is selected and no attempt to cut between vertebrae is necessary since the bones are soft. The skin is pushed cranially and a pair of angled cuts are made with scissors or a scalpel blade to create a dorsal and ventral tail flap. The flaps are closed with a single cruciate suture of absorbable suture (chromic catgut). The tourniquet is released and pressure over the tail is applied until bleeding stops.

Postoperative considerations

Complications are uncommon when the technique is performed properly and in appropriately aged animals. Premature removal of the suture (by the dam) may result in exposure of the caudal vertebrae and predispose to infection and substantial scar formation. Failure to push the skin cranially to create adequate tissue coverage of the tail end may result in scar formation also. Scar formation may require revision if it is unsightly or painful.

Cosmetic otoplasty

Cosmetic otoplasty or ear cropping is performed to meet breed standards for some dogs as requested by certain owners or breeders (Table 11.4). The authors include this information for completeness and express no opinion as to its endorsement. Otoplasty is performed best in young dogs about 9–10 weeks of age unless otherwise indicated. These dogs should have begun their vaccination programme and should be screened for coagulopathies. This is particularly important in the Dobermann which has a high incidence of von Willebrand's disease.

Ear cropping is not technically difficult to perform but is a very exacting procedure with a high propensity for complications that cause the owners to consider the result unacceptable. The authors recommend that a surgeon wishing to begin performing these procedures should seek advice and guidance from someone with considerable experience and success.

References

Kusba, J.K. (1988) Speaking out. *Journal of the American Hospital Association*, **24**, 262.

Rife, J.N. (1988) Deep digital flexor tendonectomy: An alternative to amputation onchyectomy for declawing cats. *Journal of the American Animal Hospital Association*, **24**, 73–76.

Smeak, D.D. (1989) Anti-drool cheiloplasty: Clinical results in six dogs. *Journal of the American Animal Hospital Association*, **25**, 181–185.

Tobias, K.S. (1994) Feline onchyectomy at a teaching institution: A retrospective study of 163 cases. *Veterinary Surgery*, **23**, 274–280.

Table 11.4 AKC ear-cropping guidelines

Breed	Age	Length of trim
Boston Terrier	6 months	As long as possible
Boxer	9 weeks	$2\frac{1}{2}$ in (63–4 mm) to $2\frac{3}{4}$ in (70 mm)
Dobermann Pinscher	9 weeks	$2\frac{3}{4}$ in (70 mm)
Great Dane	9 weeks	$3\frac{1}{2}$ in (89 mm) to $3\frac{3}{4}$ in (95 mm)
Miniature Pinscher	12 weeks	$1\frac{3}{4}$ in (44–5 mm)
Schnauzer – Minature	12 weeks	2–$2\frac{1}{2}$ in (51–64 mm)
Schnauzer – Standard	9 weeks	$2\frac{1}{2}$ in (63–4 mm)

Musculoskeletal disorders

The causes of lameness in puppies vary according to breed and age (Tables 12.1 and 12.2). Lameness in kittens is a less common problem than in puppies and is usually the result of trauma, although some developmental problems are encountered.

Arthropathies

Shoulder joint

Osteochondritis dissecans

Osteochondrosis is a developmental condition in which there is failure of normal endochondral ossification. The normal process of differentiation of cartilage cells and bone formation is disrupted. When it occurs at the bone end, the articular cartilage may be abnormally thickened. The chondrocytes in the deeper layers of the articular cartilage necrose and the surrounding cartilage matrix fails to mineralize.

Osteochondritis dissecans (OCD) is a form of osteochondrosis, the cause of which is multifactorial and poorly understood. Implicated factors include overnutrition, rapid growth rate, hormonal influence, genetics and trauma (Slater *et al.*, 1992). Thickening of the articular cartilage may cause separation between the calcified and non-calcified layers, which creates a cartilage flap. If the separation communicates with the

Table 12.1 Causes of forelimb lameness in puppies

Causes of forelimb lameness in a young large-breed dog
Shoulder osteochondritis dissecans
Elbow osteochondritis dissecans
Fragmented coronoid process
Ununited anconeal process
Panosteitis
Trauma (fracture or tendon disruption)
Hypertrophic osteodystrophy
Arthritis (infectious, inflammatory or immune-mediated)
Bone cyst
Sesamoid bone degeneration

Causes of forelimb lameness in a young small-breed dog
Congenital shoulder luxation
Congenital elbow luxation
Arthritis (infectious, inflammatory or immune-mediated)
Trauma (fracture or tendon disruption)

Table 12.2 Causes of hindlimb lameness in puppies

Causes of hindlimb lameness in a young large-breed dog
Hip dysplasia
Stifle osteochondritis dissecans
Hock osteochondritis dissecans
Panosteitis
Trauma (fracture or tendon disruption)
Hypertrophic osteodystrophy
Arthritis (infectious, inflammatory or immune-mediated)
Bone cyst
Sesamoid bone degeneration

Causes of hindlimb lameness in a young small-breed dog
Legg–Calvé–Perthes
Patellar luxation
Arthritis (infectious, inflammatory or immune-mediated)
Trauma (fracture or tendon disruption)

joint surface the synovial fluid has access to the subchondral bone and causes synovitis and pain. Articular cartilage does not undergo repair, hence it will only heal if the cartilage flap is reattached or removed. Loose cartilage flaps may fragment and become free in the joint. Cartilage fragments may be completely absorbed or be nourished by the synovial fluid and become loose bodies called joint mice. Alternatively, the cartilage fragments may attach to the synovium, become vascularized and ossify. If the cartilage flap is surgically removed, the articular cartilage defect will heal by ingrowth of granulation tissue which transforms into fibrocartilage.

Clinical signs

The shoulder, elbow, hock and stifle of young (5–10 months), large, rapidly growing large- and giant-breed dogs are most commonly affected (Whitehair and Rudd, 1990; Slater *et al.*, 1991; Weinstein *et al.*, 1995b). Males are affected more often than females. The condition is bilateral in most affected dogs, although one joint may be clinically worse. Affected dogs may be asymptomatic or show mild to severe lameness. Disuse muscle atrophy of the affected limb occurs with chronic lameness. Permanent lameness due to secondary degenerative joint disease (DJD) may occur.

Manipulation of the affected joint elicits pain. Crepitus and reduced range of motion may also be present. Joint effusion and joint capsule thickening may be detected in some affected elbow, hock and stifle joints.

Diagnosis

Diagnosis of OCD is based on clinical signs and physical examination findings in characteristic breeds (Table 12.3). The diagnosis is confirmed by radiographic findings including an irregular subchondral surface, a focal defect in the subchondral bone and sclerosis of the bone underlying the defect. Cartilage flaps or free fragments

Table 12.3 Clinical and radiographic features of osteochondritis dissecans (OCD)

Location	Clinical features	Radiographic features	Comments
Shoulder	Mild to moderate forelimb lameness, worse after exercise	Irregular radiolucent subchondral defect of the caudal aspect of the humeral head is best seen on the mediolateral radiographic view, but oblique views may be required	Shoulder is most common site of OCD. May develop tenosynovitis if a piece of fragmented cartilage enters the biceps tendon sheath. Seroma is the most common postoperative complication. Prognosis is excellent if minimal degenerative joint disease (DJD) is present
Elbow	Unilateral or bilateral forelimb lameness in 4–10 month-old dog	Defect or flattening of medial humeral condyle on craniocaudal view Dogs > 9 months old may have osteophytes on anconeus and radial head	Common site. Defect may be related to pressure from medial coronoid process. Prognosis is fair to poor. Progressive DJD is expected
Hock	Subtle hindlimb lameness with hyperextension of the hock in 5–48 month-old dog	Most commonly a radiolucent or flattened area on medial trochlear ridge of the talus on craniocaudal view. Can be on the lateral trochlear ridge (lateral or oblique view). Joint space may be widened	Uncommon site. Rottweilers appear to be predisposed (Wisner *et al.*, 1990; Beale *et al.*, 1991; Montgomery *et al.*, 1994). Reattachment of large cartilage flaps may be considered to avoid joint instability (Aron and Gorse, 1991; Dew and Martin, 1992). Prognosis is fair to guarded
Stifle	Insidious onset of lameness which may be undetected if condition is bilateral. May have a crouched stance	Radiolucent defect of the lateral femoral condyle seen on mediolateral and craniocaudal views. Occasionally occurs on medial condyle	Uncommon site. Prognosis is fair to guarded. Prognosis is more favourable if lesions are small and treated early, but DJD is progressive

(joint mice) may be identified if they are mineralized. DJD may be apparent with chronic OCD. An arthrogram (water-soluble contrast) may be necessary to identify some cartilage flaps or joint mice (van Bree, 1993). Radiographs should be made of both joints to check for bilateral disease. The history and clinical signs of elbow and shoulder OCD are similar, so both joints may need to be evaluated in some cases. Arthroscopy and magnetic resonance imaging can also be used to identify cartilage defects (Person, 1989; Van Ryssen, 1992; van Bree *et al.*, 1993; Van Ryssen *et al.*, 1993).

Treatment and surgical technique

If the radiographic lesion is an incidental finding and not supported by clinical signs, altering the diet to control rate of growth and exercise restriction may be indicated. In some cases, the lesion resolves spontaneously. Conservative treatment can be attempted if the dog is less than 7 months of age and has mild lameness. Conservative treatment includes 4–6 weeks of cage confinement and non-steroidal anti-inflammatory drug (NSAID) therapy.

The treatment of choice for clinically affected dogs is surgical removal of any cartilage flaps or joint mice. Subchondral bone curettage or forage (drilling multiple small holes into the subchondral bone with a Kirschner wire or small pin) is indicated to stimulate fibrocartilage growth. Any loosely attached cartilage at the periphery of the lesion is removed with a bone curette and the joint is thoroughly lavaged to remove any free fragments.

Surgical approaches

Shoulder OCD is approached through craniolateral, caudolateral or caudal approaches (Piermattei, 1993). Both the caudolateral and caudal approaches allow visualization of the caudal aspect of the humeral head (Fig. 12.1). The humerus must be internally rotated to

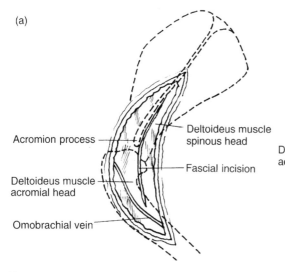

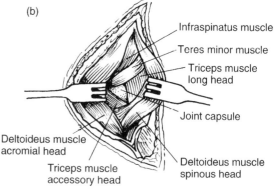

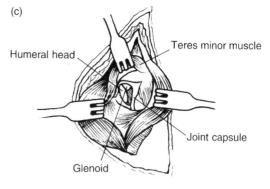

Figure 12.1 Caudolateral approach to the shoulder. The dog is positioned in lateral recumbency with the affected leg up. (a) A curvilinear incision is made through the skin and subcutaneous tissue from the middle of the scapula to the midpoint of the humeral shaft. The fascia is incised over the division between the acromial and scapular portions of the deltoideus muscle from the spine of the scapula to the level of the omobrachial vein. (b) Blunt dissection is continued between the two parts of the deltoideus muscle. A muscular branch of the axillary nerve and caudal circumflex humeral vessels lie in this area. Dorsocranial retraction of the teres minor muscle provides exposure of the joint capsule. (c) The joint capsule is incised parallel to the rim of the glenoid, avoiding the subscapular vessels and the axillary nerve.

(a)

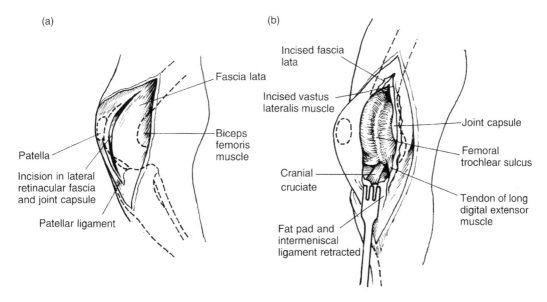

(b)

Incised fascia
lata

Incised vastus
lateralis muscle

Fascia lata

Biceps
femoris
muscle

Joint capsule

Patella

Femoral
trochlear sulcus

Incision in lateral
retinacular fascia
and joint capsule

Cranial
cruciate

Patellar ligament

Fat pad and
intermeniscal
ligament retracted

Tendon of long
digital extensor
muscle

Figure 12.2 Lateral parapatellar approach to the stifle. (a) The skin incision is made from the distal quarter of the femur, along the lateral aspect of the patella and extending to the tibial crest. The fascia is incised a few millimetres lateral to the patellar tendon and patella and extends from the tibial plateau to the distal femur. A stab incision is made in the joint capsule at the tibial plateau. One blade of the scissors is inserted into the incision and the capsule is cut proximally. At the mid patellar level the incision may be angled caudally to avoid cutting through the vastus lateralis muscle. (b) The patella is luxated. If it is difficult to luxate, the incision may be extended proximally.

view the entire caudal aspect of the humeral head. To close the surgical wound, the joint capsule is sutured with interrupted sutures of 3/0 absorbable material. The two parts of the deltoideus are apposed. The fascia, subcutaneous tissue and skin are closed routinely.

Stifle OCD is approached through a standard lateral parapatellar approach (Fig. 12.2; Piermattei, 1993). The joint capsule and fascia may be closed in one or two layers. Closure of the subcutaneous tissue and skin is routine.

Elbow OCD is approached through a medial arthrotomy (Fig. 12.3). An osteotomy of the medial humeral epicondyle may be used but is usually not necessary (Probst *et al.*, 1989; Piermattei, 1993).

Hock OCD is approached through a medial or lateral arthrotomy (Beale and Goring, 1990; Goring and Beale, 1990; Piermattei, 1993). Osteotomy of the medial malleolus can be used but is more technically demanding and usually not necessary (Beale *et al.*, 1991).

Postoperative considerations and prognosis

Postoperative care includes restricted activity

with leash walking only for 3–4 weeks. Swimming is excellent physiotherapy once skin sutures have been removed. The prognosis varies with anatomical location (Table 12.3), size of the lesion and severity of DJD at the time of treatment (Smith *et al.*, 1985; Montgomery *et al.*, 1989b; Rudd *et al.*, 1990; van Bree, 1994; Weinstein *et al.*, 1995a).

Congenital shoulder luxation

Medial shoulder luxation may be a developmental or congenital problem in small-breed dogs such as the Miniature Poodle, Chihuahua, Fox Terrier, Dachshund and Pomeranian. Congenital medial shoulder luxation is often bilateral. Dogs with congenital shoulder luxations usually have a number of predisposing anatomical abnormalities. The glenoid cavity may be shallow, malformed or hypoplastic. The humeral head may be flattened. The tendons surrounding the shoulder joint may be stretched or ruptured. The joint capsule is usually intact and lax, but may be ruptured (Vaughan and Jones, 1969).

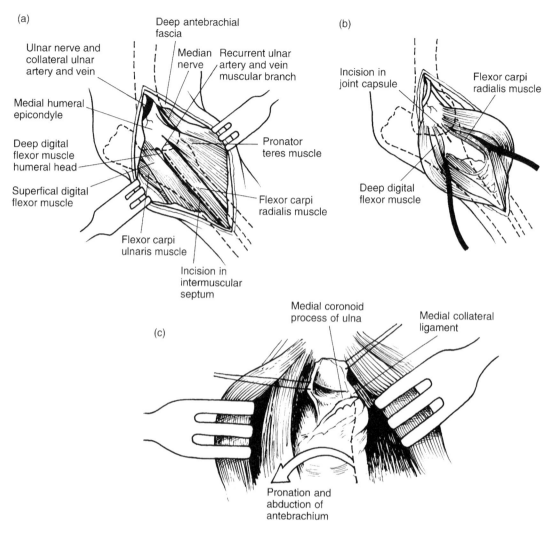

Figure 12.3 Medial arthrotomy of the elbow. (a) To perform a medial arthrotomy a skin incision is made from the epicondyle to the proximal quarter of the antebrachium. The incision is continued through the fascia avoiding the median nerve cranially and the ulnar nerve caudally. The flexor carpi radialis and deep digital flexor muscles are bluntly separated. (b) The muscles are retracted to expose the joint capsule. The joint capsule is incised parallel to the muscles and retracted. (c) The joint capsule incision may need to be extended cranially. Although transection of the medial collateral ligament is avoided, it may be performed if necessary. Firm pronation and abduction of the antebrachium may be necessary to visualize the medial humeral condyle and coronoid process of the ulna.

Clinical signs

Affected dogs usually present at 3–8 months of age with a history of lameness of several months' duration. Intermittent or chronic, weight-bearing or non-weight-bearing lameness is reported. There may be disuse atrophy of the shoulder and forelimb. The leg is carried in flexion with the elbow adducted and the lower limb rotated outwards.

Physical examination of the shoulder may demonstrate crepitus on flexion and extension but pain may or may not be elicited. The greater tubercle is palpated medially relative to the acromion process of the scapula and there may be decreased range of motion, particularly in extension.

Diagnosis

Clinical signs and physical examination are usually diagnostic, but radiographs are indicated to assess the conformation of the glenoid and humeral head and to assess for fractures. DJD may be present, as well as erosion of the medial glenoid rim. Stress radiographs may be necessary to demonstrate instability of the joint (Puglisi *et al.*, 1988).

Treatment and surgical techniques

Congenital luxations are usually not amenable to closed reduction due to malformations of the glenoid and humeral head. Closed reduction may be feasible when the condition is diagnosed early (Read, 1994), but surgical reduction is usually indicated in dogs with lameness. Medial wearing of the labrum of the glenoid, chondromalacia on the lateral aspect of the humeral head or DJD reduces the long-term success of surgical stabilization. If the articular surfaces are not eroded, the joint may be stabilized by suturing the joint capsule and the subscapularis tendon using mattress sutures. However, biceps tendon transfer is generally more successful (Hohn *et al.*, 1971; Vasseur, 1983). Procedures to stabilize and preserve the joint are performed through a craniomedial approach to the shoulder (Fig. 12.4). Biceps tendon transfer is generally more effective than capsulorrhaphy or transfer of the supraspinatous. However, biceps tendon transfer is ineffective if the glenoid surface is small, convex, severely deformed or excessively worn, and shoulder arthrodesis or excision arthroplasty is indicated. Amputation may also be considered.

Joint capsule imbrication with prosthetic capsulorrhaphy

After the joint has been inspected via a craniomedial approach (Fig. 12.4), the medial aspect of the joint is closed by plication of the joint capsule and medial glenohumeral ligament using mattress or cruciate absorbable sutures. The tendon of insertion of the subscapularis muscle is advanced as far cranially as possible and sutured near the insertion of the deep pectoral muscle on the greater tubercle. The deep pectoral muscle is sutured to the origin of the superficial pectoral muscle. The superficial pectoral muscle is sutured to the acromial head of the deltoideus muscle and the deep brachial fascia. The brachiocephalicus muscle is sutured to the brachial fascia. The subcutaneous tissue and skin are closed separately.

Medial transfer of biceps brachii tendon

A craniomedial approach is made to the shoulder joint and the transverse humeral ligament is transected over the biceps tendon to allow mobilization of the tendon from the bicipital groove (Fig. 12.4). A partial osteotomy is made in the lesser tubercle elevating a crescent-shaped bone flap which is used to entrap the biceps tendon (Fig. 12.5). Closure is the same as that described for joint capsule imbrication (Fig. 12.6).

Medial transfer of part of supraspinatus insertion

A craniomedial approach is made to the joint (Fig. 12.4) and a partial osteotomy is made in the greater tubercle. The osteotome is placed on the crest of the greater tubercle and directed so the medial line of the cut parallels the humeral border of the transverse humeral ligament. Laterally the osteotomy is immediately cranial to the insertion of the infraspinatus tendon. The tendon of the supraspinatus is carefully split by using dorsal and medial traction on the severed tubercle with sharp dissection parallel to tendon fibres.

The tendon fibres are split far enough to allow the distal end with the free portion of the greater tubercle to reach the region of the lesser tubercle. Cortical bone is removed over the lesser tubercle and the greater tubercle is attached to this decorticated area using Kirschner pins and tension band wire.

The deep pectoral muscle is sutured to the fascia and periosteum over the lesser tubercle and transverse humeral ligament. The superficial pectoral muscle is sutured to the cranial border of the deltoideus muscle. The brachiocephalicus muscle, subcutaneous tissue and skin are closed routinely.

Arthrodesis

Combined craniolateral and cranial approaches to the shoulder joint are performed with osteotomics of the acromial process and the greater tubercule (Piermattei, 1993). The biceps tendon

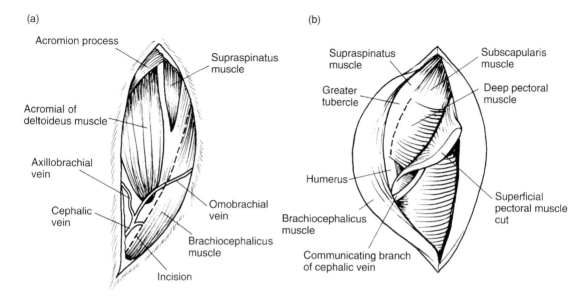

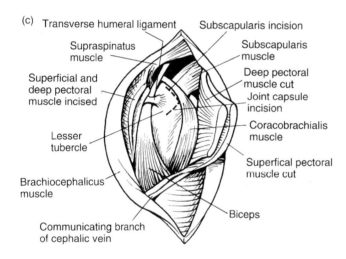

Figure 12.4 Craniomedial approach to the shoulder. (a) The dog is placed in dorsal recumbency. A craniomedial incision is made over the shoulder joint through the skin and subcutaneous tissues. The fascia on the border of the brachiocephalicus muscle is incised in order to retract the brachiocephalicus muscle laterally. The superficial and deep pectoral muscles, the supraspinatus muscle and the distal communicating branch of the cephalic vein are exposed. (b) The limb is externally rotated and the insertion of the superficial pectoral muscle is transected from its proximal border distally to the cephalic vein. The insertion of the deep pectoral muscle is incised completely from its attachments on the greater and lesser tubercles of the humerus. (c) The fascia between the deep pectoral muscle and the tendinous fold of the supraspinatus muscle is incised to allow medial retraction of the pectoral muscles. The tendon of the coracobrachialis muscle may be incised near its insertion. The insertion of the subscapularis muscle is detached from the lesser tubercle and retracted (Piermattei, 1993). The tendon of insertion of the subscapularis is often torn at its insertion and may have retracted, making it difficult to identify (Brinker *et al.*, 1990). The joint capsule is inspected and torn portions of the capsule are identified. The joint capsule should be incised parallel to the medial rim of the glenoid cavity and the joint should be inspected.

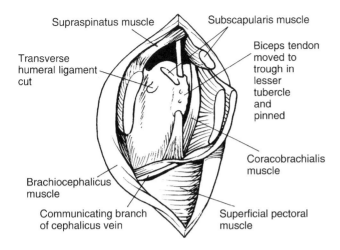

Figure 12.5 Transfer of biceps brachii. A bone flap is elevated leaving the periosteum intact cranially to act as a hinge. A small trough of bone is curetted from the lesser tubercle under the bone flap to accommodate the tendon. The luxated joint is reduced and the bicipital tendon is positioned in the trough under the bone flap. The bone flap is fixed over the tendon using two 0.045-in Kirschner wires or a 2.7-mm screw with a spiked Teflon washer (Hohn *et al.*, 1990).

is detached from the supraglenoid tubercle. Cartilage and bone are removed from the humeral head and the glenoid to create flat surfaces. The two bone ends should contact with the shoulder joint at a functional angle of about 105° (Brinker *et al.*, 1990). The greater tubercle of the humerus is removed using a saw or rongeurs to provide an area of good contact for a bone plate. A small intramedullary pin or Kirschner wire is driven from the cranial humerus into the glenoid to maintain reduction

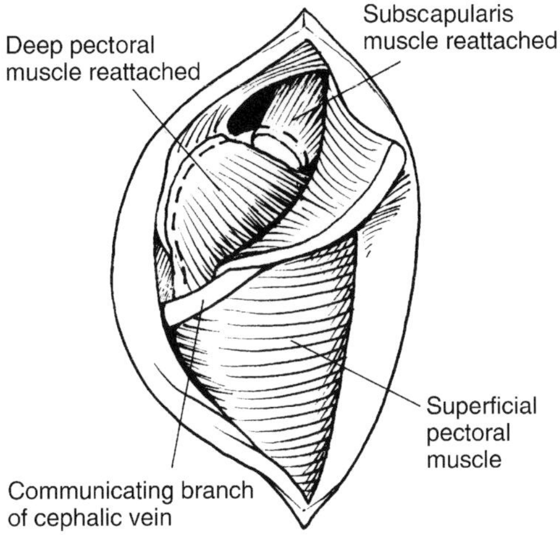

until a plate can be contoured to fit the cranial surface of the humerus and the cranial base of the scapular spine (Fig. 12.7).

A reconstruction plate is easier to contour than a conventional plate and some torsion is needed to make the plate fit the junction of the spine and the body of the scapula. The plate should be positioned under the suprascapular nerve. It is preferable to position at least one screw in lag fashion from the scapula to the humerus in order to compress the two cut surfaces. The small pin may be removed and cancellous bone graft should be placed around the bone ends. The biceps tendon is sutured to the supraspinatus muscle fascia or attached to the humerus medial to the plate using a bone

Figure 12.6 Closure with imbrication. The joint capsule is imbricated with mattress sutures of absorbable material. The deep pectoral muscle is advanced and sutured to the origin of the superficial pectoral muscle. The superficial pectoral muscle is advanced and sutured to the fascia of the acromial head of the deltoideus muscle. The subscapularis is sutured to the proximal border of the deep pectoral muscle and to any available humeral periosteum or fascia.

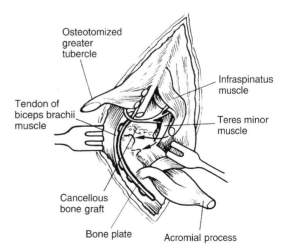

Figure 12.7 Shoulder arthrodesis. Bone plate is contoured and placed to provide rigid stabilization. Autogenous cancellous bone is placed around the osteotomy site.

screw and spiked washer. The greater tubercle is attached to the humerus lateral to the plate using a lag screw or divergent pins. The acromial process and the remaining soft tissues are closed routinely.

Excision arthroplasty

A craniolateral approach is made to the shoulder joint using an osteotomy of the acromial process and tenotomics of the biceps, infraspinatous and teres minor muscles (Piermattei, 1993). The suprascapular nerve is identified and the caudal circumflex humeral artery must also be protected. A glenoid ostectomy is performed with an osteotome or high-speed pneumatic surgical bur. The ostectomy is made obliquely with the medial edge longer than the lateral. An ostectomy may also be performed on the humeral head. The base of the scapular spine is notched to allow the suprascapular nerve to be displaced proximally. The infraspinatus is reattached. The teres minor muscle is pulled medially to pass between the bone ends and is sutured to the biceps tendon and medial joint capsule. Any available joint capsule is sutured to the teres minor muscle and biceps tendon. This interposition of soft tissues should promote the formation of a fibrous false joint. It may be necessary to wire the acromial process more proximally on the scapular spine to reduce the laxity in the deltoideus muscles (Brinker *et al.*, 1990).

Forequarter amputation

Forequarter amputation may be used as a salvage procedure. The technique used is the same as that for adult animal and has been well described (Daly, 1990).

Postoperative considerations and prognosis

Following prosthetic capsulorrhaphy or tendon relocation the forelimb is placed in a Velpeau sling for 2 weeks and exercise is restricted for 4–8 weeks. Passive physiotherapy may be required to restore range of motion after the sling has been removed.

Prognosis depends on the severity of the problem. Closed reduction with immobilization generally has a poor prognosis due to the high rate of reluxation. Dogs that undergo open reduction and internal stabilization of the joint generally recover full weight-bearing. If the glenoid has abnormal size and shape, the surgical stabilization will usually fail and excision arthroplasty or arthrodesis is indicated. Arthrodesis may have a guarded prognosis for larger dogs.

Postoperative management of arthrodesis

The shoulder is placed in a spica splint for 4 weeks following arthrodesis. The splint may be removed once there is radiographic evidence of bony union, which should occur between 6 and 12 weeks postoperatively. After the splint is removed gradual return to function is allowed over a 4 week period. Scapular motion will compensate for loss of motion in the shoulder joint, resulting in minimal functional disability (Fowler *et al.*, 1988; Vasseur, 1990).

Postoperative management after excision arthroplasty

The limb is not immobilized and leash walking is encouraged. Increased vigorous activity is recommended after 2 weeks in order to stimulate fibrosis. There may be a slight limp and atrophy of the shoulder muscles (Bruecker and Piermattei, 1988; Franczuszki and Parkes, 1988), but prognosis for pain-free function is good, especially in smaller dogs (Franczuszki and Parkes, 1988).

Elbow joint

Fragmented medial coronoid process

Fragmented medial coronoid process (FCP) occurs primarily in large- and giant-breed dogs. There may be a genetic predisposition in the German Shepherd Dog, Rottweiler, St Bernard and Bernese Mountain Dog. The aetiology of FCP is unclear. The condition may be a form of osteochondrosis, or may be related to joint incongruity. The condition may occur concomitantly with ununited anconeal process (UAP) or OCD of the distal humerus. The cranial half of the coronoid process may be fragmented or, more commonly, only the lateral part of the process immediately adjacent to the radius is fragmented. The fragmented process may abrade the opposing humeral articular cartilage. This is termed a kissing lesion and may be difficult to distinguish from OCD of the distal humerus.

Clinical signs

The primary clinical sign is forelimb lameness developing between 6 and 12 months of age, although there may an abnormal gait if the condition is bilateral. Pain and crepitation may be elicited during joint manipulation. In chronic cases, there may be joint effusion and joint thickening with atrophy of the limb muscles.

Diagnosis

Diagnosis is based on physical examination and radiographic findings. FCP is difficult to diagnose radiographically since it is uncommon to see the fragmented process. Radiographic signs include elbow joint incongruity and evidence of DJD. There may be sclerosis of the subchondral bone of the trochlear notch, best observed on oblique projections. The earliest sign of DJD is osteophytes on the anconeal process. Later in the disease osteophytes are seen on the cranial radial head and the medial humeral condyle. Computed tomography is more accurate than plain-film radiography and may enable the diagnosis to be made earlier in the course of the disease (Carrig *et al.*, 1981; Carpenter *et al.*, 1993).

Treatment and surgical technique

Exploratory surgery is indicated in dogs thought to have FCP if other causes of lameness have been ruled out. However, medical management has also been advocated (Bouck, 1995). In some cases, surgery is needed to make a definitive diagnosis (Henry, 1984; Lewis *et al.*, 1989). The surgical approach is a medial elbow arthrotomy (Fig. 12.3). The coronoid region is carefully inspected for loose pieces. The fragmented coronoid is often still attached by fibrous tissue and may be identified by noting a fissure line in the articular cartilage. A periosteal elevator may be used to free the fragmented coronoid. The humeral condyle is inspected for an OCD or a kissing lesion, which appears on articular cartilage of humerus where the FCP would contact. Kissing lesions may be impossible to differentiate from OCD lesions, but are generally located slightly more laterally. OCD lesions should be treated by removing the cartilage flap and curettage to bleeding bone. Surface wear of cartilage with no associated flap requires no treatment. The joint is thoroughly flushed before closing.

Postoperative considerations and prognosis

Activity should be restricted for 3–5 weeks. The response to surgery is unpredictable, and the prognosis is fair to poor. Removal of the coronoid process does not prevent development of DJD (Huibregtse *et al.*, 1994; Tobias *et al.*, 1994) and the progression of DJD is variable.

Ununited anconeal process

UAP occurs primarily in large-breed dogs and is more common in males than females. German Shepherd Dogs, Basset Hounds and English Bulldogs are predisposed to UAP. It occurs bilaterally in 20–35% of affected dogs. The bone of the anconeus and olecranon form from separate centres of ossification. Normally the anconeal process and the olecranon fuse by 4–5 months of age. If this bony union does not occur, the anconeal process is considered to be ununited.

The aetiology of UAP is unclear. The condition may be a form of osteochondrosis or factors such as joint incongruity and genetics may play a role. In chondrodystrophied breeds such as the Basset Hound and Bulldog, UAP may be caused by distal subluxation of the anconeal process as a result of asynchronous growth of the radius and ulna.

Clinical signs

Affected dogs show subtle to severe lameness between 6 and 12 months of age. The lameness may be intermittent or continuous and can be exacerbated by exercise. On physical examination, pain and crepitation may be elicited by manipulating the elbow. In chronic cases, there may be joint effusion and joint thickening with atrophy of the limb muscles secondary to progressive DJD. A decreased range of motion may also be apparent.

Diagnosis

Diagnosis is based on clinical signs and physical examination and is confirmed radiographically. A flexed mediolateral radiographic projection will demonstrate a radiolucent line between anconeal process and ulna, and is considered diagnostic in dogs older than 5 months. Signs of DJD may also be present and are similar to those seen with FCP. It is important to radiograph both elbows to identify bilateral disease.

Treatment and surgical technique

If the dog is less than 5 months of age it may be treated conservatively with cage rest for 4 weeks to allow bony union. For chondrodystrophoid breeds, the fractured anconeal process may heal at 4–5 months of age if the radioulnar ligament is cut to free the ulna from the distal pull of the radius. Ulnar osteotomy has also allowed the anconeal process to heal in some cases (Sjostrom, 1995). If the anconeal process is displaced and unstable, excision is recommended. Although surgical stabilization with a lag screw may be performed (Fox *et al.*, 1996), it is contraindicated in the presence of joint incongruency, an abnormally shaped anconeal process or remodelling changes.

Surgical removal of the anconeal process is the treatment of choice. A lateral approach is made to the caudolateral compartment of the elbow joint. A curved skin incision is centred caudal to the lateral epicondyle. The lateral head of the triceps is elevated to expose the anconeus muscle. The anconeal muscle and attached joint capsule are incised along their caudal attachment to the lateral humeral condyle. The joint is inspected and the anconeal process grasped with Allis tissue forceps or fragment forceps. It may be necessary to use a scalpel or periosteal elevator to free the anconeal process from its fibrous attachments (Fig. 12.8).

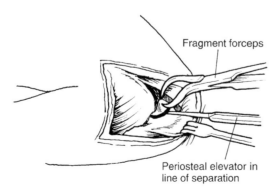

Fragment forceps

Periosteal elevator in line of separation

Figure 12.8 Surgical removal of ununited anconeal process.

The joint is thoroughly lavaged before routine closure.

Postoperative considerations and prognosis

Activity should be restricted for 2–4 weeks. Prognosis for UAP is good if minimal DJD is present (Roy *et al.*, 1994). The DJD may require management with NSAIDs (Table 12.8). In severely affected dogs, arthrodesis may be indicated to preserve limb function.

Elbow dysplasia

Elbow dysplasia is the term which describes the three developmental disorders which can occur in this joint (OCD, UAP, FCP). It is thought to have polygenetic inheritance (Padgett *et al.*, 1995). Osteochondrosis has been proposed as an aetiology for all three disorders. Another proposed aetiology for elbow dysplasia is abnormal development of the ulnar trochlear notch or asynchronous radius and ulnar growth causing incongruity between the articular surfaces of the proximal ulna and the distal humerus (Wind, 1986; Wind and Packard, 1986). One, two or all three of these lesions may occur within the same joint, and DJD develops secondary to joint incongruity or fragment movement. Prognosis varies with the degree of degenerative change. Early surgical intervention (before 9 months of age) to remove loose fragments carries a favourable prognosis, but DJD is a progressive problem. Dogs with both FCP and UAP have the worst prognosis and may have a lameness which is unresponsive to anti-inflammatory drugs by 4–5 years of age. However, if the problem is not diagnosed until the dog is mature, the fragments have usually stabilized and surgery may only exacerbate the DJD.

Congenital elbow luxation

Congenital elbow luxation occurs most commonly in small-breed dogs but has also been described in large-breed dogs. It has not been described in cats. The condition may be hereditary (Bingel and Riser, 1977; Milton *et al.*, 1979; Gurevitch and Hohn, 1980; Milton and Montgomery, 1987) and other skeletal deformities, especially ectrodactyly, may occur concomitantly (Bingel and Riser, 1977; Montgomery and Tomlinson, 1985). Congenital elbow luxation is associated with anatomical deformities of the joint resulting in a lateral luxation, although there is one report of a medial congenital elbow luxation (Montgomery *et al.*, 1993). Agenesis or hypoplasia of the medial collateral ligament will destabilize the joint and allow the proximal radius and ulna to rotate and subluxate. Hypoplasia of the coronoid and anconeal processes of the ulna and a shallow humeral trochlear notch can also contribute to joint instability.

Clinical signs and diagnosis

Three relatively distinct types of elbow luxation have been described based on radiographic appearance (Kene *et al.*, 1982; Table 12.4). Diagnosis is based on physical examination and radiographs.

Table 12.4 Congenital elbow luxation

Luxation	Radiographic appearance	Clinical signs	Surgical considerations
Type I humeroradial luxation	Caudolateral displacement of the radial head with relatively normal positioning of the ulna. The radius and ulna change with time. The articular surface of the radial head is convex, the proximal radius curves laterally, proximal ulna curves cranially, shallow trochlear notch, aplasia or hypoplasia of the anconeal and medial coronoid processes. The distal ulnar physis is sometimes abnormal, which suggests that retarded ulnar growth may be a factor in this condition	More common in large breeds. Affected puppies may appear normal or have mild supination of the antebrachium. The puppy may have a normal gait or a moderate lameness. The carpus may have a valgus deformity and the luxated radial head may be seen as a bony protuberance on the lateral aspect of the elbow (Chambers, 1993)	Conservative management may be attempted if the condition is not severe. Radiographs should be made at 2–3 week intervals to evaluate elbow joint congruity and continued long bone growth. Surgical reduction and stabilization are required when the humeroradial joint is completely luxated
			In young dogs, an oblique radial osteotomy is made to allow manipulation of the proximal radius. The humeroradial joint is reduced and the lateral collateral ligament and joint capsule are imbricated with non-absorbable suture material (Komtebedde and Vasseur, 1993). If the distal ulnar physis is abnormal, concurrent ulnar osteotomy should be considered. The limb should be placed in a supportive bandage for 2–3 weeks. The procedure is similar for older dogs (3–6 months). A wedge of bone may be removed from the proximal radius to align the radial head with the articular surface of the lateral humeral condyle. The radial osteotomy is stabilized with a bone plate or small pins (DeCamp, 1995). Alternatively, the radius can be fixed to the ulna (Campbell, 1979). If there is collateral instability, a prosthetic collateral ligament can be constructed using two screws and non-absorbable suture material. The limb is maintained in a carpal flexion bandage for 2–3 weeks to allow passive movement of the elbow. Restricted activity is recommended for 1–2 months. The prognosis is less favourable for older dogs
			Options for surgical correction of radial head luxation in older dogs include radial ostectomy (Chambers, 1993), reduction of the radial head and fixation of the proximal radius (Johnson, 1995)

Table 12.4 (continued)

Luxation	Radiographic appearance	Clinical signs	Surgical considerations
Type II humeroulnar luxation	Internal rotation (up to 90°) of the ulna causing displacement of the humeroulnar joint. Radial head is rotated but the radioulnar joint is relatively unaffected. Proximal ulna may be deformed as in type I and conforms with the convex surface of the lateral humeral epicondyle. Proximal radius is normal. Radiographic evaluation reveals lateral displacement and internal rotation of the proximal ulna. The radial head is in a relatively normal position but the radial neck is narrowed. Degenerative joint disease is usually not apparent	Most common in small breeds (Yorkshire Terrier, Boston Terrier, Miniature Poodle, Pekinese, Miniature Pinscher, Pomeranian, Pug and Chihuahua). Also reported in Cocker Spaniel, English Bulldog, Shetland Sheepdog, Collie and mixed breeds. The puppies are usually presented between 3 and 22 weeks of age for a limb deformity or for lameness. This type of elbow luxation is usually bilateral and the degree of deformity is variable. The gait ranges from normal to a non-weight-bearing lameness. The limb may be non-functional with the elbow held in partial flexion and the antebrachium pronated (Withrow, 1977; Campbell, 1979; Milton and Montgomery, 1987). The front legs may almost cross if the condition is bilateral. Skin ulcerations can develop on the caudomedial aspect of the elbow and antebrachium if the limb bears weight. Palpation reveals lateral displacement of the olecranon and triceps tendon. The range of motion is restricted, especially in extension, but there is usually no pain or crepitus associated with manipulation of the joint (Stevens and Sande, 1974; Bingel and Riser, 1977; Milton *et al.*, 1979)	If the condition is not severe and the dog can function without pain, conservative management may be indicated. The main objective of surgical correction is to preserve limb function rather than to reconstruct the joint completely. If surgical correction is attempted, the dog should be as young as possible. The joint should be anatomically reduced to decrease secondary growth abnormalities, which can result in joint incongruity and secondary degenerative changes. The age of the dog primarily determines the appropriate surgical procedure. Closed reduction may be attempted for dogs under 4 months old but open reduction is required in older animals
Type III humeroulnar and radioulnar luxation	Similar to type II but there is also cranioproximal luxation of the radial head		

Treatment and surgical technique

Dogs less than 4 months of age with type II luxation usually have minimal degenerative changes which allow closed reduction and stabilization of the elbow. The puppy is anaesthetized and the limb is aseptically prepared. Pressure is applied to the lateral aspect of the olecranon with counterpressure on the medial humerus in order to force the olecranon medially and caudally into the olecranon fossa. Caution is required to avoid fracturing the olecranon. Reduction is maintained using a transarticular pin or a modified external fixator. To perform transarticular pinning, one or two Kirschner wires or small Steinmann pins are driven from the caudal aspect of the olecranon into the humeral condyles while maintaining the elbow in a normal standing angle (Withrow, 1977). The pins are cut flush with the skin and left in place for 2–3 weeks. To use a modified external fixator, two small pins are placed transversely in the distal humeral condyle and the olecranon. A padded splint is put on the caudal aspect of the antebrachium. Elastic bands are placed from the lateral olecranon pin to the medial humeral pin, lying across the padded splint (Milton *et al.*, 1979; Milton and Montgomery, 1987).

Puppies with severe elbow deformities or chronic changes require open reduction and stabilization. A caudolateral approach is made to the elbow (Piermattei, 1993). An ulnar osteotomy may be performed distal to the trochlear notch to improve exposure or aid in reduction of the joint. A lateral releasing incision, capsulotomy, desmotomy the lateral collateral ligament or anconeus myotomy may be required to facilitate reduction (Campbell, 1979; Milton and Montgomery, 1987). The joint is inspected and the trochlea can be revised, if necessary, by deepening it with a scalpel blade to achieve a more congruent fit (DeCamp, 1995). If the congruency between the trochlea and trochlear notch is good, lateral release and medial imbrication of the joint capsule (Campbell, 1971; Milton *et al.*, 1979), combined with transposition of the olecranon process distally or a derotational osteotomy of the proximal ulna, will usually maintain reduction. The joint is stabilized by small transarticular pins or Kirschner wires from the ulna to the humeral condyles (Johnson, 1995). Alternatively, the ulna can be fixed to the proximal radius with pin or screw fixation if the dog is not in a rapid growth phase (i.e. not between 4–8 months of age; Milton *et al.*, 1979; Gurevitch and Hohn, 1980). Other techniques used to maintain reduction include external fixation and collateral ligament reconstruction (Campbell, 1971; 1979; Milton and Montgomery, 1987). If surgical stabilization does not result in a functional limb, arthrodesis or amputation is required (Bingel and Riser, 1977; Milton *et al.*, 1979; Gurevitch and Hohn, 1980; Brinker *et al.*, 1990).

Postoperative considerations and prognosis

For closed reduction and stabilization, the fixator is removed after 1 week and activity is restricted for 4–6 weeks. After open reduction the limb is placed in a splint for 2–3 weeks, at which time the pins are removed. Exercise should be restricted for several months after surgery. The prognosis for return to normal function is guarded. Complications include reluxation, infection and physeal arrest. Some degree of DJD is expected even if the joint is sucessfully reduced. Development of the joint may not be normal, but early corrective surgery may provide satisfactory function for young puppies. Radial head excision, arthrodesis or amputation should be considered for severely affected older dogs (Chambers, 1993). The prognosis is guarded if the repair is delayed and the bony changes are severe.

Hip joint

Legg–Calvé–Perthes

Legg–Calvé–Perthes disease (aseptic or avascular necrosis of the femoral head) is a disease reported in miniature and toy dog breeds, particularly the Manchester Terrier, Miniature Pinscher, Poodle, Lakeland Terrier, West Highland White Terrier, Pug and Cairn Terrier. There is no sex predilection in dogs (Lewis *et al.*, 1992; Gambardella, 1993). It may be hereditary, although the aetiology is unclear. Ischaemic necrosis of the femoral capital epiphysis with femoral head and neck collapse results in joint incongruity and degenerative changes in the hip joint. Right and left legs are affected with equal frequency but it occurs bilaterally only 12–17% of the time (Gambardella, 1993).

Clinical signs

Clinical signs appear between 3 and 13 months of age with an insidious onset of lameness in one rear leg. The lameness may be mild at first and progress to non-weight-bearing lameness over 6–8 weeks. In some dogs, the onset is apparently sudden. Pain and crepitus are elicited upon abduction or extension of the hip. Manipulation may demonstrate a restricted range of motion of the coxofemoral joint. Mild to severe atrophy of the hindlimb muscles may be present.

Diagnosis

Diagnosis is based on physical examination and confirmed by radiographs. Early radiographic changes include decreased density of the epiphysis and sclerosis and thickening of the femoral neck. As the disease progresses foci of radiolucency are seen in the epiphysis and irregular densities in the metaphysis. Later changes include increased joint space, flattening or deformation of the femoral head due to collapse and fragmentation and a thickened femoral neck. The femoral head and neck may appear as an irregular mass of bone with multiple radiolucencies and fractures. Chronically affected dogs will show signs of severe DJD.

Treatment and surgical technique

Cage confinement, good nutrition and analgesia may be indicated in dogs with minimal clinical signs and no radiographic changes in the contour of the femoral head (Gibson *et al.*, 1990). An Ehmer sling is contraindicated because severe muscular atrophy will develop, along with early degenerative changes in the distal femoral articular cartilage (Wallace and Olmstead, 1995). Confinement is indicated until the radiolucent changes in the femoral head are resolved, usually 4–6 months. Although a few dogs will recover with conservative management, surgery is indicated if there is no improvement after 1 month or if the femoral head collapses. Excision of the femoral head and neck is performed and is considered to be the treatment of choice for most dogs.

Surgical procedure – femoral head and neck excision

Approach to the hip
The dog is placed in lateral recumbency with the affected limb up. The limb should be prepared from the hock to dorsal and ventral midline. It is preferable to hang the limb during preparation and use a sterile stockinette on it while draping to allow for limb manipulation during surgery. A craniolateral approach is made to the hip (Piermattei, 1993; Fig. 12.9).

Excision of the femoral head and neck
The round ligament, if intact, is cut blindly with Mayo scissors or a scalpel blade. The hip is externally rotated and luxated. The entire femoral head and neck should be visible. Any remaining muscle or joint capsule on the femoral neck should be removed with a periosteal elevator so the entire cranial aspect of the

femoral neck and the medial edge of the greater trochanter are exposed. The hip is externally rotated so the stifle is pointing straight up towards the ceiling. The lesser trochanter is palpated on the medial aspect of the femur. The ostectomy can be performed with an oscillating saw or an osteotome and mallet. Gigli wire is not recommended because it is difficult to control the location of the cut and is more traumatic to nearby soft tissues.

The osteotome is positioned along a line which extends from the lesser trochanter to the medial edge of the greater trochanter (Fig. 12.10). The handle of the osteotome should be tilted slightly cranially (towards the dog's shoulders). If the osteotome is positioned perpendicular to the table, it will result in incomplete excision of the caudal aspect of the femoral neck. Once the leg and the osteotome are properly positioned, the entire femoral head and neck is removed with a few sharp strokes of the mallet. The femoral head and neck is grasped with fragment forceps and any joint capsule remnants are severed. The femoral head and neck is inspected for completeness of neck excision. Any bony projections or irregularities at the osteotomy site are removed with a rongeur or bone rasp. The joint is palpated through full range of motion to ensure that it is smooth. The joint is thoroughly lavaged prior to closure.

Hip joint closure
The joint capsule should be sutured to cover the acetabulum, if possible. If a tenotomy was performed on the tendon of the deep gluteal muscle, it is repaired with one or two mattress sutures of absorbable suture. The vastus lateralis muscle is sutured to the deep gluteal with absorbable mattress sutures. The fascia lata is sutured to the superficial gluteal and the biceps femoris with one simple continuous line of sutures. The subcutaneous tissue and skin are closed routinely.

Ancillary interpositional procedures
A number of surgical procedures have been described to try to pad the area between the proximal femur and acetabulum. This includes muscle flaps using deep gluteal or biceps femoris, fat grafts and joint capsule. The simplest technique is to suture the remaining joint capsule together over the acetabulum. Alternatively, a partial-thickness biceps femoris

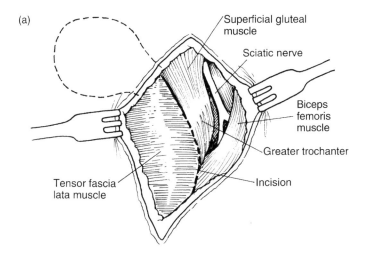

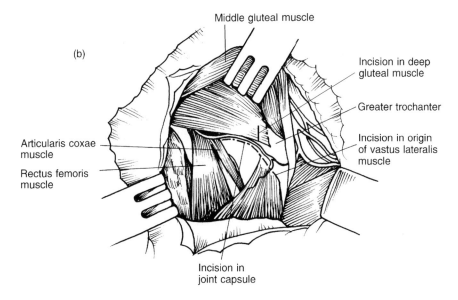

Figure 12.9 Approach to the hip. (a) The skin incision is centred slightly cranial to the greater trochanter. Proximally it is within several centimetres of dorsal midline and it extends to the proximal third of the femur. The subcutaneous tissue is sutured to the stockinette. The incision is continued through the subcutaneous layer of fat to expose the tensor fascia lata and superficial gluteal muscles. An incision is made in the fascia lata along the cranial border of the biceps femoris muscle, and continued proximally along the cranial border of the superficial gluteal muscle. (b) The tensor fascia lata muscle is retracted cranially, and the biceps femoris and superficial gluteal muscles are retracted caudally. Self-retaining retractors are helpful to maintain exposure. The middle gluteal muscle is retracted dorsally to reveal the deep gluteal muscle tendon of insertion. This tendon can either be elevated from the joint capsule or a partial tenotomy can be performed by transversely transecting aproximately one-third of the tendon. The proximal aspect of the vastus lateralis may be elevated from the femoral neck with a periosteal elevator. The joint capsule is incised near its attachment on the femoral neck.

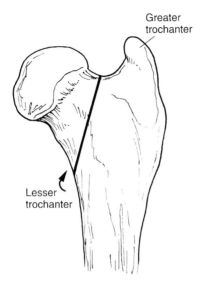

Figure 12.10 Angle for ostectomy of femoral head and neck, viewed from anterior aspect.

muscle flap can be raised from the cranial aspect of the muscle. It is then passed through the joint from caudal to cranial and sutured to the surrounding tissue to maintain it in this position. There is no evidence that these techniques improve long-term clinical outcome (Mann *et al.*, 1987; Remedios *et al.*, 1994). However, they may improve limb use in the early postoperative period (Prostredny *et al.*, 1991).

Postoperative considerations and prognosis

Physiotherapy is critical to restore muscle strength and limb function. Passive range-of-motion exercise should be initiated on the second or third postoperative day. This should be performed for 15 minutes three to four times a day. Buffered aspirin may be administered as needed. Warm packs placed on the limb prior to physiotherapy may help relax the muscles. In addition to the passive therapy, active use of the limb should be encouraged. Swimming is an excellent activity, but leash walks may also be used. When the dog is using the limb well the passive exercise can be discontinued. Most dogs will start using the limb within 5 weeks and return to normal function within 4 months.

If the surgery is performed appropriately and the owners carry out the physiotherapy, the long-term prognosis for pain free function is good to excellent (Berzon *et al.*, 1980). If a dog with Legg–Calvé–Perthes disease is untreated, severe muscle atrophy and DJD will develop.

Hip dysplasia

Hip dysplasia is a developmental disease reported in both dogs and cats. An increased frequency is observed in large, fast-growing dog breeds, especially German Shepherd Dogs and Rottweilers (Popovitch *et al.*, 1995; Smith *et al.*, 1995; Weinstein *et al.*, 1993a). However, it can be seen in any breed of dog and also in pure-bred cats. Both sexes are affected equally. The aetiology is unclear and development of hip dysplasia is a multifactorial condition involving genetic, environmental and nutritional factors (Rettenmaier and Constantinescu, 1991; Kealy *et al.*, 1992; 1993; Smith *et al.*, 1995; Table 12.5). Hip dysplasia is polygenetic so selective breeding can reduce the prevalence of hip dysplasia in a breed. Breeding phenotypically normal animals does not guarantee that their offspring will be free of hip dysplasia, but parents with disease-free hips are more likely to have sound offspring.

Dogs that develop hip dysplasia have normal hips at birth. Increased stress on an immature joint can affect the phenotypic manifestation of hip dysplasia. There must be strong, well-balanced muscle support of the pelvic region to maintain proper joint congruity. Increased angles of inclination (coxa valga) and anteversion are sometimes seen in dogs with hip dysplasia (Fig. 12.11), and can alter the stresses within the joint. Whether the cause of hip dysplasia is related to the supporting soft tissues or bony conformation, the main feature of hip dysplasia is joint laxity with femoral head subluxation (Lust *et al.*, 1993). The consequences of femoral head subluxation include erosion of the articular cartilage, synovitis, swelling of the teres ligament which may stretch and eventually rupture, and abnormal concentration of forces on the dorsal rim of the acetabulum causing microfractures with subsequent loss of acetabular shape. Later changes include osteophyte formation, remodelling of the femoral head and neck, remodelling of the acetabulum and progressive DJD.

Clinical signs

The age of onset, severity of clinical signs and progression of hip dysplasia vary between

Table 12.5 Nutritional factors and their role in hip dysplasia

Nutritional factors	*Recommendations for feeding*
High caloric intake influences hip dysplasia – but it has not been proven whether carbohydrate, protein or fat are most important	Feed a good-quality commercial adult maintenance dog food once the puppy is weaned
Dogs with weight gain above the standard curve for the breed have higher incidence and severity of hip dysplasia	Limit feed both by time restriction and volume restriction, adjusting intake as needed to result in a lean, slow-growing puppy
Vitamin supplementation may contribute to osteochondrosis. Excess calcium may promote osteochondrosis, retained cartilage cores, radius curvus and stunted growth	Do not supplement the diet

animals. The first clinical signs are often noted between 4 and 12 months of age and include decreased activity, lameness exacerbated by exercise, swaying and unsteady gait or 'bunny-hopping', difficulty rising or jumping, and reluctance to go up or down stairs. These clinical signs may spontaneously resolve for months to years until there is significant DJD. Signs associated with DJD include a chronic, slowly progressive onset of lameness, acute lameness after

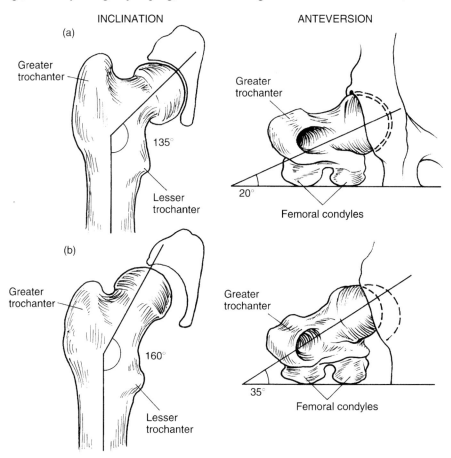

Figure 12.11 Angles of inclination and anteversion. (a) Normal angle of inclination is 135–145°. Normal anteversion is 20–25°. (b) Both angles of inclination and anteversion may be increased in dogs with hip dysplasia.

strenuous exercise, stiffness or lameness which is worse immediately after rising, pain on hip manipulation, palpable hip joint crepitation, forelimb muscle hypertrophy due to transfer of weight to forequarters, atrophy of pelvic musculature, waddling gait due to a shortened stride and reluctance to stand or walk. Some animals remain asymptomatic.

Diagnosis

Diagnosis is based on clinical signs, physical examination and radiographic signs. A complete examination is indicated to rule out neurologic or concurrent orthopaedic diseases. Approximately one-third of affected animals also have shoulder or stifle problems. Some puppies have hip joint pain (associated with microfractures, collapse of subchondral bone, microtears in the joint capsule or ligaments or early DJD), but laxity is usually the primary problem. It is important to distinguish the degree of laxity present from that of a normal puppy. There are several methods to identify hip laxity and all are best performed on a sedated dog (Table 12.6).

Radiographs must be made with the animal under sedation or anaesthesia since accurate positioning is required. The standard radiographic view is made with the dog in dorsal recumbency with rear limbs extended and parallel to each other, stifles rotated so patellae are centred in the trochlear groove, and a symmetrically positioned pelvis. The ventrodorsal view should include the last two lumbar vertebrae and both stifles. The severity of clinical signs does not correspond to the severity of radiographic changes (Table 12.7). Stressed radiographic positioning techniques may be used to quantitate joint laxity (Smith *et al.*, 1990; 1993; Heyman *et al.*, 1993)

Treatment and surgical techniques

Treatment is based on consideration of the stage of the disease, whether the animal is a working dog, the severity of clinical signs and the owner's financial situation. The goals of treatment for young animals with joint laxity include pain relief and decreasing the progression of degenerative changes. The goals for treatment of animals with chronic DJD include pain relief and restoration of function.

Conservative management may be used alone, prior to surgery or as an adjunct to surgery. Exercise is restricted and attempts made to maintain lean body weight. Non-weight-bearing exercise (i.e. swimming) may be beneficial to maintain muscle mass and joint function without undue stress on the joint. Maintaining a warm environment or application of warm compresses may help relieve discomfort. A variety of different drugs can be used to make the animal more comfortable (Wallace and Olmstead, 1995; Table 12.8).

Animals with severe osteoarthritis may not respond adequately to conservative therapy so surgery must be considered. The appropriate surgical procedure depends on whether the goal is to prevent the development of DJD, relieve pain or salvage function (Table 12.9).

Table 12.6 Examination for hip laxity

Methods of palpating hip laxity	Description of procedure
Ortolani's sign (angle of reduction)	With the dog in dorsal recumbency, grasp the stifle and position the femur perpendicular to the floor. Push down firmly on the stifle (if the hip is lax, it will now be subluxated) and slowly abduct the limb while maintaining pressure on the stifle. The hip joint will reduce with a motion that may be felt and heard. This is the angle of reduction
Barlow's sign (angle of subluxation)	After performing the Ortolani sign, adduct the limb and the femoral head can be felt to subluxate. This is the angle of subluxation
Barden test (lateral displacement)	With the dog in lateral recumbency, place one hand lightly on the greater trochanter. Use the other hand to grasp the thigh as far proximally as possible and lift it laterally without abducting the limb. The greater trochanter can be felt to rise if the joint is lax

Table 12.7 Radiographic changes with hip dysplasia

Normal radiographic findings	Early radiographic changes	Later radiographic changes
Acetabulum is a deep C shape	Poorly developed acetabulum appears as widening of the normal tight C shape and decreased acetabular depth	Shallow acetabulum
Joint space between femoral head and acetabulum has even width	Incongruent joint surfaces and uneven joint space width	Osteophytes at sites of joint capsule attachment on the acetabular rim and femoral neck
Curvature of the femoral head and the cranial acetabular margin form concentric circles	Widening or wedging of the cranial third of the joint space	Wearing away or remodelling of craniodorsal acetabulum
Fovea capitis may be observed as a flattened area on the femoral head in some projections	Subluxation of the femoral head	Remodelling and irregular shape of femoral head
At least 60% of the femoral head is covered by the dorsal acetabular margin	Less than 60% of the femoral head is covered by the acetabulum	Subluxation or luxation of the femoral head
Breed variations of normal conformation must be considered, especially in chondrodysplastic breeds	Sclerotic white line on femoral neck indicates enthesiophyte formation	Thickening of femoral neck with resultant short appearance

Table 12.8 Drugs for conservative management of dogs with hip dysplasia

Drug	Examples	Comments
Non-steroidal anti-inflammatory drugs (NSAIDs)	Buffered aspirin (10–25 mg/kg PO t.i.d. or b.i.d.) Phenylbutazone (1 mg/kg divided PO t.i.d. up to 15 mg/kg PO t.i.d. max. 800 mg/24 hours no more than 2 weeks' treatment) Meclofenamic acid 1.1 mg/kg PO s.i.d. for 2 weeks, then every other day for 2 weeks Carprofen 1–2 mg/kg PO b.i.d.	Aspirin is the drug of choice. If not effective, try one of the other NSAIDs. Use the lowest effective dose. Side-effects include gastrointestinal irritation, renal toxicity, abnormal platelet function. Carprofen appears to have the least side-effects
Joint fluid modifiers	Polysulphated glycosaminoglycans (PSGAGs), e.g. Adequan (1–4 mg/kg IM once or twice weekly) Hyaluronic acid	Chondroprotective. Dosages and side-effects are not well-documented. Anecdotal reports that they help, but has not been proven (DeHaan *et al.*, 1994)
Corticosteroids	Prednisone p.o. Depot injection of methy prednisolene acetate intra-articularly	Contraindicated with NSAIDs. Side-effects include degradation of cartilage matrix and progression of degenerative joint disease. Use lowest effective dose. Not desirable for long-term treatment

Table 12.9 Surgical procedures for hip dysplasia

Procedure	Objective	Indication/patient selection	Prognosis	Comments
Pectineal myectomy	Temporary pain relief. Technique: excise pectineal muscle or tendon (Wallace and Olmstead, 1995)	Dogs with taut pectineus when legs are abducted	Variable period of pain relief. Degenerative joint disease (DJD) progresses and lameness returns within months. Few complications	Inexpensive and simple procedure
Triple pelvic osteotomy	Improved joint congruency to prevent DJD. Technique: cut ilium, ischium, and pubis to create a free segment containing the acetabulum which is rotated laterally to improve femoral head coverage (Slocum and Devine, 1987)	Joint should have minimal DJD, reasonable acetabular depth and the femoral head may be subluxated but not luxated	Good to excellent. May still have abnormal conformation or gait. Complications include sciatic neuropathy, implant failure, infection and progressive DJD but are not common (Remedios and Fries, 1993)	Need cage rest for 6–8 weeks post-operatively. Can perform bilaterally
Intertrochanteric osteotomy	Correct angle of inclination or torsion to prevent DJD. Technique: remove bone wedge between greater and lesser trochanters and stabilize in improved position (Walker and Prieur, 1987)	Young dog with increased angle of inclination or anteversion and normal acetabulum with minimal DJD	Good prognosis. (Braden *et al.*, 1990). Complications include infection, implant failure and progression of DJD	Restricted activity for 4–8 weeks post-operatively
Femoral head and neck excision	Salvage limb function and relieve pain. Technique: remove femoral head and neck to allow a false joint to form (see Legg–Calvé–Perthes)	Dogs with severe DJD who no longer respond to conservative management and are not total hip replacement candidates	Good to excellent. Large dogs, obese dogs and dogs with significant muscle atrophy may not do as well. Complications are rare and include lameness, functional limb shortening, muscle atrophy and decreased hip extension	Postoperative physiotherapy is important. May have residual gait abnormalities due to limb-shortening and decreased range of motion
Biocompatible osteoconductive polymer shelf arthroplasty	Form shelf over acetabulum to improve joint stability	Dogs with shallow acetabulum and subluxation	Progressive DJD is expected. Complications include sciatic neuropathy, broken implants, seroma and chronic draining tracts non-responsive to antimicromials	Not osteoconductive and may cause foreign-body reaction (Trevor *et al.*, 1992; Oakes, 1996)

Table 12.9 (continued)

Procedure	Objective	Indication/patient selection	Prognosis	Comments
Total hip replacement	Salvage limb with normal function and no pain. Technique: requires some type of advanced training. Cemented or cementless systems are available (Olmstead, 1995a)	Dogs with severe DJD who no longer respond to conservative management. Must be skeletally mature (> 10–12 months). Bones must be large enough for implants (> 13.5 kg)	Prognosis is good to excellent. Most dogs only need one hip replaced even if severe DJD is present in both. Complications include infection, aseptic implant-loosening, hip luxation and sciatic neuropraxia (Massat and Vasseur, 1994; Olmstead, 1995b)	Rule out any concurrent problems (cruciate rupture, neurological deficit, bone tumour). Dog should not have any active infections or susceptibility to infections (pyoderma, otitis, cystitis, gingivitis, etc.). Post-op care includes cage rest for 1 month and gradual return to normal activity over 2–3 months

Stifle joint

Patellar luxation

Congenital or developmental medial patellar luxation occurs in small and toy-breed dogs, commonly poodles, Yorkshire Terriers, Chihuahuas, Pomeranians and Pekinese. Medial patellar luxation also occurs in cats and in large-breed dogs (Houlton and Meynink, 1989; Remedios *et al.*, 1992; Hayes *et al.*, 1994). Medial patellar luxation is often bilateral. Concurrent bony abnormalities include a flattened trochlear ridge of the distal femur, lateral bowing of the distal femur and internal rotation and medial bowing of the proximal tibia. These abnormalities result in genu varum or an S-shaped appearance of the limb from a craniocaudal view and result in malalignment of the stifle extensor mechanism (the quadriceps muscles, patella, trochlear groove, straight patellar tendon and tibial tuberosity). Abnormalities of the hip (coxa vara, decreased anteversion) may also be involved. The bony abnormalities may be a cause or an effect of patellar luxation.

Lateral patellar luxations are uncommon. They are most often diagnosed in large or giant breeds and are often associated with severe limb deformities characterized by coxa valga, excessive anteversion of the femoral neck, hypoplasia of the vastus medialis, medial bowing of the femur and tibia and external rotation of the foot. These dogs often have concurrent hip dysplasia. Lateral patellar luxation is usually bilateral and apparent by 5–6 months of age.

Clinical signs

The severity of patellar luxation varies and may be described using a grading system (Table 12.10).

Puppies with grade III or IV luxation may have an abnormal gait as soon as they start walking.

Puppies or mature dogs with grade II or III luxation may have abnormal or intermittent lameness all their lives. The condition is usually non-painful and many animals are asymptomatic. A characteristic skipping lameness is often reported, especially with grade II luxations. The dog will suddenly carry the leg (when patella luxates), shake or flex it a few times (until patella reduces) and then bear weight again. Animals with grade III or IV medial patellar luxations may be severely lame with a crouching or bow-legged stance (genu varum). Animals with lateral patellar luxations may have a knock-kneed stance (genu valgum). An acute onset of lameness in a mature dog can be due to worsening DJD or concurrent ruptured anterior cruciate ligament. The severity of the deformities may progress with time. The

Table 12.10 Grading of patellar luxations

Grade	Clinical findings	Concurrent abnormalities with medial patellar luxation
I	Patella can be manually luxated while the stifle is extended, but it spontaneously reduces. Animal is asymptomatic or has infrequent lameness	
II	Patella is easily luxated. May luxate when the stifle is flexed and reduce when the stifle is extended or remain luxated until manually reduced. Animal has intermittent lameness. May progress to grade III	May have medial tibial torsion with deviation of the tibial crest and tibial bowing
III	Patella is permanently luxated but can be manually reduced with the stifle in extension. May walk in crouched position, with stifle semi-flexed because of inability to extend the stifle. May be asymptomatic or mildly to severely lame	Usually have more severe bony deformities of the proximal tibia and distal femur. Trochlear groove may be shallow or flattened. Quadriceps mechanism is displaced medially. May be predisposed to anterior cruciate ligament rupture
IV	Patella is permanently luxated and cannot be reduced. May walk crouched or carry the limb. If not corrected early, severe bony and ligamentous deformities develop which may not be reparable	Tibial tuberosity may be rotated medially by 60–90°. Trochlear groove may be absent. Quadriceps mechanism is displaced medially. May be predisposed to anterior cruciate ligament rupture

movement of the patella in and out of the trochlear groove may cause erosions of the patellar and trochlear articular cartilage.

Diagnosis

Diagnosis is based on physical examination. Radiographs may be used to evaluate bony deformities (curvature of femur or tibia), depth of the trochlear groove and severity of DJD.

Treatment and surgical technique

Indications for surgery are not clear but are generally based on consideration of the animal's age, grade of luxation and severity of clinical signs. Although surgery is rarely indicated for animals with grade I luxations, the client should be aware that the abnormalities could progress, especially if the animal is quite young. Puppies and kittens with clinical lameness and grade II, III or IV luxations are generally surgical candidates. The more severe patellar luxations should be surgically corrected as early as possible to prevent further cartilage erosion and the progression of bony and ligamentous deformities.

The goal of surgery is to stabilize the patella in the trochlear groove and align the extensor mechanism. The selection of procedures is based on the intraoperative assessment of the stifle and the surgeon's experience. There are a number of procedures which can be used alone or in various combinations (Table 12.11).

Postoperative considerations and prognosis

A supportive bandage may be used for 7–10 days in very active animals. Passive physiotherapy or swimming is recommended, especially if a sulcoplasty was performed. Complications include reluxation and overcorrection which require further surgery. The prognosis is generally good for animals with grade II or III luxations. Grade IV patellar luxations may be given a good prognosis if they are corrected before the animal is 4–6 months old, but beyond that age the prognosis is guarded.

Other joints

Temporomandibular dysplasia/luxation

Temporomandibular dysplasia has been described predominantly in young Basset Hounds but has also been reported in Irish Setters, Weimaraners, Dalmatians and Boxers. The condyloid process of the mandible is more oblique than normal, allowing the contralateral coronoid process to slip out of the coronoid fossa and engage the zygomatic arch (Lantz and Cantwell, 1986).

Table 12.11 Surgical procedures to correct patellar luxation

Procedure	Indication
Desmotomy (Fig. 12.12)	This releases the tension on the patella which is generated by the contracted joint capsule and other soft tissues. Recommended for all patellar luxations
Trochleoplasty: Sulcoplasty (Fig. 12.13), Wedge recession (Fig 12.14) Chondroplasty (Fig. 12.15)	One of the three types of trochleoplasty is required if the trochlear groove is too shallow. May not be needed for some grade II luxations, but usually required for grade III and IV luxations
Tibial tubercle transposition (Fig. 12.16)	Recommended if the tibial tuberosity is not in alignment with the trochlear groove on the cranial aspect of the limb. It is often needed for animals with grade II luxations, and almost always necessary for grade III and IV luxation
Tibial antirotational suture (Fig. 12.17)	May be used instead of transposing the tibial tuberosity for young animals with remodelling potential
Patellar antirotational suture (Fig. 12.18)	Helpful for added stability of the patella but usually not needed
Imbrication (Fig. 12.19)	Tightens the soft tissues. It is usually helpful to perform a lateral imbrication while closing the wound for a medial patellar luxation
Femoral osteotomy	Used in grade IV patellar luxations when there is severe angular deformity of the distal femur and the other techniques are not sufficient. Wedge osteotomy of the femur requires special equipment and training
Stifle arthrodesis	May be used to preserve limb function for severe patellar luxations in which surgical correction has failed or is not possible

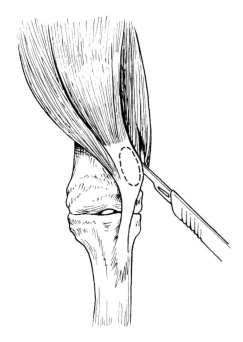

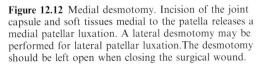

Figure 12.12 Medial desmotomy. Incision of the joint capsule and soft tissues medial to the patella releases a medial patellar luxation. A lateral desmotomy may be performed for lateral patellar luxation.The desmotomy should be left open when closing the surgical wound.

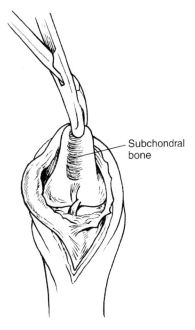

Figure 12.13 Trochlear sulcoplasty. Articular cartilage and subchondral bone are removed with a rongeur or high-speed bur. About half the patella should ride above the newly formed trochlear ridges.

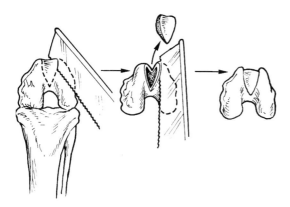

Figure 12.14 Wedge recession. A V-shaped wedge of cartilage and bone is removed from the centre of the trochlea with a hobby saw. The recess is deepened by removing additional bone from the recess's lateral edge. The replaced wedge sits more deeply (is recessed) within the trochlea. This procedure preserves the hyaline cartilage surface of the trochlea.

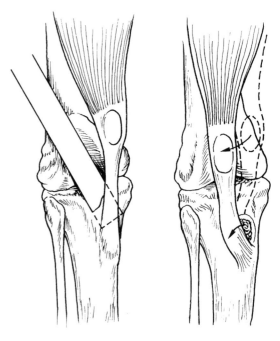

Figure 12.16 Tibial tuberosity transposition. The tuberosity is cut at the base with bone cutters or osteotome and shifted until it is in proper alignment with the rest of the extensor mechanism. It is stabilized with two K wires.

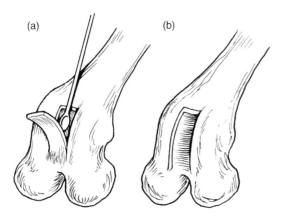

Figure 12.15 Chondroplasty. (a) A cartilage flap is outlined with a scalpel blade and sharply elevated from the trochlear groove with a periosteal elevator. Subchondral bone is removed using a rongeur or bone curette. (b) The cartilage flap is replaced. It is not necessary to stabilize the flap. This procedure preserves hyaline cartilage but can only be performed on young animals (< 6 months).

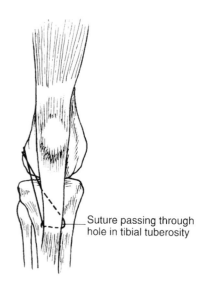

Suture passing through hole in tibial tuberosity

Figure 12.17 Tibial antirotational suture. Heavy suture is placed around the fabella and through a hole made in the tibial tuberosity.

(a)

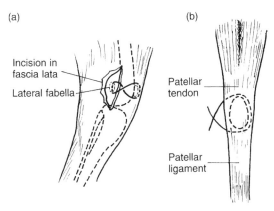

Incision in
fascia lata

Lateral fabella

(b)

Patellar
tendon

Patellar
ligament

Figure 12.18 Patellar antirotational suture. Heavy suture
is passed around the lateral or medial fabella and around
the patella.

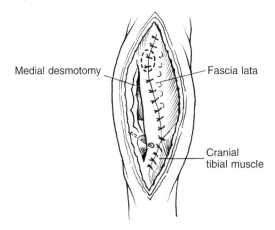

Medial desmotomy

Fascia lata

Cranial
tibial muscle

Figure 12.19 Imbrication. The joint capsule or fascia is
inverted or overlapped with mattress sutures to increase
tension on the soft tissues. It is done laterally in the case
of a medial luxation. Note the desmotomy was left open.

Clinical signs and diagnosis

The coronoid process catches on the zygomatic
arch to cause open-mouth-locking which lasts
for several seconds or until the jaw is manually
reduced. The laterally shifted coronoid process
causes a pronounced facial protuberance.

Treatment and surgical technique

The luxation is reduced by hyperextending the
jaw while placing inwards pressure on the displaced mandibular condyle. Jaw locking can be
prevented by excising part of the zygomatic
arch. Two dogs with temporomandibular dysplasia unassociated with lateral displacement
of the coronoid process have also been
described. Mandibular condylectomy was suc-

cessful in preventing open-mouth jaw-locking
and temporomandibular joint pain in these
dogs (Bennett and Prymak, 1986).

Septic arthritis

Closed-joint infections may develop secondary
to bacteraemia from a remote infection such as
maternal uterine or mammary gland infections,
omphalophlebitis (*Pasteurella multocida*
common in kittens), streptococcal pharyngitis
with retropharyngeal lymph node abscess or
juvenile pyoderma.

Clinical signs

Septic arthritis is usually monoarticular or pauci-
articular rather than polyarticular. Affected
joints (commonly hip, stifle, shoulder and
elbow) are warm, swollen and painful. The
animal is lame or non-weight-bearing and is
often pyrexic.

Diagnosis

The diagnosis is confirmed by evaluation of the
synovial fluid. Characteristic features of the
synovial fluid include haemorrhage, excess protein (4–5 g/dl), presence of bacteria on Gram
stain and elevated neutrophil count (40–
$100 \times 10^3/\mu l$) (Smith, 1993). Neutrophils may
be ruptured and degranulated. Blood culture
medium should be used to facilitate culture of
the synovial fluid (Montgomery *et al.*, 1989a).
If bacteria cannot be cultured from the joint,
bacteria identified in blood or urine cultures
are considered representative of the joint infection. Radiographic changes include evidence of
soft-tissue swelling and joint effusion with thickened synovial membrane and slightly widened
joint space. In late stages, periosteal proliferation is observed adjacent to the joint space and
bone lysis, joint surface irregularity and subluxation may be apparent.

Treatment and surgical technique

Fluid therapy may be necessary for animals that
are systemically ill. NSAIDs may be used to
treat fever and pain. Antimicrobial therapy
should be begun immediately after arthro-
centesis. A broad-spectrum bactericidal drug
such as a cephalosporin is indicated pending bacterial culture and sensitivity results. Although
fluoroquinolones are potent broad-spectum

antimicrobials, they should be avoided in young animals due to their adverse effects on articular cartilage.

Open-joint lavage is performed if there is no response to 72 hours of conservative treatment. The leg is prepared for aseptic surgery and an arthrotomy is performed. Lavage with a sterile isotonic saline or lactated Ringer's solution is performed to remove cellular debris and enzymes, and to reduce joint pressure and preserve epiphyseal vascularity. The arthrotomy is closed; however, for severe infections, drains may be placed to allow postoperative flushing, or the joint may be managed as an open wound.

Postoperative considerations and prognosis

Parenteral antimicrobials and daily aseptic bandage changes are recommended for the first week. Oral antibiotic therapy should be continued for at least 4 weeks. Puppies or kittens with multiple joint involvement die or do poorly despite appropriate therapy. These animals often have concurrent pneumonia, hepatic abscess, pyelonephritis or other organ involvement (Schrader, 1995). Prognosis is better for monoarticular bacterial arthritis.

Complications of septic arthritis include osteomyelitis, joint ankylosis and secondary DJD.

Other arthropathies

There are a variety of nonseptic arthropathies which may affect paediatric animals, some of these are listed in Table 12.12.

Table 12.12 Characteristics of selected arthropathies

Agent	Signs and diagnostic tests	Treatment
Rickettsia (Rocky mountain spotted fever, *Ehrlichia*)	Any age. Fever, anorexia, depression. Acute lameness with several joints affected. Inflamed synovial fluid ($30–50 \times 10^3$ cells/μl, 60–80% non-degenerative neutrophils, 4–5 mg/dl protein). Serological titres (Schrader, 1995)	Doxycycline (5–10 mg/kg PO b.i.d. or s.i.d. for 7–10 days)
Spirochaetal (Lyme disease)	Usually 1–4 years of age. Fever and anorexia. Acute onset of lameness which is shifting and episodic. Inflammatory response in synovial fluid. Serial serological titres (Schrader, 1995)	Doxycycline (10 mg/kg PO s.i.d. for 21–28 days) or amoxicillin (22 mg/kg PO b.i.d. for 21–28 days)
Viral (post viral or post vaccination, calicivirus in cats, feline infectious peritonitis (FIP))	The incidence of arthropathy associated with acute viral diseases is unknown in animals. A condition has been described in dogs which resembles human post viral arthritides (Pedersen *et al.*, 1989). It is characterized by a sterile, generalized inflammatory joint disorder in young dogs between 6 and 10 months of age. Signs include fever, lameness and stiff joints. Duration of the arthritis varies from several days to a month or more. Synovial fluid is thin, cloudy, yellow-tinged, and contains large numbers of neutrophils but no bacteria An arthropathy has been reported in 6–12 week-old kittens (Pederson *et al.*, 1983). Signs include fever, stiffness, lameness and pain with manipulation of the muscles and joints. They recover after 2–4 days. Two or more strains of calicivirus can be recovered from the blood during the acute phase of the illness. This condition can also occur following vaccination with live calicivirus vaccines A mild to moderate synovitis has been reported in cats with the effusive form of FIP (Pedersen *et al.*, 1989). Some cats with FIP may have synovial inflammation but show no signs of lameness or stiffness A sterile inflammatory polyarthritis can occur in dogs and cats as an uncommon sequela to vaccination (Pedersen *et al.*, 1989). It is usually associated with live virus vaccines	If the condition persists for more than a few days, corticosteroids may be beneficial Usually self-limiting. In humans, it is usually not treated unless it persists for more than 5 days and then corticosteroids may be administered

Table 12.12 (continued)

Agent	Signs and diagnostic tests	Treatment
Systemic lupus erythematosus	Tends to affect medium to large-breed dogs from 2 months to 12 years of age. Also affects cats. Often have polyarthritis. Chronic inflammation may lead to degenerative joint disease. Other signs may be present and depend on the body system involved. Diagnosis is difficult and criteria include Coombs-positive, skin lesions, haemolytic anaemia, thrombocytopenia, proteinuria, glomerulonephritis, myocarditis, positive lupus erythematosus preparation, antinuclear antibody and anticellular antibody tests (Goring and Beale, 1993)	Immunosuppressive doses of prednisone or other drugs such as cyclophosphamide or azathioprine
Rheumatoid arthritis	Rare. Primarily affects distal joints of small or toy-breed dogs from 8 months to 9 years of age. Signs include fever, anorexia and lethargy. Intermittent shifting lameness may progress to swollen, painful, crepitant joints. Joints are usually symmetrically involved. Joint instability may cause difficulty walking. Radiographs show collapsed joint space, fibrosis or bony ankylosis with soft-tissue calcification (Goring and Beale, 1993)	Chemotherapy with corticosteroids and cytotoxic drugs. Synovectomy may reduce synovial catabolic enzymes but complete synovectomy is difficult. Joint arthrodesis may be performed when the joints are luxated or dysfunctional due to destruction of supporting structures and articular cartilage erosion
Erosive polyarthritis of Greyhounds	Affects young Greyhounds from 3 to 30 months of age. No aetiological agent has been identified and antinuclear antibody tests, rheumatoid factor tests and lupus erythematosus cell preparations are negative (Huxtable and Davis, 1976; Woodard *et al.*, 1991). *Mycoplasma spumans* was isolated from the joint fluid of one affected Greyhound (Barton *et al.*, 1985). It most commonly affects the proximal interphalangeal, carpal, tarsal, elbow and stifle joints. The synovial fluid is yellow, cloudy and contains fibrin tags. Signs range from swollen joints to acute illness with anorexia, weight loss, depression and pyrexia. Affected dogs may be reluctant to walk due to severe joint pain. Peripheral lymph nodes may be enlarged. Radiographic changes include synovial effusion, periarticular soft-tissue swelling and narrowing of the joint space. It is similar to rheumatoid arthritis but not as severe and most closely resembles idiopathic non-erosive polyarthritis of dogs	It is treated as other immune-mediated arthritides with glucocorticoids and other cytotoxic drugs. However, neither these drugs nor antibiotics, non-steroidal anti-inflammatory drugs or polysulphated glycosaminoglycans have induced remission and prognosis is poor
Periarteritis nodosa	Rare (Altera and Bonasch, 1966). It is an inflammatory condition of small arteries. It has been reported in Beagles, Boxers and German Shorthaired Pointers. Affected dogs often have meningitis, pauciarthritis, cyclical fever and severe neck pain. The neck pain is the most prominent sign and may be debilitating. Episodes often last 3–7 days followed by days or weeks of normality. With time the periods of remission are longer and the episodes are less severe. Recovery is usually complete in weeks to months. The disease tends to be more severe in Bernese Mountain Dogs and prolonged glucocorticoid therapy may be required. The most severe form of the disease occurs in Akitas and they often have polyarthritis. Young Akitas are the most severely affected and the least responsive to chemotherapy. Periarteritis nodosa has been reported in the cat, but it may look very similar to the non-effusive form of FIP	

Table 12.12 (continued)

Agent	Signs and diagnostic tests	Treatment
Polyarthritis–polymyositis syndrome	Young adults (> 1 year). Polyarthritis–polymyositis syndrome is an immune-mediated, non-erosive polyarthritis in young dogs. Spaniels are overrepresented. Clinical signs include stiffness, swelling and pain of multiple joints. There is also muscle pain and contracture, muscle atrophy and pyrexia. Serum antinuclear antibody and rheumatoid factor levels are negative. There are elevated leukocyte counts in the synovial fluid, and histopathological evaluation of synovial tissue is consistent with chronic inflammation. Evaluation of muscle biopsies reveals some areas of atrophy and other areas of active inflammation. Radiographic changes are the same as with other non-erosive, immune-mediated arthropathies	Response to treatment with cyclophosphamide and prednisone is inconsistent. Some respond poorly and others make a complete recovery (Bennett, D. and Kelly, D.F., 1987)
Heritable polyarthritis of Akitas	A clinical syndrome has been reported in Akitas less than 1 year of age. It is thought to be hereditary. Clinical signs include pyrexia, polyarthritis, myalgia, peripheral lymphadenopathy and meningitis (Dougherty *et al.*, 1991)	Affected dogs may not respond to immunosuppressive therapy, but improvement is seen in some dogs following aggressive anti-inflammatory or immunomodulatory therapy (Dougherty *et al.*, 1991)

Disorders of bone and tendons

Limb deformities

Pes varus

Pes varus is an angular limb deformity which occurs in Dachshunds. A genetic aetiology has been suggested but not confirmed. Although there is no history of trauma there is asymmetrical closure of the distal tibial physis leading to a varus angulation of the distal tibia. Clinical signs may be apparent at 5–6 months of age. Surgical correction is recommended to align the joints and prevent severe tarsal osteoarthritis. Surgical correction is accomplished by an oblique osteotomy and stabilization with an external fixator as described for radial angular deformities (Johnson *et al.*, 1989; see section on physeal disorders, below).

Genu recurvatum

Genu recurvatum is a developmental deformity causing hyperextension of the stifle and hock. Initially the stifle can be passively flexed but the flexor muscles are too weak to function normally. As the condition becomes chronic, the limb is fixed in hyperextension and presents as a type of quadriceps contracture. If the dog is presented before the limb becomes stiff it may be treated by maintaining the limb in flexion by use of an external fixator. Two external fixator pins are placed in the femur and two in the tibia. Two single clamps and a connecting bar are secured laterally on the femur and the same is done on the tibia. Rubber bands are used between the two connecting bars to flex the stifle. The device may be maintained for 1–2 weeks and the dog should be monitored carefully (Johnson, 1995). The prognosis is fair.

Hyperextension of the tibiotarsal joint

Hyperextension of the tibiotarsal joint is often seen in association with hip dysplasia, particularly in Chow Chows, St Bernards and Newfoundlands. It may be a compensatory mechanism in that it allows for a lengthening of the stride when hip joint extension is limited. There is no specific treatment other than that for hip dysplasia.

Hyperextension has also been described as a developmental problem in some puppies (Egger and Freeman, 1985). This has been treated by lengthening the Achilles tendon or placing a transarticular pin across the tibiotarsal joint for 2 weeks (Smith, 1976). If left untreated the tarsal joint can be severely traumatized.

Carpal subluxation

Carpal subluxation or laxity has been described in young dogs. The Dobermann and Great Dane seem to be overrepresented. It has also been reported in Golden Retrievers, German Shepherd Dogs, Black and Tan Hounds, and Chinese Shar-Peis (Alexander and Earley, 1984).

Clinical signs and diagnosis

The puppies show carpal laxity by 3 months of age and walk on the limb but maintain the carpus in a valgus position with hyperextension of the radiocarpal joint. The problem is usually bilateral, although one limb may be more severely affected. The aetiology is unknown but lack of exercise and smooth flooring may be factors (Shires *et al.*, 1985). Stressed radiographic views will reveal mild subluxation of the radiocarpal joint but no bony changes.

Treatment and prognosis

Treatment involves mild exercise on a surface with good traction to stimulate increased muscle tone and strengthen the supportive structures (Shires *et al.*, 1985). Splinting or casting of the limb is contraindicated because some stress is needed on the tendons and ligaments to promote strengthening. Recovery may vary from days to months and some dogs are euthanized if the problem is severe.

Dysostoses

Dysostosis is a congenital bony malformation. Some of these conditions are described in Table 12.13.

Swimmer puppies and kittens

Swimmer is a term applied to young animals that are unable to stand by 2 weeks of age. The limbs are maintained in an abducted position and attempts to walk result in a paddling motion. The aetiology is unknown but environmental conditions such as confinement in an area with poor traction may be factors. A genetic influence is also possible as some dams will produce more than one litter of swimmer puppies. Polyarthrodysplasia or instability of the proximal limb joints has been reported (Fox, 1964). Various myopathies may result in signs similar to those of a swimmer puppy and may need to be ruled out. Osteopetrosis of Dachshunds is a congenital disorder that can cause a syndrome which is clinically similar to the swimmer puppy syndrome (Riser and Frankhauser, 1970). If the condition is not corrected, the thoracic cavity tends to become dorsoventrally compressed and widens laterally. This change may be permanent, but progression may be prevented by hobbling the legs. The affected animals will usually begin to walk over a 2–4-week period as the muscles strengthen. Treatment includes housing the puppies on a surface with good traction and monitoring caloric intake to prevent obesity. The prognosis is good if treatment is instituted before 3–4 weeks of age.

Table 12.13 Dysostoses

Disorder	Definition and characteristic appearance	Treatment
Apodia	Congenital absence of the foot with transverse (amelia) limb defect. Rare (Schneck, 1974; Schultz and Watson, 1995)	None
Radial aplasia	The radius is absent and the ulna may become shorter and of larger diameter than normal. Subluxation or luxation of the humeroulnar and ulnarcarpal joints may be apparent on radiographs. Pull of the extensor muscles causes varus and flexor deformities of the carpus which may be permanent as the muscles become contracted (Lewis and Van Sickle, 1970). May be genetic (Alonso *et al.*, 1982), environmental or both	Replacing the radius with an autogenous rib may provide some limb function but does not alleviate elbow and carpal problems (Pederson, 1968). Both the elbow and carpal joints can be arthrodesed, but the resulting pegleg may not be very useful. Amputation can also be performed to alleviate soft-tissue trauma to the weight-bearing surface or for cosmetic reasons (Chambers, 1993). Light-weight animals may learn to walk on their hindlimbs

Table 12.13 (continued)

Disorder	Definition and characteristic appearance	Treatment
Ectrodactyly	Ectrodactyly is the separation of the medial and lateral portions of the limb. The separation occurs between any of the metacarpal bones and may include separation of the soft tissues. One to four digits with their respective metacarpal bones may be missing or the metacarpal bones may be hypoplastic. The respective carpal bones may be severely hypoplastic or absent. The region has an unusual appearance because of complete cleavage between the remaining digits up to the level of the carpus. Absence of carpal and metacarpal bones results in severely deficient or absent articulations at the carpus. The carpal region may be unable to support weight. The abnormal biomechanics of the carpus may also cause elbow incongruency (Chambers, 1993). Hypoplasia of the radius or ulna can also occur. Ectrodactyly may be associated with congenital elbow luxation and contracture of the soft tissues and digits (Carrig *et al.*, 1981; Montgomery and Tomlinson, 1983). Although it is usually unilateral in the dog, it may be bilateral and it is more commonly bilateral in the cat (Carrig *et al.*, 1981). It is heritable in cats with variable expression of a dominant gene	Reconstruction of the manus and carpal arthrodesis may be performed to salvage limb function, but amputation may be considered as the primary treatment for cosmetic reasons or if severe degenerative joint disease is present (Chambers, 1993). If the bone structure is intact and the elbow is functional, it is reasonable to perform carpal arthrodesis (Keller and Chambers, 1989) and reconstruct the manus. The adjacent metacarpal bones are wired together to unite the segments. The skin is closed dorsally and palmarly (Johnson, 1995). Prognosis for function depends on the severity of the deformity
Polydactyly	Polydactyly is the presence of one or more extra digits. In dogs and cats the extra digit most commonly occurs on the medial aspect of the foot. It is an autosomal dominant trait with variable expressivity in the cat. A similar inheritance pattern appears to occur with multiple dewclaws in the dog. There are no clinical problems associated with polydactyly although the extra digit may be predisposed to trauma. A syndrome of multiple defects, including syndactyly and polydactyly, has been reported to be lethal to males in a family of Australian Shepherd Dogs (Sponenberg and Bowling, 1985)	
Syndactyly	Syndactyly is the soft-tissue or bony union of two or more digits, and has been described as simple or complex, respectively. It may occur spontaneously or as a heritable condition. Since syndactyly rarely causes clinical problems it is infrequently reported in the veterinary literature. There is one report of simple syndactyly causing lameness due to excessive stretching of the skin which was resolved by surgical separation of the digits (Richardson *et al.*, 1994)	
Anury	Anury is the absence of a tail. It is most common in breeds that customarily have their tails docked. It is thought to have a multifactorial inheritance. Some dogs may also have lack of development of the rectococcygeus and levator ani muscles resulting in faecal staining (Hall *et al.*, 1987)	

Osteopetrosis

Osteopetrosis is a rare congenital and familial developmental abnormality which has been reported rarely in the dog. It is characterized by retardation of resorption and remodelling of the endochondral and membranous bone so the bones are abnormally dense (Riser and Frankhauser, 1970). Non-regenerative anaemia has been reported in association with osteopetrosis (Lees and Sautter, 1979; O'Brien *et al.*, 1987). Radiographic evaluation reveals uniformly dense bone with no distinction between cortical and cancellous bone in the epiphysis, metaphysis and diaphysis (Riser and Frankhauser, 1970). The length and shape of the long bones are normal. Affected neonates had difficulty crawling and were unable to adduct the limbs to stand (Riser and Frankhauser, 1970). Treatment is symptomatic.

Osteochondrodysplasias (Table 12.14)

Table 12.14 Characteristics of types of osteochondrodysplasia

Disorder	Definition and characteristic appearance
Achondroplasia	Retarded endochondral ossification of long bones results in limb-shortening, flared metaphyses, small foramen magnum, depressed nasal bridge and shortened maxilla. Typical breeds include Bulldogs, Boston Terrier, Pug, Pekinese, Japanese Spaniel and the Shih Tzu (Jezyk, 1985). Bulldogs may also have wedge or hemivertebrae (see Chapter 10). Elbow and patellar luxations may also occur, possibly due to increased joint laxity. Downwards displacement of the proximal ulna may occur, resulting in fractured anconeal process. It is an incompletely dominant autosomal trait in dogs
Hypochondroplasia	Similar to achondroplasia but less severe and characterized by limb-shortening and a normally shaped skull. The limbs may also be deformed due to disproportionate growth. Breeds include Dachshunds, Welsh Corgis, Dandie Dinmont Terriers, Scottish Terriers, Australian Silky Terriers, Skye Terriers, Basset Hounds and Beagles. These breeds may have problems with intervertebral disc disease and elbow dysplasia. Also reported sporadically in other breeds, including Cocker Spaniel, Poodles, German Shepherd Dogs and mixed-breed dogs (Beachley and Graham, 1973; Jezyk, 1985)
Chondrodysplasia punctata	Chondrodysplasia punctata is characterized by stippled epiphyses. Multiple epiphyseal dysplasia with stippled epiphyses has been described in Beagles but it is not clear whether this was chondrodysplasia punctata or multiple epiphyseal dysplasia. Poodles with pseudoachondroplasia also have stippled ephyses (Jezyk, 1985)
Chondrodysplasia (dwarfism, dyschondrosteosis, chondrodystrophy)	Dwarfism has been reported in the Scottish Terrier, Alaskan Malamute, Samoyed, Labrador Retriever, English Pointer, Norwegian Elkhound, Great Pyrenees and Scottish Deerhound (Fletch *et al.*, 1973; Carrig *et al.*, 1988; Breur *et al.*, 1989; Braden, 1993; Bingel and Sande, 1994)
	The defects usually involve the metaphyseal region of long bones. Deformities may be present in the axial skeleton as well. Animals may have difficulty walking due to skeletal deformities. Radiographic evaluation may reveal a widened physeal line, retained endochondral core and irregularities in normal ossification. The long bones are shortened and may be bowed. The radius and ulna may be more severely affected due to asynchronous growth. Chondrodysplasia has been described as a simple autosomal recessive trait in the Great Pyrenees which results in abnormalities of cartilage and bone growth and development with defects in the growth of the tubular bones and the spine. The puppies were abnormal at birth and failed to gain weight at the same rate as their littermates. The limbs, trunk and muzzle were shorter than normal. At 8 weeks of age the vertebral bodies were poorly ossified and the metaphyses of all long bones were flared. Epiphyseal ossification was normal
	An autosomal recessively inherited chondrodysplasia with variable expression of dwarfism has been described in Alaskan Malamutes. There is delayed endochondral bone formation, so it is more evident in long bones. Affected dogs have lateral bowing of the forelimbs, enlarged carpal joints and valgus deformity of the carpus but are not usually lame. Radiographic evaluation at 3–12 weeks of age will demonstrate flattening of the metaphysis of the distal radius and ulna. It is associated with spherocytes and membrane abnormalities (Fletch *et al.*, 1973)

Table 12.14 (continued)

Disorder	Definition and characteristic appearance
	A syndrome characterized by ocular and skeletal dysplasia has been reported in Labrador Retrievers, German Shepherd Dogs and Samoyeds (Carrig *et al.*, 1977; Meyers *et al.*, 1983). An autosomal recessive mode of inheritance has been suggested in Labrador Retrievers and Samoyeds. This syndrome is characterized by shortening of bones of the appendicular skeleton and abnormal joint development. Ocular changes also occur, including cataracts, retinal dysplasia and rhegmatogenous retinal detachments (Carrig *et al.*, 1988). Female Samoyeds are often more severely affected than males
Osteogenesis imperfecta	Collagen synthesis defects result in bone fragility. Limb-shortening and deformities may be present at birth. Affected animals may have multiple fractures, blue sclera and translucent teeth (Jezyk, 1985; Cohen and Meuten, 1990)
Multiple cartilaginous exostoses (osteochondromatosis)	Osteochondroma is an uncommon benign, proliferative disease of bone and cartilage. Osteochondroma refers to a monostotic lesion, while osteochondromatosis, or multiple osteocartilaginous exostosis, denotes polyostotic involvement. The cause is unknown but may be heritable in dogs (Gee and Doige, 1970; Chester, 1971; Doige, 1987). Osteochondromatosis also occurs in cats, but they are usually young adults and live less than a year after onset of signs due to the progressive nature of the disease in cats. It is associated with feline leukaemia virus in cats (Turrel and Pool, 1982). It occurs predominantly in younger dogs during the normal period of endochondral bone formation. It is characterized by multiple ossified protrusions from the cortical surfaces of the vertebrae, the ribs, the metaphyseal region of long bones or the pelvis (Gambardella *et al.*, 1975; Prata *et al.*, 1975; Santen *et al.*, 1991; Jacobson and Kirberger, 1996). The lesions may be single or multiple and may be seen on any bone except the skull. Single lesions grow until skeletal maturation is complete. Dogs may have lameness or paresis but most dogs have a firm mass with no clinical signs. Radiographically, they are pedunculated or sessile lesions which blend with the cortical surface of the bone. Sequential radiographic studies or bone biopsy may be needed to differentiate it from malignant neoplasia. Treatment is usually unnecessary unless the mass is causing a compressive neurological deficit or mechanical interference with overlying tendons or ligaments. If the mass is compressing the spinal cord, a decompressive laminectomy with resection of the growth is indicated. The exostosis can recur with inadequate removal. The prognosis depends on the number, location and surgical accessibility of lesions. Prognosis is usually good, although cartilaginous exostosis has been reported to transform into osteosarcoma or chondrosarcoma (Doige *et al.*, 1978). Continuous or renewed growth past the time of skeletal maturity should be considered to be a malignant condition
Pseudoachondroplasia	Autosomal recessive form of this disease has been reported in Miniature Poodles. It is characterized by dwarfism and enlarged, stiff joints which make locomotion difficult. Radiographic abnormalities include stippling and patchy densities of the epiphyses in juvenile animals and short, severely malformed bones in adults (Jezyk, 1985; Riser *et al.*, 1980)
Endochondromatosis	Hyaline cartilage is formed instead of bone at the growth plates (Krauser, 1989). It leads to angular deformities, pathological fractures and lameness (Matis *et al.*, 1989)
Zinc-responsive chondrodystrophy	Zinc-responsive chondrodysplasia is a form of dwarfism which is most commonly seen in Alaskan Malmutes and other northern breeds. The legs are short and bowed, expecially the forelimbs. Affected animals also have mild normochromic, haemolytic anaemia. Recommended zinc requirements are 0.11 mg/kg for an adult and 0.22 mg/kg for a growing dog. Affected dogs need to be supplemented with dietary zinc at approximately four times the normal recommended level. Most dry dog foods based on corn grain and soybean meal contain phytin or calcium. Phytin binds zinc and calcium impairs zinc absorption, so dogs on such a diet need twice the calculated amount of zinc. Zinc sulphate (150 mg) or 250 mg zinc gluconate provides about 35 mg zinc. Zinc overdosage is characterized by anorexia, vomiting, diarrhoea and fever (Newton and Bierly, 1989)

Chondrodysplasia is an inherited trait which causes abnormal cartilage or bone growth and development. It is thought to cause early cessation of chondrogenesis in the physes and results in shortening of the long bones, especially the radius and ulna. Shortening of the radius and ulna have no proven pathogenic sequelae, but elbow and carpal arthropathies occur in some cases. Many breeds with this syndrome have been bred intentionally and resultant conformational abnormalities are considered to be normal for these animals. Chondrodystrophy in other breeds, such as the Alaskan Malamute, German Shepherd Dog and Samoyed, is considered undesirable. Endo-chondral ossification defects in these breeds are associated with defects in other organ systems (Fletch *et al.*, 1975). Chondrodystrophic animals have angular limb deformities with altered articular cartilage surfaces which predispose the joints to degenerative changes.

Mucopolysaccharidosis

Mucopolysaccharidosis is a class of inherited metabolic diseases which occur in humans, and have been documented in dogs and cats (Haskins *et al.*, 1983; Jezyk, 1985; Newton and Bierly, 1989) (Table 12.15). Each form of this lysosomal storage disease is due to a defect in

Table 12.15 Mucopolysaccharidosis

Mucopolysaccharidosis	Breeds	Clinical signs	Diagnostic features
Type I α_L-iduronidase deficiency (autosomal recessive)	Dog: Plott Hounds Cat: domestic cat	Dog: dwarfed with swollen, painful joints and progressive motor deficits. Corneal clouding and progressive visual deficits. Glossoptosis Cat: enlarged body and head, short ears, wide-spaced eyes and broad nose. Diffuse corneal clouding. Mitral insufficiency. Hindlimb gait abnormality, joint pain	Dog: Urine: excessive dermatan and heparan sulphate Fibroblasts: deficient in α_L-iduronidase activity Lymphocytes: increased granulation Radiographs: epiphyseal dysgenesis and periarticular bony proliferation Cat: Urine: excessive dermatan and heparin sulphates Tissues: α_L-iduronidase-deficient Radiographs: bilateral coxofemoral subluxation, fusion and widening of cervical vertebrae, mild pectus excavatum
Type VI aryl-sulphatase B deficiency (autosomal recessive)	Dog: Dachshunds Cat: Siamese	Dwarfism, facial abnormalities, severe skeletal abnormalities, multiple neurological deficits and retinal atrophy	Urine: dermatin sulphate is 90 times normal. High mucopolysaccharide Leukocytes: inclusion bodies. Mucopolysaccharide granules in lymphocytes and neutrophils Radiographs: similar to hypovitaminosis A (bridged vertebrae, broad and irregular long bone epiphyses, bony proliferation around joints)
Type VII β-glucuronidase deficiency	Dog: mixed-breed	Large head with shortened maxillae and protruding mandible Progressive hindlimb paresis	Radiographs: platyspondylia, caudal breaking of vertebrae and generalized epiphyseal dysplasia

a different lysosomal enzyme involved with the degradation of glycosaminoglycans. The result is an inability to metabolize aminoglycans properly such as heparin, chondroitin and keratan sulphates, so abnormalities occur in tissues which are rich in these substances (cartilage, connective tissue, cornea).

Metabolic disorders

Panhypopituitarism (pituitary dwarfism)

Panhypopituitarism (growth hormone deficiency or hyposomatotropism) has been reported in dogs and cats. Hypothyroidism, hypoadrenocorticism and hypogonadism may also be present. Panhypopituitarism causes retardation of skeletal maturation resulting in uniform shortening of the forelimbs and hindlimbs. Affected animals have a soft, woolly haircoat or bilaterally symmetrical alopecia and mental dullness (DeBowes, 1987). Clinical signs become apparent around 2–3 months of age, but affected animals may not be presented until 1 year of age for stunted growth or dermatological abnormalities. A presumptive diagnosis is made from the signalment (breed, age, sex and description), history, physical examination and routine laboratory studies that rule out other causes of small stature. Growth hormone stimulation tests are needed for definitive diagnosis. Treatment requires administration of growth hormone (bovine or porcine 0.3 IU/kg PO divided into two to three doses per week). The long-term prognosis is poor, despite therapy. Most animals die by 3–8 years of age (average 4 years) as a result of infections, degenerative diseases or neurological dysfunction.

Congenital hypothyroidism

Congenital hypothyroidism has been described in dogs and cats, but it is rare. Boxers may be predisposed. Congenital or juvenile-onset hypothyroidism is due to iodine organification defect, thyroid dysgenesis or deficient dietary iodine uptake. Secondary (pituitary) hypothyroidism can be due to congenital malformation of the pituitary. Affected animals are disproportionately dwarfed with short limbs and a large head with myxoedematous facial features (Jezyk, 1985; Greco *et al.*, 1991). Epiphyseal dysgenesis is seen in most of the animals. The long bones are shorter and wider than normal with metaphyseal flaring. Vertebral bodies are malformed and thoracolumbar kyphosis is common. Affected animals are lethargic and have a juvenile haircoat. The lethargy responds to lavothyroxine, but the bony abnormalities are permanent.

Congenital primary hyperparathyroidism

Primary hyperparathyroidism has been reported in puppies, but is very rare. By 2 weeks of age the puppies had stunted growth, muscle weakness and polyuria/polydipsia (Thompson *et al.*, 1984).

Nutritional disorders

There are a number of nutritional imbalances which can cause musculoskeletal abnormalities. Some of these nutritional disorders are summarized in Table 12.17.

Secondary nutritional hyperparathyroidism

Nutritional hyperparathyroidism is caused by dietary imbalances that result in compensatory increase in parathyroid hormone (PTH) levels. Congenital renal insufficiency can also cause secondary hyperparathyroidism. Diets having inadequate calcium, excess phophorus with inadequate or normal calcium or inadequate cholecalciferol (vitamin D_3) are implicated (Table 12.16). It is most common in young animals, especially kittens that are fed all-meat or all-grain diets or diets supplemented with abnormal ratios of calcium and phosphorus. These diets result in subtle hypocalcaemia and subsequent stimulation of the parathyroid to release PTH. PTH mobilizes calcium from the skeleton or inhibits bone mineralization in young animals. Animals may be affected at any age, although young animals are affected much more quickly than mature animals.

Clinical signs

Affected animals usually present with pathological fractures or they may be lame or reluctant to move due to bone pain. They may have bowed long bones, compression fractures in metaphyseal and epiphyseal areas, deformation of the pelvis and vertebrae and greenstick fractures of long bones. Vertebral compression fractures

Table 12.16 Diets which cause nutritional hyperparathyroidism

Causes of nutritional secondary hyperparathyroidism
Inadequate dietary calcium
Excess dietary phosphorus with normal or decreased calcium
Inadequate vitamin D
Excess calcium binders (mineral oil)

can result in pain or neurological deficits. Major limb joints may undergo ankylosis.

Diagnosis

Diagnosis is based on history, clinical signs, blood chemistries and radiographic findings. Laboratory findings include a low to normal serum calcium, a normal to high serum phosphorus, elevated serum alkaline phosphatase and increased plasma PTH. Radiographic changes include thin cortices and generalized loss of bone density of long bones. Radiographic evaluation of the mandible and maxilla may show resorption of the alveolar bone and loss of the lamina dura dentes. Pathological fractures may be present in various bones.

Treatment and surgical technique

The diet must be modified. A diet containing a calcium : phosphorus ratio of 2 : 1 (normal 1.2 : 1) is fed for 8–12 weeks until the pathologic fractures are healed (Cavanagh and Kosovshy, 1993). Growing puppies require approximately 500–600 mg calcium/kg body weight/day, and kittens require approximately 200–400 mg/kg body weight (Cavanagh and Kosovshy, 1993). Confinement for at least 4 weeks is required to reduce further self-injury. The pathological fractures are treated as needed. Corrective osteotomies of long bone deformities can be considered once the skeleton is adequately mineralized. Healed pelvic fractures may require surgical intervention if obstipation does not respond to medical management or if dystocia is a potential problem.

Postoperative considerations and prognosis

The prognosis is good unless severe skeletal deformities have occurred.

Hypervitaminosis D

Hypervitaminosis D is a rare disorder caused by excessive intake of vitamin D resulting in hypercalcaemia with normal or elevated serum phosphorus due to increased bone resorption and increased gastrointestinal absorption. It is usually due to a high intake of cod liver oil or dietary vitamin supplementation. Signs include anorexia, polydipsia, polyuria, vomiting, muscle weakness and lameness (Kallfelz and Dzanis, 1989). Radiographic changes include generalized osteoporosis and dystrophic calcification. Mineralization of soft tissues can cause damage to the kidneys, gastrointestinal tract and heart. Severe renal damage can result in secondary hyperparathyroidism. Treatment is to remove the source of excessive vitamin D. Complete removal of vitamin D may be required until liver stores are depleted. Steroid therapy may help control the hypercalcaemia. Proper dietary intake of vitamin D, calcium and phosphorus can reverse the bony problems, but resolution of soft-tissue calcification is slow and will probably be incomplete. The prognosis is guarded.

Hypovitaminosis D

Hypovitaminosis D (rickets) is rare. Vitamin D is required for normal absorption of calcium from the intestine. If vitamin D is deficient in the diet, or the animal is not exposed to sunlight there may be inadequate calcium available for mineralization of the growth plates. Excessive chronic administration of oral mineral oil can cause malabsorption of vitamin D. The result is abnormal bone growth. Clinically, it is similar to nutritional hyperparathyroidism (Kallfelz, 1987). Radiographic signs are also similar to hyperparathyroidism. In addition to the decreased bone density and pathological fractures, the growth plates may appear wider than normal and cartilage cores may be seen in the metaphysis. Long bones may be shortened and have abnormal curvature. Treatment is to feed a balanced commercial diet or correct environmental problems. Vitamin D supplementation is usually not indicated because commercial pet foods contain more than minimal recommended amounts of vitamin D (Kallfelz and Dzanis, 1989). The fractures should be treated. The prognosis is good unless the growth plate abnormalities or fractures are severe.

Hypervitaminosis A

Hypervitaminosis A occurs after prolonged intake of diets high in vitamin A, hence clinical signs are generally seen in mature animals (Seawright and English, 1967), typically cats between 2 and 5 years of age. Hypervitaminosis A is caused by consumption of a diet composed principally of raw liver or by oversupplementation with vitamin A. In kittens, long bone growth may be severely retarded. There may be osteoporosis of the diaphysis with flaring of the metaphysis (Clark, 1970). The primary lesions in chronic cases are exostoses of the cervical vertebrae (Clark, 1970). This results in lethargy, sensitivity to palpation of the neck and an unkempt haircoat due to decreased grooming. The thoracic vertebrae can be affected in some animals, causing spinal rigidity with a compensatory gait and posture (Kallfelz and Dzanis, 1989). Bony proliferations around the joints can cause painful ankylosis. Dystrophic calcification similar to vitamin D toxicity, and inhibited endochondral ossification has also been reported. Treatment is to remove the source of vitamin A from the diet. Adult cats will show clinical improvement and reversal of most signs except those relating to ankylosis. Bony changes will not progress and some remodelling may occur, but epiphyseal damage is irreversible. The prognosis is guarded.

Overnutrition

Nutrition may affect the expression of some inherited disorders including coxa valga, panosteitis, hip dysplasia, hypertrophic osteo-

Table 12.17 Nutritional disorders causing musculoskeletal abnormalities

Disorder	Cause	Clinical signs	Treatment
Overnutrition	Excessive intake of calories and protein. Excessive calcium intake	Osteopetrosis, hip dysplasia, osteochondritis dissecans, panosteitis, cervical spondylomyelopathy, hypertrophic osteodystrophy	Limit caloric intake and feed balanced diet. Growth deformities may self-correct or require surgery
Nutritional secondary hyper-parathyroidism	Dietary imbalance of calcium and phosphorus; all-meat or all-grain diet, excessive mineral oil	Lameness, loss of bone density with pathological fractures, neurologic deficits if there are spinal fractures. Bowing of long bones. Joint ankylosis	Supplement Ca : P at 2 : 1 until bone healed, then 1.2: 1. Limit activity. Repair fractures as needed
Hypovitaminosis D	Vitamin D-deficient diet or lack of sunlight	Similar to hyperparathyroidism, but less severe. May also have widened metaphyses, retained cartilage cores and shortened, curved bones	Supplement vitamin D or increase sunlight exposure
Hypervitaminosis D	Dietary supplementation with vitamin D or cod liver oil	Anorexia, vomiting, polyuria/polydipsia, muscle weakness, soft-tissue mineralization	Remove source of excessive vitamin D
Hypovitaminosis C	Not proven to exist in dogs and cats as they can synthesize vitamin C in the liver	Vitamin C deficiency has been suggested as a causative factor for hypertrophic osteodystrophy and hip dysplasia, but has not been verified	
Hypovitaminosis A	Decreased intake of vitamin A. Very rare	Lame. Shortened, thickened long bones and abnormal skull development (Bennet, 1976)	Vitamin A (200 IU/kg body weight) added to balanced diet containing 1250–2500 IU vitamin A/kg dry matter
Hypervitaminosis A	Raw liver diet or diets supplemented with vitamin A	Lethargy, retarded bone growth, dystrophic calcification. Exostosis of cervical vertebrae and joint ankylosis	Remove source of vitamin A from the diet

Ca = Calcium; P = Phosphorus

dystrophy (HOD)-like syndrome, OCD and cervical spondylomyelopathy (Table 12.17; Hedhammer *et al.*, 1974). It is not recommended to force a puppy's growth by feeding excessive amounts of nutrients or vitamins. Large, fast-growing dogs fed a highly palatable diet *ad libitum* or receiving dietary supplements are at risk. Diets restricted to a maximum of twice maintenance are recommended. Puppies fed restricted diets will reach normal adult height (Hazewinkel, 1993).

Infectious disorders

Osteomyelitis

Acute haematogenous osteomyelitis may be seen in young animals as a result of haematogenous spread of infection from any source, commonly omphalitis. Septicaemia causes formation of infective emboli which enter the nutrient arteries of long bones and become trapped in the small arteries of the metaphysis at the level of the physis. If a portion of the infected metaphysis is intra-articular, septic arthritis can result. Rarely, epiphysitis occurs as a result of exogenous or endogenous pathogens.

Clinical signs

Fever, lethargy and lameness of the affected limb are typical. Multiple sites of infection are possible so a thorough physical examination should be performed. Animals with epiphysitis have a warm and swollen physeal region.

Diagnosis

Diagnosis is based on physical examination, radiographs and joint cytology. Radiographic evaluation may not reveal any bony changes with acute infection. After 2–3 weeks, lysis and new bone production may be apparent in the metaphysis. Haematology reveals leukocytosis. If the animal is pyrexic, blood cultures may be taken. Joint fluid from fluctuant areas may be aspirated. Cytology shows large numbers of neutrophils which may be toxic, ruptured and degranulated. Joint fluid is also submitted for bacterial culture and sensitivities.

Treatment and surgical technique

If there is a region of abscess, it should be opened, drained and flushed. A broad-spectrum antibiotic such as a cephalosporin should be administered intravenously until culture and sensitivity test results are available. The appropriate oral antibiotic should be administered for 4 weeks. Limb immobilization can have a deleterious effect on the articular cartilage, but activity should be restricted until the region is healed (Nunamaker, 1985; Smith, 1993).

Postoperative considerations and prognosis

Prognosis for epiphysitis is generally good. In some cases premature growth plate closure can occur (Braden, 1993).

Idiopathic disorders

Canine panosteitis

Panosteitis is a common spontaneous but self-limiting inflammatory disease of the long bones (Lewis *et al.*, 1992; Muir *et al.*, 1996b). Panosteitis primarily affects large- and giant-breed dogs. German Shepherd Dogs appear to be predisposed. The aetiology is unclear but proposed aetiologies have included infection, metabolic disease, endocrine dysfunction, allergy, autoimmune mechanisms, parasitism and hereditary factors. Panosteitis has also been reported in young dogs with von Willebrand's disease and haemophilia A (Dodds, 1978; Grondalen *et al.*, 1991). Males are reportedly affected four times more commonly than females, although authors disagree on whether a sex predilection exists (Barrett *et al.*, 1968; Bohning *et al.*, 1970). The pathophysiology relates to degeneration of bone marrow adipocytes which results in osteoid formation within the medullary cavity. The medullary trabecular bone is then remodelled and the adipose bone marrow is regenerated. The bones commonly affected (in order) are the ulna, radius, humerus, femur and tibia. Affected dogs are usually between 5 and 12 months of age and the condition usually resolves by 18–20 months of age. However, it has been reported in dogs as young as 2 months and as old as 5 years (Bohning *et al.*, 1970).

Clinical signs

Affected dogs are presented for an acute onset of lameness unrelated to trauma. In females it may be associated with the first oestrus. The lameness may resolve spontaneously within days to weeks and then occur in a different limb. Pain can be elicited on deep palpation of the diaphysis of the affected long bone. The dog may be mildly to severely lame in one or more limbs and the lameness may be accompanied by fever, anorexia or lethargy. Haematology is usually normal although eosinophilia may be present (Barrett *et al.*, 1968; Cotter *et al.*, 1968; Bohning *et al.*, 1970). There is no consistent relationship between the severity of radiographic changes, the amount of pain elicited on palpation and the degree of lameness (Bohning *et al.*, 1970).

Diagnosis

Radiographic findings confirm the diagnosis. In early stages of disease, there may be no visible changes or there may be some radiolucency at the nutrient foramen. Most commonly there is increased intramedullary radiopacity, usually most prominent at the nutrient canal. The increased opacity results in a mottled or patchy appearance. The endosteal surface may be indistinct and thickened and a mild periosteal reaction may be present. Radiographic changes lag behind clinical signs and affected bones become radiographically normal once the disease has resolved.

Treatment and surgical technique

Treatment is symptomatic. NSAIDs may provide some analgesia and decrease the lameness. Limited activity may also be beneficial.

Postoperative considerations and prognosis

The prognosis is excellent for return to normal function within several weeks to several months.

Hypertrophic osteodystrophy

HOD is a rare condition of unknown aetiology (Table 12.18; Teare *et al.*, 1979; Schulz *et al.*, 1991; Lewis *et al.*, 1992; Malik *et al.*, 1995; Muir *et al.*, 1996a). The condition primarily affects young (2–8 months old) large- and giant-breed dogs (Watson *et al.*, 1973). Males are affected

Table 12.18 Aetiologies of hypertrophic osteodystrophy

Excessive dietary protein and energy
Vitamin and mineral oversupplementation
Bacterial or viral infection (distemper)
Heredity

more commonly than females (Grøndalen, 1976). Typical breeds include Great Danes, Boxers, German Shepherd Dogs and Weimaraners but it has been reported in other breeds, including terriers.

Clinical signs

HOD is characterized by swelling and pain of the metaphyseal region of long bones, although other bones may be affected as well. The condition is usually bilaterally symmetrical and may affect all four limbs. The distal radius, ulna and tibia are most often affected and hyperthermia and pain are noted upon palpation of these regions. Lameness may range from mild to severe, and the puppies may refuse to stand. The lameness may be episodic. Fever (up to 106° F or 41.1° C), anorexia and depression may develop. Diarrhoea, ocular or nasal discharge, footpad hyperkeratosis and tooth enamel hypoplasia have also been reported. Complete blood count may be normal or show leukocytosis or mild anaemia. Mild disease may resolve in 7–10 days but multiple relapses can occur (Grøndalen, 1976). Death has been reported in a few cases.

Diagnosis

Diagnosis is based on clinical signs and confirmed by radiographs of the affected limbs. An irregular radiolucent line (double physeal line) is observed in the metaphyses of affected long bones parallel to the normal radiolucent physeal line. The physis may appear normal or irregularly widened. Later in the course of the disease, the radiolucent line is no longer visible but a more radiodense line is present in the reparative region. Subperiosteal new bone formation may be present at the metaphysis and this may form a collar of bone if the new bone formation is extensive. Although there is usually no problem with premature physeal closure, permanent bony changes and growth deformities can occur. Similar changes have also been reported in the costochondral junctions and vertebrae, and periosteal proliferation may occur on the mandible (Newton and Bierly, 1989). In some cases, HOD may resemble craniomandibular osteopathy.

Treatment and surgical technique

Hypertrophic osteodystrophy is usually self-limiting and mildly affected dogs recover within a few weeks. The episodic nature of the condition makes anecdotal response to various treatments suspect. Treatment requires supportive care with proper nutrition, fluid therapy and analgesics. Enteral nutrition and intravenous fluid therapy may be necessary if the puppies are anorexic and dehydrated. The preferred analgesic is buffered aspirin at a dose of 10–25 mg/kg PO t.i.d. Corticosteroids may be used in severe cases, but caution should be used because of the possible infectious causes of HOD. In severe cases, antimicrobials are used and blood cultures may be indicated. Recumbent puppies should be turned every 2–4 hours to prevent hypostatic pulmonary congestion, and should be on a well-padded area to prevent decubital ulcers. Correction of angular deformities may be needed in some cases.

Postoperative considerations and prognosis

Prognosis is related to disease severity – good for mildly affected dogs, poor for severely affected dogs. Diaphyseal deformities can be severe but are usually not debilitating. In rare cases death may occur related to prolonged recumbency, prolonged anorexia or pyrexia. Euthanasia may be warranted in severely affected dogs.

Bone cyst

Bone cysts are rare, benign, fluid-filled lesions of unknown aetiology in the dog and cat (Table 12.19). This discussion is directed towards unicameral cysts.

Clinical signs

Bone cysts may be asymptomatic unless they are large or cause a pathological fracture. Clinical signs include joint stiffness, lameness, pain and swelling, especially if a pathological fracture has developed.

Diagnosis

Diagnosis is based on clinical signs and confirmed by radiographic findings. Characteristic

Table 12.19 Characteristic features of bone cysts

Bone cysts	Location	Fluid	Age of animal	Comments
Aneurysmal	Vertebrae, elbow, zygomatic arch	Blood	Adult, but has been reported in 6-month-old dog (Pernell *et al.*, 1992).	Invasive. Complete resection or irradiation indicated. Poor prognosis (Bowles and Freeman, 1987; Shiroma *et al.*, 1993)
Subchondral	Between physis and articular cartilage of long bones	Serous		Rare – one report in a 10-month-old Labrador (Basher *et al.*, 1988)
Unicameral, monostotic or polyostotic	Metaphysis or diaphysis of long bones	Serous or serosanguineous	5–15 months	Tend to be large-breed dogs. Polyostotic cysts have been associated with polyostotic fibrous dysplasia (bone is replaced by fibrous matrix of immature bone) and may be inherited in Dobermanns (Carrig and Seawright, 1969; Schrader *et al.*, 1983) Good prognosis

Table 12.20 Differential diagnoses for bone cysts

Abscess
Enchondroma
Polyostotic fibrous dysplasia
Non-ossifying fibroma
Malignant bone or cartilage neoplasia

radiographic findings include an expansile radiolucent area in the metaphyseal region of a long bone. Cortical thinning and pathological fracture may be apparent. The lesion may appear active if a pathological fracture results in callus formation (Table 12.20).

Treatment and surgical technique

Solitary bone cysts in young dogs may heal spontaneously, especially following a pathological fracture. Surgical drainage of the fluid, curettage and autogenous cancellous bone grafting may be indicated to promote healing and prevent bony deformity or pathological fracture (Schrader *et al.*, 1983). Bone biopsy is indicated to confirm the diagnosis.

Postoperative considerations and prognosis

The limb should be immobilized until the bone heals. Prognosis is good if the cyst does not interfere with a growth plate.

Retained cartilaginous cores

Retained cartilaginous cores is a rare condition of young large- and giant-breed dogs. Possible aetiologies suggest that it is secondary to overnutrition, that it is a form of osteochondrosis causing delayed endochondral ossification at the physis, or that it is a result of abnormal chondrocytes or loss of vascularization to the central metaphysis (Riser and Shirer, 1965; Hazewinkel *et al.*, 1985). The condition is characterized by hypertrophied endochondral cartilage which persists bilaterally in the ulnar metaphysis and may retard the overall length of ulna. Retained cartilaginous cores has also been reported in other bones, including the lateral femoral condyle. Asymmetrical delayed distal femoral growth results in medial bowing of the femur, genu valgum and lateral patellar luxation (Riser *et al.*, 1969).

Clinical signs

There may be no clinical signs unless a limb deformity begins to develop.

Diagnosis

Diagnosis is based on radiographic findings. The ulna has an inverted cone or 'candlestick' region of radiolucency in the distal metaphysis. The ulna may be shortened resulting in deformities of the antebrachium which can include valgus, external rotation and cranial bowing of the radius (Riser and Shirer, 1965; O'Brien *et al.*, 1971).

Treatment and surgical technique

Dietary restriction for puppies on a high plane of nutrition is indicated (Riser and Shirer, 1965; Johnson, 1981). The dog should be monitored weekly for growth deformities. If the deformities are progressing in a young dog with retained cartilage core in the distal ulna, an ulnar ostectomy with autogenous fat graft should be performed to release the radius and allow it to grow straight. When growth deformities are severe, corrective osteotomy may be indicated.

Postoperative considerations and prognosis

The prognosis is guarded for dogs with growth deformities.

Craniomandibular osteopathy

Craniomandibular (mandibular periostitis, temporomandibular osteodystrophy or lion jaw) is a rare disease that most commonly affects the Scottish, West Highland White and Cairn Terriers. It has also been reported in the Boston Terrier, Boxer, Labrador Retriever, Great Dane, English Bulldog and Dobermann (Smith *et al.*, 1985; Riser, 1993). It may be an autosomal recessive trait in West Highland White Terriers.

Clinical signs

Clinical signs include discomfort or difficulty in chewing or opening the mouth (usually noticed when the dog is 3–7 months of age). This may be accompanied by an intermittent fever (up to 104°F or 40°C) for 3 or 4 days which recurs every 10–14 days until the dog is over 8 months old (Riser, 1993). The pain diminishes and the fever occurs less frequently as the dog nears skeletal maturity. If the mandibular rami fuse with the bullae it may prevent movement of the jaw (Riser, 1993). Malnutrition may be a problem if the dog is unable to eat. Other clinical signs include lethargy, anorexia, salivation, lymphadenopathy, weight loss and temporal and masseter muscle atrophy. The condition is seldom fatal but progresses until the dog is 11–13 months of age when the pain disappears and the bony changes stop or regress.

Diagnosis

Diagnosis is based on physical examination findings of a bilaterally thickened mandible, up to twice its normal size (Riser, 1993). The angular processes of the mandible and the tympanic bullae are often so enlarged that the mouth cannot be fully opened, even with sedation. Skull radiographs show bilateral, symmetrical bony proliferations of the mandible and ossification may also be seen in the adjacent soft tissues, especially near the angular process of the mandible. The bony lesions do not extend rostral to the region of the middle mental foramen. New bone may fill and expand the tympanic bullae. There may be partial or complete ankylosis of the temporomandibular joint. Abnormal bone may also be seen associated with the flat bones of the skull or the long bones resulting in a presentation similar to HOD. The new bone proliferation decreases after 7–8 months of age and as much as half of the proliferative bone may be resorbed by 11–13 months of age (Riser, 1993).

Treatment and surgical technique

The treatment of this disease is primarily supportive care. Attempts to remove the proliferative bone around the temporomandibular joint surgically have not been successful (Pool and Leighton, 1969). Buffered aspirin may provide some pain relief. Nutritional support is important and may require surgical placement of a feeding tube until the proliferative changes stop or regress.

Postoperative considerations and prognosis

Animals that survive may have impaired jaw function, but can usually maintain normal nutritional status once the disease regresses. Euthanasia may be indicated in severe cases.

Sesamoid bone degeneration

Fracture of the volar sesamoid bones of the metacarpophalangeal and metatarsophalangeal joints is a problem of racing Greyhounds; however, a degenerative disease has been described in young large-breed dogs, particularly Rottweilers. The aetiology is unknown, but trauma is a possible cause and it is unclear whether sesamoid fractures and degenerative disease of the sesamoids are related conditions (Robins and Read, 1993). It usually affects the sesamoids of second and seventh digits and may be asymptomatic or result in lameness (Vaughan and France, 1986; Atilola, 1989; Weinstein *et al.*, 1995b). The affected joint may be thickened and effusive. Palpation of the joint may elicit pain and crepitus. It is important to rule out other causes of lameness in the affected limb because of the high incidence of other orthopaedic problems in young large-breed dogs.

Radiographic changes include evidence of DJD and periarticular calcified bodies of variable size, number and location. Restricted activity may resolve the lameness associated with sesamoid disease. If the lameness persists, surgical removal of the affected sesamoids is indicated (Robins and Read, 1993). After placing a tourniquet on the affected limb, an incision is made directly over the affected sesamoid bone. The annular ligament is incised near the affected bone, allowing the superficial and deep flexor tendons to be retracted (Bennett and Kelly, 1985). The bone is dissected from the surrounding tissues and the wound is closed in layers. The foot is bandaged for 1 week and exercise is restricted for 2 weeks. The lameness usually resolves within 1 month of surgery.

Traumatic disorders

Physeal disorders

Physeal disorders are usually caused by trauma and result in conformational abnormalities of the limbs including shortened limbs, angular deformities, rotational defects and abnormal joint congruency. The severity of the condition depends on the degree to which the growth plate contributes to the total bone growth, the age and breed of the animal, the type of injury, the involvement of infection and the method of surgical repair if the physis was fractured. Growth disorders involving the radius or ulna cause asynchronous growth which can result in severe limb deformities, especially if the animal is very young at the time of injury.

Premature physeal closure

Premature closure of the distal ulnar physis is the most common physeal disorder in young dogs. The conical shape of this physis causes it to be traumatized more easily, although a traumatic event is not always identified. Premature physeal closure has a recessive mode of inheritance in Skye Terriers (Lau, 1977) and may be associated with osteochondrosis, delayed endochondral ossification or nutritional deficiencies in larger breeds. Premature physeal closure is usually unilateral, but is bilateral in about 15% of cases. Premature closure of the proximal or distal physis of the radius or ulna can cause problems associated with asynchronous growth of these bones, but premature closure of the physes of other long bones is often not clinically significant.

Clinical signs

Lameness or noticeable angulation of the limb are the first signs. Premature closure of the distal ulnar physis causes the ulna to be shortened. The radius continues to grow, resulting in a cranial bowing and external rotation of the radius with carpal valgus. In addition, distal displacement of proximal ulna may result in subluxation of the elbow. This can fracture the anconeal process or eventually cause DJD (Fig. 12.20).

Symmetrical closure of the proximal or distal radius is uncommon and results in a short, straight radius with elbow joint subluxation as the radius is pulled distally. Premature closure of the distal radius usually occurs as a partial closure of the physis caudolaterally. The medial portion continues to grow, resulting in a valgus deformity of the carpus. However, the distal radius can also have a partial closure medially, resulting in varus angulation of the carpus (Fig. 12.21).

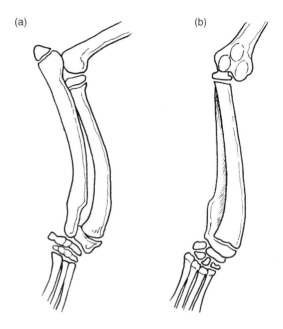

Figure 12.20 Premature closure of the distal ulna results in valgus, cranial bowing and external rotation of the antebrachium. Lateral (a) and cranial view (b).

Diagnosis

Diagnosis is based on clinical signs and radiographic evaluation. If the opposite limb is normal, radiographs should be made for comparison.

Treatment and surgical techniques

Treatment depends on the age of the animal and the severity of the deformity (Table 12.21 and Table 12.22). The treatment goal for an immature animal is to allow as much growth as possible to encourage natural correction of angular deformities. The treatment goal for a mature animal is to correct the deformity while preserving limb length.

Partial ulnar ostectomy

For a unilateral partial ulnar ostectomy, the affected limb and the ipsilateral flank are prepared for aseptic surgery and the dog is positioned in lateral recumbency with the affected side up. For a bilateral ulnar ostectomy, both limbs and the abdomen are prepared for surgery and the dog is positioned in dorsal recumbency. The skin incision is made over the middle to

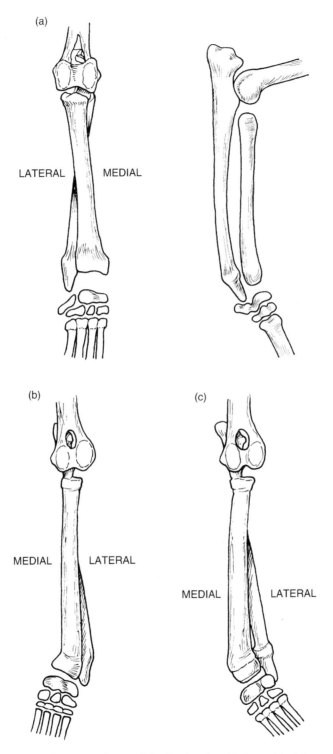

Figure 12.21 Premature closure of the distal radius. (a) Symmetrical closure
resulting in radial carpal joint malarticulation and elbow subluxation.
(b) Asymmetrical closure medially resulting in a varus deformity.
(c) Asymmetrical closure laterally resulting in a valgus deformity.

Table 12.21 Surgical procedures for puppies and kittens with closure of the distal ulnar physis

Condition	Procedures	Goal	Technique
Immature animal with growth potential	Partial ulnar ostectomy with free fat graft	Segmental ostectomy of the ulna allows the radius to grow unimpeded. Angular deformity may self-correct depending on severity and timing of surgery. If ulna heals before animal's growth has stopped, a second ostectomy may be required. If the angular deformity does not self-correct sufficiently, a corrective osteotomy may be indicated	See text
Animals that are mature or near maturity	Corrective osteotomies: Oblique (opening-wedge) osteotomy Cuneiform (closing-wedge) osteotomy Reverse-wedge osteotomy Radial dome osteotomy	Corrects angular and rotational deformities while maintaining limb length. Before performing a corrective osteotomy, radiographs are evaluated to determine the greatest point of curvature of the radius, and to evaluate the congruency of the elbow and carpus. Autogenous cancellous bone graft is required, usually taken from the proximal humerus of the affected limb	See text

Table 12.22 Surgical procedures for puppies and kittens with premature radial physeal closures

Indications	Procedure	Goal	Technique
Immature animal with premature closure of caudolateral portion of distal radial physis	Resection of closed physis	Allows unrestricted growth of the normal part of the physis	Remove closed section of physis and place autogenous fat graft to prevent bony bridging (Vandewater and Olmstead, 1983). Computed tomography may help define affected region of physis
Immature animal with symmetrical complete premature closure of the proximal or distal radius	Partial radial ostectomy with free fat graft	Allows unrestricted growth of the radius and ulna, and restores elbow congruity	An approach is made to the mid diaphyseal region of the radius. A 1–2 cm segment of bone is removed using an oscillating saw or osteotome. A free autogenous fat graft is placed in the defect to prevent bony union. Release of tension on the proximal and distal radius may allow re-establishment of normal elbow and carpus congruency. As the radius is the primary weight-bearing bone in the antebrachium, a splint or supportive bandage is recommended. Once the animal is mature, an autogenous cancellous bone graft may be indicated to ensure bony union of the radius
Immature animal with symmetrical complete premature closure of the proximal or distal radius	Radial osteotomy with continuous distraction	Allows unrestricted growth of the radius and ulna, and restores elbow congruity	A mid diaphyseal radial osteotomy is made. An external fixator is applied to the radius using a turnbuckle distractor on the connecting bars. Alternatively an Ilizarov distractor may be applied (Elkins *et al.*, 1993). Optimal distraction is 1 mm per day divided into two to four increments (Yanoff *et al.*, 1992). Adjustments can be made based on the growth rate of the contralateral radius and the ipsilateral ulna

Table 12.22 (continued)

Indications	Procedure	Goal	Technique
Immature animal with symmetrical complete premature closure of the proximal or distal radius	Partial ulnar ostectomy	Corrects humeroradial luxation, but does not restore limb length or improve varus or valgus deformities (Shields Henney and Gambardella, 1990)	Technique is the same as described in the text. If the ulnar segments do not spontaneously distract, the interosseous membrane should be broken down. This procedure may be done on the proximal ulna to allow visualization of the joint. If done proximally an intramedullary pin is placed to counteract the pull of the triceps (Gilson *et al.*, 1989)
Mature animal with symmetrical complete premature closure of the proximal or distal radius	Transverse lengthening osteotomy	Provides normal radial length and elbow congruency and improves limb function	Proximal and distal external fixation pins are placed in the radius. A transverse mid diaphyseal radial osteotomy is performed and distracted using a Gelpi retractor until length is restored. While holding the radius in distraction, medial and lateral connecting bars are placed with empty clamps. At least two more pins are placed in each radial segment. An autogenous cancellous bone graft is obtained for placement at the osteotomy site. Bone plating may be used for fixation instead of an external fixator (Olson *et al.*, 1981; Vandewater and Olmstead, 1983)
			Postoperative radiographs are made to evaluate pin placement and the position of the radial head. If the radial head is not contacting the humerus, tension can be placed on the proximal radius by using an external fixator pin in the proximal olecranon. The clamps on the proximal radius are loosened and elastic bands are placed between the most proximal radial pin and the ulnar pin. In 24–36 hours the elbow is radiographed. If the articulation is correct, the elastic bands and ulnar pin are removed and the fixator pins are tightened (Mason and Baker, 1978)
Mature animal with symmetrical complete premature closure of the proximal or distal radius	Stairstep osteotomy of the radius	Provides normal radial length and elbow congruency and improves limb function	A stairstep osteotomy is created in the mid diaphyseal radius and the osteotomy is distracted. A lateral approach is made to the elbow to evaluate whether the radial head is contacting the humerus. The longitudinal portions of the stairstep are compressed using lag screws. A bone plate and screws are then used to stabilize the osteotomy. Autogenous cancellous bone graft is placed in the osteotomy gap (Vandewater and Olmstead, 1983)
Nearly mature animal with symmetrical complete premature closure of the proximal or distal radius	Radial dome osteotomy	Corrects valgus deformity while maintaining radial length. Cannot correct severe rotational and valgus deformities (MacDonald and Matthiesen, 1991)	A partial ulnar ostectomy is performed. A dome-shaped osteotomy is made in the distal radial metaphysis. The distal section of radius is rotated to achieve normal angulation. The limb is placed in a cast or splint for 4–5 weeks

distal ulna over the lateral aspect of the bone. The fascia is incised between the tendon of the lateral digital extensor muscle cranially, and the tendon of the ulnaris lateralis muscle caudally (Piermattei, 1993). The fascia and musculature are retracted to allow removal of a 1–2-cm segment of the ulna. The segment of bone with its associated periosteum is removed using an oscillating bone saw or bone cutters (DeCamp *et al.*, 1986). If humeroulnar subluxation is present, the ostectomy may be performed more proximally to facilitate joint reduction (Gilson *et al.*, 1989).

A 2–3 cm skin incision is made in the flank region. A large section of subcutaneous fat is dissected free and placed in the ostectomy gap. Alternatively, if the dog is in dorsal recumbency a small approach can be made in the abdomen to resect part of the falciform ligament or omentum for placement at the ostectomy site. The subcutaneous and skin wounds are closed over the donor site and the ostectomy site.

Oblique or opening-wedge osteotomy
The simplest technique, and the only one which preserves or increases limb length, is an oblique osteotomy using external fixation. First a distal ulnar osteotomy or partial ostectomy is performed as described previously. Then a centrally threaded external fixator pin is placed in the proximal radius so it is parallel to the joint surface of the radial head and is within the transverse plane of the proximal radius. A second centrally threaded pin is placed in the distal radius so it is parallel to the distal radial joint surface and within the lateral transverse plane of the distal radius. The distal radius is approached at the point of greatest curvature. A radial osteotomy is made parallel to the distal radial joint surface using an oscillating bone saw. The radius and ulna are repositioned so the two pins are parallel and in the same lateral transverse plane, eliminating any angular or rotational deformity. Connecting bars with empty clamps are placed on the lateral and medial aspect of the limb. Two additional pins are passed through the proximal segment of the radius. At least one additional pin should be placed in the distal segment. It may not be possible to pass all of the pins through to the opposite connecting bar. An autogenous cancellous bone graft is placed at the radial osteotomy site before closing the surgical wounds. Radiographs are made to assess pin placement and

joint alignment. If small angular or rotational deformities exist they may be corrected by adjusting the external fixator.

Cuneiform or closing-wedge osteotomy
To perform a cuneiform osteotomy the radiographs must be carefully examined to determine the correct angles needed. On the craniocaudal radiograph, two lines are drawn at the region of greatest radial curvature. The first line is parallel to the proximal radial articular surface and the second line is parallel to the distal radial articular surface. These lines will intersect at the lateral cortex of the radius at the point of greatest curvature, and identify the shape and amount of bone to be removed to correct the angular deformity. Similar lines are drawn on the lateral radiograph to determine the amount of bone to be removed to correct cranial bowing.

A ulnar osteotomy or partial ulnar osteotomy is performed. The radial osteotomy is performed following the angles determined by the preoperative radiographic assessment. The wedge is removed and the radial osteotomy gap is reduced; this should correct the cranial bowing and the angular and rotational deformities. The region is compressed and stabilized using a bone plate or external fixator (Newton *et al.*, 1975; Forell and Schwarz, 1983).

Reverse-wedge osteotomy
The cuneiform osteotomy may result in significant loss of bone length. If this is a concern, a reverse-wedge osteotomy may be performed to reduce the amount of bone removed from the radius. A wedge size is determined as described for the cuneiform osteotomy. The osteotomy is performed removing half of the predetermined wedge size. The wedge is rotated 180° and replaced at the osteotomy site. The radial osteotomy and wedge are stabilized using a bone plate (Newton, 1974).

Radial dome osteotomy
The radial dome osteotomy can be used to correct angular limb deformities resulting from closure of the distal ulnar or distal radial physis. After performing a partial distal ulnar ostectomy, a dome-shaped osteotomy is made in the distal radial metaphysis at the region of maximal deformity. The osteotomy is performed by drilling holes in the radius until it is weak enough to break the distal segment free. The distal fragment is rotated to correct the malalignment.

A splint or cast is applied for 4–5 weeks. This procedure does not shorten the radius, but it is only useful in two-dimensional corrections. Animals with severe external rotation and valgus deformities require one of the previously mentioned osteotomies (MacDonald and Matthiesen, 1991).

Postoperative considerations and prognosis

Postoperative radiographs of a partial ulnar or radial ostectomy, or partial physeal resection should be made to document the location and extent of the ostectomy. Postoperatively the limb is placed in a soft padded bandage for 2–3 weeks. The limb should be evaluated monthly to assess elbow conformation, growth of the long bones, correction of the angular deformity and bridging of the ostectomy. If the ostectomy site bridges before the animal is skeletally mature, the surgery may need to be repeated. If angular or rotational deformities are still present when the dog is mature, corrective osteotomy may be necessary. A potential complication of partial ulnar or radial ostectomy is synostosis (bony bridging) of the radius and ulna (MacPhearson and Johnson, 1992). Synostosis causes lameness and contributes to asynchronous growth of the radius and ulna. Treatment of synostosis requires removal of the bridging callus and a dynamic ulnar ostectomy may be needed to restore normal elbow articulation.

Postoperative care of the corrective osteotomies includes limited activity and monthly radiographs to assess bone healing. The implants are removed after bony union.

The prognosis for premature closure of the distal ulnar physis is good if corrective surgery is performed promptly. Animals with mild deformities may only need an ulnar ostectomy, but if the deformities are moderate to severe, a corrective osteotomy is also indicated. Animals with moderate to severe deformities which are not corrected may develop DJD that is severe enough to impair normal function (Shields Henney and Gambardella, 1989; Morgan and Miller, 1994).

Physeal fractures

Physeal fractures are classified based on their radiographic appearance (Llewellyn, 1976;

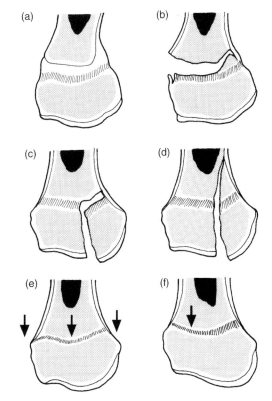

Figure 12.22 Classification of physeal fractures. (a) Salter I fracture is a separation through the physis. (b) Salter II fracture occurs through part of the physis and part of the metaphysis. (c) Salter III fracture occurs through part of the physis and part of the epiphysis. (d) Salter IV fracture occurs through the metaphysis and epiphysis, crossing the physis. (e) Salter V fracture is a crushing injury to the physis. (f) Salter VI fracture is a crushing injury to part of the physis, resulting in asymmetrical damage.

Fig. 12.22). The forces on a physis are primarily traction, pressure or a combination of both. Traction physes are located where muscles insert or originate. Traction physes generally contribute little to long bone length so premature closure of these physes is usually not a problem. Examples of traction physes include the supraglenoid tubercle, olecranon, greater trochanter, tibial tuberosity and tuber calcanei. Traction physes often sustain Salter type I fractures. Pressure physes are located at the ends of long bones and contribute to the majority of long bone growth. Commonly fractured pressure physes include the humeral condyle, the femoral condyle and the femoral head (Table 12.23).

Table 12.23 Characteristic features of physeal fractures

Location	Comments
Proximal humeral fractures	Salter–Harris type I or II fractures occur most commonly and can be stabilized with k wires. If the animal is near maturity, a screw may be used
Humeral condylar fractures	Salter–Harris type IV fractures are common in the distal humerus. Angular limb deformities are not reported. Most humeral growth is from the proximal physis so loss of length from the distal humerus is usually not significant
Proximal radius	Salter–Harris type I or II are most common types, but these are rare fractures
Distal radius	Salter–Harris type I or V are most common. There is likely to be a concurrent distal ulnar fracture
Distal ulna	Salter–Harris type V or VI is most common and can result in severe angular limb deformities
Capital physeal fractures	Salter–Harris type I fracture of the proximal femoral physis is also called a slipped capital physis. In the immature animal, the physis is weaker than the surrounding bone and ligamentous structures so the physis will fracture secondary to trauma that would cause the hip to luxate in a mature animal. This fracture is repaired with open reduction and internal fixation using multiple small pins or a compression screw. Comminuted fractures or failed fracture repair can be treated by femoral head ostectomy (Gibson *et al.*, 1991). Closure of this physis can result in a shortened femoral neck
Femoral condylar fractures	Salter–Harris type I and II are common. Symmetrical damage to the physis can result in a shortened femur which is usually compensated for by extension of the stifle. Asymmetrical closure is rare but causes femoral angulation if it occurs. Monitor for quadriceps contracture if soft-tissue trauma is extensive
Proximal tibia	Salter–Harris type I and II are most common. This is an uncommon fracture site
Distal tibia	Salter–Harris type I and II are most common. Most tibial growth is from the proximal physis so this rarely results in deformity

Treatment and surgical techniques

Acceptable methods of stabilization for physeal fractures include external coaptation or internal fixation. Some Salter I and II fractures can be reduced closed and maintained with a cast or splint. External coaptation does not affect physeal growth. However, most physeal fractures require open reduction and internal fixation. The method of fracture fixation can affect the growth of the physis and the severity of subsequent growth deformities. Bone plates or external fixation that bridge the physis will prevent normal bone growth. Implants that pass through the physis have the potential to damage that part of the physis. Threaded pins or screws which cross the physis will prevent continued growth. Smooth pins or Kirschner wires that cross the physis will allow continued growth, especially if the pins are perpendicular to the physis rather than oblique to it. If an animal is close to skeletal maturity, inhibition of continued growth may not be a major concern. Premature closure may occur as a result of the initial trauma regardless of the method of repair. Traction physes are often repaired using a tension band wire as there is often a strong muscle pull on the fracture fragment and premature closure is usually not a clinical problem (Hauptman and Butler, 1979).

Postoperative considerations and prognosis

In general, the prognosis for physeal fracture healing is good if they are treated rapidly and properly. The prognosis for continued growth from the physis depends on the severity of damage to the physis. The prognosis tends to be worse with a higher Salter–Harris classification, so crushing injuries to the physis carry the poorest prognosis. Salter IV, V and VI fractures are more likely to result in closure regardless of the treatment. Whether delayed or arrested growth results in significant deformity depends on the degree to which the growth plate contributes to the total bone growth, and the age and breed of the animal. Radiographs should be evaluated every 2–3 weeks until bony union of the fracture, at which time implants may be removed. This is followed by monthly evaluations of the traumatized limb and the contralateral limb for 2–3 months to monitor for impaired growth.

Tendon disruptions (Table 12.24)

Trauma may result in various tendon disruptions in any age animal. Some of the tendon disruptions which are more likely to be seen in immature animals are described in Table 12.24.

Myopathies

Myopathies are uncommon in small animals and most are secondary to peripheral nerve disease rather than primary myopathies. Most primary myopathies in young animals are congenital or hereditary (Table 12.25). Myopathies are usually characterized by muscle weakness and exercise intolerance. The gait is often abnormal because of muscle weakness or stiffness, and strength may return after rest. Diagnosis is based on signalment, signs, serum creatine phosphokinase, electromyogram and muscle biopsy.

Table 12.24 Tendon disruptions

Disruption	Clinical signs and diagnosis	Treatment and prognosis
Avulsion of the origin of the biceps brachii tendon	Occurs primarily in young large-breed dogs (4–8 months of age). Acute onset of a weight-bearing lameness and pain on flexion and extension of the shoulder. Diagnosis is based on clinical signs and radiographs. On radiographs, an avulsed segment of bone (the supraglenoid tubercle) may be seen (Bloomberg, 1995)	Surgical reattachment of the tendon using a pin and tension band or screw. External coaptation with the shoulder extended and the elbow flexed for 2 weeks. Physiotherapy and restricted exercise are required for another 3–4 weeks. The prognosis is good with sucessful fixation
Avulsion of the proximal epiphysis of the olecranon with the triceps tendon	Diagnosis is based on clinical signs and radiographs. An avulsed fragment of bone proximal to the olecranon may be detected on radiographs. Need to differentiate from ruptured triceps tendon (Gilmore, 1984)	Reattachment of the olecranon epiphysis using a pin and tension band or screw Coaptation of the limb for 2 weeks with physiotherapy and restricted exercise for another 3–4 weeks. Prognosis for return to function is good; however, joint motion may be restricted (Anson and Betts, 1989)
Disruption of the tendon of origin of the long digital extensor	Tendon avulsion occurs primarily in immature, large-breed dogs. Avulsion causes mild weight-bearing lameness and pain on manipulation of the affected stifle are apparent. Lateral soft-tissue swelling may be present. Diagnosis is based on clinical signs and radiographs. Radiographs may show avulsed bone and cartilage near the extensor fossa of the lateral femoral condyle, best observed on the lateral projection. In a very young dog, the portion of bone may consist primarily of cartilage and not be visible on the radiograph. Rule out cranial cruciate rupture and stifle osteochondritis dissecans. Diagnosis is confirmed by exploratory arthrotomy	For avulsion, surgical reattachment of the avulsed segment using bone screws is the treatment of choice. If the bony portion is too small or for chronic injuries, the bone fragment may be left in place or excised. A fresh bed is prepared on the lateral femoral condyle and the avulsed segment is wired or stapled in place. If no bone is present, the tendon can be sutured to the joint capsule near its point of penetration. Fixation requires support with a splint, cast or coaptive dressing. This can be removed after 2 weeks. Gradual return to function over 3–4 weeks after the coaptation is removed is advised. Prognosis for return to function after acute injuries is good to excellent
	Tendon displacement occurs in young dogs during flexion and extension of the stifle. Displacement causes chronic, mild, weight-bearing lameness. Diagnosis is based on clinical signs and radiographs. Palpation during extension and flexion of the stifle allows detection of the tendon moving in and out of the muscular groove. Rule out cranial cruciate rupture and stifle osteochondritis dissecans	For displacement, surgical stabilization of the tendon is performed by reconstruction of the supporting retinacular tissue, use of a staple to make a roof over the tendon, or tenotomy and transplantation of the tendon to the craniolateral aspect of the proximal tibia (as a last resort). Prognosis is variable and depends on the degree of displacement and surgical repair required (Bloomberg, 1995)

Table 12.24 (continued)

Disruption	Clinical signs and diagnosis	Treatment and prognosis
Avulsion and calcification of the flexor tendons of the medial epicondyle	Young dogs between 5 and 8 months of age may develop traumatic avulsion of the tendinous orgin of the humeral head of the flexor carpi ulnaris or the superficial digital flexor muscles. The avulsed bone fragment has a periosteal blood supply so it may grow and become much larger than the original epicondylar defect. Signs include acute forelimb lameness. Joint effusion and pain on palpation are present initially but diminish rapidly	Treatment is exploratory surgery by blunt dissection through the muscle to remove all the bone fragments. Rest is recommended for 3 weeks postoperatively. Prognosis is good if all fragments are removed

Table 12.25 Characteristic features of myopathies affecting puppies and kittens

Myopathies	Clinical signs	Diagnosis	Treatment
Myopathy of Labrador Retrievers (2–6 months)	Generalized muscle stiffness, especially with cold or stress. Exercise intolerance, bunny-hopping. Improves with rest. Signs stabilize at 6–12 months of age, but megaoesophagus has been reported in mature dogs. May be acceptable pets (Kramer *et al.*, 1981)	Signalment and clinical signs. Abnormal EMG. Muscle biopsy (decreased type 2 myofibres)	Diazepam 5 mg PO t.i.d. or q.i.d. for stiffness. Avoid cold weather
Sex-linked myopathies: Irish terriers, Golden Retrievers, Samoyed, Rottweiler, Belgian Groenendaeler Shepherd (6–8 weeks) cats (12 months)	Dog: stiff gait or bunny-hop, difficulty swallowing, enlarged tongue, atrophy of temporal muscles. Appendicular muscles may be atrophied or hypertrophied. Stunted growth. Die of cardiac failure due to cardiomyopathy; mildly affected dogs may live several years (Wentworth *et al.*, 1972; Kornegay, 1984; Presthues and Nordstoza, 1989; van Ham *et al.*, 1993)	Abnormal EMG. Muscle biopsy (fibre necrosis and regeneration or fibrosis) (Cardinet and Holliday, 1979)	No treatment. Quinidine or procainamide may help temporarily
	Cat: Slowly progressive onset. Stiff, rigid neck. Adduction of hocks. Symmetrical enlargement of muscles. Lumbar kyphosis with a peculiar hunched gait. Reduced cardiac contractility and biventricular enlargement (Vos *et al.*, 1986; Robinson, 1992; Malik, 1993)		
Congenital myotonia: Chow Chow, West Highland White Terrier, Laborador Retriever, Samoyed, Staffordshire Terrier, Cocker Spaniel (2–3 months)	Abduction of forelimbs, stiff gait, bunny-hop, arched back. Gait improves with exercise but exacerbated by cold. Hypertrophy of all skeletal muscles, expecially proximal appendicular muscles, also tongue and anal sphincter. Muscle tone is normal at rest. Dysphagia may be observed. The disease is not progressive (Duncan and Griffiths, 1983; Shires *et al.*, 1983; Hill *et al.*, 1995)	Clinical signs. A characteristic myotonic dimple persists for 30–40 s after tapping the muscle Abnormal EMG. Elevated serum creatine kinase	No known therapy. Procainamide and quinidine appear to lessen the initial weakness. Avoid prolonged exercise

Table 12.25 (continued)

Myopathies	Clinical signs	Diagnosis	Treatment
Dermatomyositis: Collies and Shetland Sheepdogs (7–11) weeks	Primary signs are related to skin lesions on the head, tail, and skin over prominent bones. Dogs with severe dermatitis may have myositis: masticatory myositis predominates with difficulty prehending, masticating and swallowing. May have bilaterally symmetrical, generalized muscle atrophy with paresis or exercise intolerance. Severely affected dogs have stiff gait with hyperreflexia. Disease usually resolves spontaneously by 1 year of age. Severely affected dogs may have dermatitis which waxes and wanes over the dog's lifetime (Hargis and Mundell, 1992)	Abnormal EMG. The masticatory muscles may be the only muscles affected. Muscle biopsy indicated for diagnosis	Corticosteriods have been used
Myasthenia gravis: congenital form is rare but has been reported in the Springer Spaniel, Jack Russell Terrier, Smooth Fox Terrier, Samoyeds, Gammel Dansk Honsehund, and cats (6–8 weeks of age)	Signs are similar to acquired myasthenia and include: premature fatigue that is relieved by rest and regurgitation due to megaoesophagus (Miller *et al.*, 1983)	Presumptive diagnosis is made from clinical signs, response to short-acting anticholinesterase (edrophonium chloride, Tensilon), decremental response to repetitive nerve stimulations and a negative serum acetylcholine receptor antibody titre	Anticholinesterase drugs. Pyridostigmine bromide syrup (1–3 mg/kg PO t.i.d. or b.i.d.). The dose is adjusted based on response. If severe megaoesophagus, neostigmine (0.04 mg/kg IM q.i.d..) Corticosteroids are not indicated since it is not immune-mediated disease. Megaoesophagus is treated by elevated feedings. Do not respond to anticholinesterase therapy as well as animals with acquired disease. Poor long-term survival (Amann, 1987)
Nemaline myopathy: kittens	Apprehension, reluctance to move and abrupt exaggerated movements with a rapid, hopping, hypermetric gait. Muscle atrophy and muscle tremors may also be present. All limbs affected but no loss of strength or balance. Depressed patellar reflexes	Normal EMG and cerebrospinal fluid Elevated serum creatine kinase	No treatment
Metabolic myelopathies pyruvate dehydrogenase defect in Clumber Spaniels. Glycogen storage disease in German Shepherd Dogs. Hyperkalaemic paralysis in 7-month-old Pit Bull Dog	These diseases are characterized by muscle weakness which worsens with exercise. Very rare	The main differential is myasthenia gravis	No specific treatment

Table 12.25 (continued)

Myopathies	Clinical signs	Diagnosis	Treatment
Nutritional myopathy (nutritional myodegeneration, white muscle disease, selenium-responsive myopathy). Due to low dietary levels of selenium, vitamin E or both, and is rare because of the commercially available balanced diets	Generalized weakness, stiff or stilted gait and difficulty rising from recumbency. Signs exacerbated with exercise. Muscles may be swollen, hot and painful. Dysphagia and sialosis may also be present. Sudden death can occur in neonates (Kaspar and Lombard, 1963; Van Vleet, 1975; Dennis and Alexander, 1982)	History of an unusual diet (large amounts of unsaturated fats) by the dam of a newborn. Diagnosis is confirmed by elevated serum muscle enzymes, abnormal EMG and histopathology of muscles of dead animals. Differential diagnosis includes infectious myopathy, congenital myopathy and swimmer syndrome	Proper diet and selenium and vitamin E replacement therapy. Prognosis is usually grave due to the involvement of cardiac, diaphragmatic and intercostal muscles
Scotty cramp: Scottish Terriers (6 weeks to 18 months)	Muscle spasms with an arched back and stiff gait, which may be exacerbated by exercise or excitement. Mildly affected dogs have only muscle rigidity of the pelvic limbs. Severely affected dogs have episodes in which all the muscles become rigid and they fall over and curl into a ball. Within minutes the dog returns to normal. It is hereditary	Diagnosis is based on clinical signs	No treatment needed for dogs with mild, infrequent signs. Modification of the environment and behaviour may help. Dogs with more severe signs may be treated with daily oral acepromazine, diazepam (0.5–1.5 mg/kg PO), primidone or phenobarbitone. Vitamin E (125 IU/kg PO s.i.d.) may reduce the frequency of attacks (Meyers and Clemmons, 1983)
Dancing Dobermann disease: 6 months to 7 years	One pelvic limb is flexed while standing. Within 3–7 months the other limb is affected so the hindlimbs are alternately flexed and extended. With progression the pelvic limb muscles atrophy and proprioception deficits develop. Signs progress over months to years but they are usually acceptable pets for many years	Normal or slightly elevated serum creatine phosphokinase. Abnormal EMG of the gastrocnemius muscles	There is no known treatment
Protozoal myositis: infection may be acquired *in utero* with onset of signs between 2 and 4 months. Toxoplasmosis is often associated with distemper infection, while *Neospora* is usually a primary pathogen	One syndrome: progressive arreflexive paraplegia, with rigid hindlimbs and firm, atrophied muscles (Core *et al.*, 1983). Another syndrome: generalized muscle weakness, poor hopping reaction and normal reflexes. In young puppies, can cause swimmer syndrome. Protozoa may also infect the central nervous system, resulting in stupor, seizures and chorioretinitis. It has been reported to cause death within 48 h of initial signs (Drake and Hime, 1967; Dubey, 1990). Hepatozoon spp. may cause myositis and periosteal bone reaction	Elevated serum creatine kinase. Muscle biopsy indicated for diagnosis. Single serum titres are unreliable and evidence of rising titres requires a long delay before results are obtained. Indirect fluorescent antibody test of serum, cerebrospinal fluid or tissue will aid in the distinguishing *Neospora caninum* from *Toxoplasma gondii*.	Clindamycin (10–40 mg/kg PO, divided t.i.d. or q.i.d.). Or trimethoprim/sulphadiazine (30 mg/kg PO b.i.d.) and pyrimethamine (0.5–1.0 mg/kg PO s.i.d. for 7–10 days) for systemic toxoplasmosis. Long-term prognosis is guarded because of other immuno-suppressive diseases or concomitant central nervous system lesions

Table 12.25 (continued)

Myopathies	Clinical signs	Diagnosis	Treatment
		Definitive diagnosis of *N. caninum* may be made at necropsy using electron microscopy and immunohistochemical methods	
Bacterial myositis (Rarely occurs)	*Leptospira icterohaemorrhagiae* causes stiff gait and muscle pain, but may also causes renal and hepatic signs. *Clostridium* spp. also cause infectious myositis (Kornegay *et al.*, 1980)	Tissue cultures	Antimicrobials selected based on culture and sensitivity. Drainage and lavage of the wound may be indicated
Parasitic myositis:	Aberrant migration of *Dirofilaria immitis* – one case of myositis of the hindlimb (Cooley *et al.*, 1987)	Muscle biopsy	
Congenital hindlimb rigidity	Marked rigidity of one or both hind limbs (Stead *et al.*, 1977)	EMG and muscle biopsy distinguish it from the rigidity of toxoplasmosis. No history of trauma	No effective treatment
Quadriceps contracture (quadriceps tie-down) Adhesions form between the quadriceps muscle and the femur after trauma Associated with inadequate fracture repair, osteomyelitis, severe trauma or overzealous tissue handling More common in young animals	Initially, the hindlimb is held with both the stifle and hock in stiff extension. The hindlimb becomes rigid and the animal may use it as a peg leg or be reluctant to bear weight. The affected limb is held cranial with respect to the other hindlimb. Later clinical signs include atrophied, taut thigh muscles which are fibrotic or adherent to the femur. May develop genu recurvatum, proximal positioning of the patella and DJD (Bardet and Hohn, 1983; 1984) Dogs younger than 3 months may develop growth disturbances throughout the limb characterized by hip luxation, bone hypoplasia, increased femoral torsion, medial patellar luxation and limb-shortening	Diagnosis is based on history and clinical signs. DJD or disuse osteoporosis may be seen on radiographs in chronic cases	Surgery to restore stifle joint mobility. Adhesions between the quadriceps muscles and the femur are broken down. Sliding myoplasty or Z-myoplasty of the quadriceps may be required (Leighton, 1981) Postoperatively, the stifle is maintained in flexion with a sling. Passive physiotherapy to improve the range of motion. The results of surgical treatment are unpredictable. If the surgery is unsatisfactory, alternatives include stifle arthrodesis or limb amputation. Prevention of this condition by careful tissue-handling and use of a flexion sling is preferable (Wilkens *et al.*, 1993)

EMG = Electromyogram; DJD = degenerative joint disease.

References

Alexander, J.W. and Earley, T.D. (1984) A carpal laxity syndrome in young dogs. *Journal of Veterinary Orthopedics*, **3**, 22–26.

Alonso, R.A., Hernandez, A., Diaz, P. and Cantu, J.M. (1982) An autosomal recessive form of hemimelia in dogs. *Veterinary Record*, **110**, 128–129.

Altera, K.P. and Bonasch, H. (1966) Periarteritis nodosa in a cat. *Journal of the American Veterinary Medical Association*, **149**, 1307–1311.

Amann, J.F. (1987) Congenital and acquired neuromuscular disease of young dogs and cats. *Veterinary Clinics of North America Small Animal Practice*, **17**, 617–639.

Anson, L.W. and Betts, C.W. (1989) Triceps tendon avulsion in a dog: surgical management and xeroradiographic evaluation. *Journal of the American Animal Hospital Association*, **25**, 655–658.

Aron, D.N. and Gorse, M.J. (1991) Clinical use of N-butyl-2-cyanoacrylate for stabilization of osteochondral fragments: preliminary report. *Journal of the American Animal Hospital Association*, **27**, 203–210.

Atilola, M. (1989) A development abnormality of the fore-sesamoids in Rottweilers – an introduction. *Veterinary Comparative Orthopedics and Traumatology*, **3**, 129–130.

Bardet, J.F. and Hohn, R.B. (1983) Quadriceps contracture in dogs. *Journal of the American Veterinary Medical Association*, **183**, 680–685.

Bardet, J.F. and Hohn, R.B. (1984) Subluxation of the hip joint and bone hypoplasia associated with quadriceps contracture in young dogs. *Journal of the American Animal Hospital Association*, **20**, 421–428.

Barrett, R.B., Schall, W.D. and Lewis, R.E. (1968) Clinical and radiographic features of canine eosinophilic panosteitis. *Journal of the American Animal Hospital Association*, **4**, 94–104.

Barton, M.D., Ireland, L., Kirschner, J.L. and Forbes, C. (1985) Isolation of *Mycoplasma spumans* from polyarthritis in a greyhound. *Australian Veterinary Journal*, **62**, 206–207.

Basher, A.W.P., Doige, C.E. and Presnell, K.R. (1988) Subchondral bone cysts in a dog with osteochondrosis. *Journal of the American Animal Hospital Association*, **24**, 321–326.

Beachley, M.C. and Graham, F.H. (1973) Hypochondroplastic dwarfism (endochondral chondrodystrophy) in a dog. *Journal of the American Veterinary Medical Association*, **163**, 283–284.

Beale, B.S. and Goring, R.L. (1990) Exposure of the medial and lateral trochlear ridges of the talus in the dog. Part I: Dorsomedial and plantaromedial surgical approaches to the medial trochlear ridge. *Journal of the American Animal Hospital Association*, **26**, 13–18.

Beale, B.S., Goring, R.L., Herrington, J., Dee, J. and Conrad, K. (1991) A prospective evaluation of four surgical approaches to the talus of the dog used in the treatment of osteochondritis dissecans. *Journal of the American Animal Hospital Association*, **27**, 221–229.

Bennett, D. (1976) Nutrition and bone disease in the dog and cat. *Veterinary Record*, **98**, 313–321.

Bennett, D. and Kelly, D.F. (1987) Immune-based non-erosive inflammatory joint disease of the dog. 2. Polyarthritis/polymyositis syndrome. *Journal of Small Animal Practice*, **28**, 891–908.

Bennett, D. and Kelly, D.F. (1985) Sesamoid disease as a cause of lameness in young dogs. *Journal of Small Animal Practice*, **26**, 567–579.

Bennett, D. and Prymak, C. (1986) Excision arthroplasty as a treatment of canine temporomandibular dysplasia. *Journal of Small Animal Practice*, **27**, 361–370.

Berzon, J.L., Howard, P.E., Covell, S.J., Trotter, E.J. and Dueland, R. (1980) A retrospective study of the efficacy of femoral head and neck excisions in 94 dogs and cats. *Veterinary Surgery*, **9**, 88–92.

Bingel, S.A. and Riser, W.H. (1977) Congenital elbow luxation in the dog. *Journal of Small Animal Practice*, **18**, 445–456.

Bingel, S.A. and Sande, R.D. (1994) Chondrodysplasia in five Great Pyrenees. *Journal of the American Veterinary Medical Association*, **205**, 845–848.

Bloomberg, M. (1995) Tendon, muscle, and ligament injuries and surgery. In: Olmstead, M.J. (ed.) *Small Animal Orthopedics*, pp. 472–499. St Louis: Mosby.

Bohning, R.H., Suter, P.F., Hohn, R.B. and Marshall, J. (1970) Clinical and radiologic survey of canine panosteitis. *Journal of the American Veterinary Medical Association*, **156**, 870–883.

Bowles, M.H.Y. and Freeman, K. (1987) Aneurysmal bone cyst in the ischia and pubes of a dog: a case report and literature review. *Journal of the American Animal Hospital Association*, **23**, 423–427.

Braden, T.D. (1993) Histophysiology of the growth plate and growth plate injuries. In: Bojrab, M.J. (ed.) *Disease Mechanisms in Small Animal Surgery*, pp. 1027–1041. Philadelphia: Lea & Febiger.

Braden, T.D., Prieur, W.D. and Kaneene, J.B. (1990) Clinical evaluation of intertrochanteric osteotomy for treatment of dogs with early-stage hip dysplasia: 37 cases (1980–1987). *Journal of the American Veterinary Medical Association*, **196**, 337–341.

Breur, G.J., Zerbe, C.A., Slocombe, R.F., Padgett, G.A. and Braden, T.D. (1989) Clinical, radiographic, pathologic, and genetic features of osteochondrodysplasia in Scottish deerhounds. *Journal of the American Veterinary Medical Association*, **195**, 606–612.

Brinker, W.O., Piermattei, D.L. and Flo, G.L. (1990) *Handbook of Small Animal Orthopedics and Fracture Treatment*. Philadelphia: WB Saunders.

Bruecker, K.A. and Piermattei, D.L. (1988) Excision arthroplasty of the canine scapulohumeral joint: report of three cases. *Veterinary Comparative Orthopedics and Traumatology*, **3**, 134–140.

Campbell, J.R. (1971) Luxation and ligamentous injuries of the elbow of the dog. *Veterinary Clinics of North America Small Animal Practice*, **1**, 429–440.

Campbell, J.R. (1979) Congenital luxation of the elbow. *Veterinary Annual*, **19**, 229–236.

Cardinet, G.H. and Holliday, T.A. (1979) Neuromuscular disease of domestic animals: A summary of muscle biopsies from 159 cases. *Annals of the New York Academy of Science*, **317**, 290–311.

Carpenter, L.G., Schwarz, P.D., Lowry, J.E., Park, R.D. and Steyn, P.F. (1993) Comparison of radiologic imaging techniques for diagnosis of fragmented medial coronoid process of the cubital joint in dogs. *Journal of the American Veterinary Medical Association*, **203**, 78–83.

Carrig, C.B., MacMillan, A., Brundage, S., Pool, R.R. and Morgan, J.P. (1977) Retinal dysplasia associated with skeletal abnormalities in labrador retrievers. *Journal of the American Veterinary Medical Association*, **170**, 49–56.

Carrig, C.B. and Seawright, A.A. (1969) A familial canine polyostotic fibrous dysplasia with subperiosteal cortical defects. *Journal of Small Animal Practice*, **10**, 397–405.

Carrig, C.B., Sponenberg, D.P., Schmidt, G.M. and Tvedten, H.W. (1988) Inheritance of associated ocular and skeletal dysplasia in Labrador retrievers. *Journal of the American Veterinary Medical Association*, **193**, 1269–1272.

Carrig, C.B., Wortman, J.A., Morris, E.L. *et al.* (1981) Ectrodactyly (split-hand deformity) in the dog. *Veterinary Radiology*, **22**, 123–143.

Cavanagh, P.G. and Kosovshy, J.E. (1993) Hyperparathyroidism and metabolic bone disease. In: Bojrab, M.J. (ed.) *Disease Mechanisms in Small Animal Surgery*, pp. 865–875. Philadelphia: Lea & Febiger.

Chambers, J.N. (1993) Developmental and congenital problems of the antebrachium and adjacent joints. In: Bojrab, M.J. (ed.) *Disease Mechanisms in Small Animal Surgery*, pp. 834–840. Philadelphia: Lea & Febiger.

Chester, D.K. (1971) Multiple cartilaginous exostoses in two generations of dogs. *Journal of the American Veterinary Medical Association*, **159**, 895–897.

Clark, L. (1970) Effect of excess vitamin A on longbone growth in kittens. *Australian Veterinary Journal of Comparative Pathology*, **80**, 625–634.

Clark, L., Seawright, A.A. and Hrdlicka, J. (1970) Exostoses in hypervitaminotic A cats with optimal calcium-phosphorus intakes. *Journal of Small Animal Practice*, **11**, 553–561.

Cohn, L.A. and Meuten, D.J. (1990) Bone fragility in a kitten: an osteogenesis imperfecta-like syndrome. *Journal of the American Veterinary Medical Association*, **197**, 98–100.

Cooley, A.J., Clemmons, R.M. and Gross, T.L. (1987) Heartworm disease manifested by encephalomyelitis and myositis in a dog. *Journal of the American Veterinary Medical Association*, **190**, 431–432.

Core, D.M., Hoff, E.J. and Milton, J.L. (1983) Hindlimb hyperextension as a result of *Toxoplasma gondii* polyradiculitis. *Journal of the American Animal Hospital Association*, **19**, 713–716.

Cotter, S.M., Griffiths, R.C. and Leav, I. (1968) Enostosis of young dogs. *Journal of the American Veterinary Medical Association*, **153**, 401–410.

Daly, W.R. (1990) Amputation of the forelimb. In: Bojrab, M.J. (ed.) *Current Techniques in Small Animal Surgery*, pp. 802–806. Philadelphia: Lea & Febiger.

DeBowes, L.J. (1987) Pituitary dwarfism in a German shepherd puppy. *Compendium on Continuing Education for the Practicing Veterinarian*, **9**, 931–938.

DeCamp, C.E. (1995) Dislocations. In: Olmstead, M.L. (ed.) *Small Animal Orthopedics*, pp. 333–359. St Louis: Mosby.

DeCamp, C.E., Hauptman, J., Knowles, G. and Reindel, J.F. (1986) Periosteum and the healing of partial ulnar ostectomy in radius curvus of dogs. *Veterinary Surgery*, **15**, 185–190.

DeHaan, J.J., Goring, R.L. and Beale, B.S. (1994) Evaluation of polysulfated glycosaminoglycan for the treatment of hip dysplasia in dogs. *Veterinary Surgery*, **23**, 177–181.

Dennis, J.M. and Alexander, R.W. (1982) Nutritional myopathy in a cat. *Veterinary Record*, **111**, 195–196.

Dew, T.L. and Martin, R.A. (1992) Functional, radiographic, and histologic assessment of healing of autogenous osteochondral grafts and full-thickness cartilage defects in the talus of dogs. *American Journal of Veterinary Research*, **53**, 2141–2152.

Dodds, W.J. (1978) Inherited bleeding disorders. *Canine Practice*, **5**, 49–58.

Doige, C.E. (1987) Multiple cartilaginous exostes in dogs. *Veterinary Pathology*, **24**, 276–278.

Doige, C.E., Pharr, J.W. and Withrow, S.J. (1978) Chondrosarcoma arising in multiple cartilaginous exostoses in a dog. *Journal of the American Animal Hospital Association*, **14**, 605–611.

Dougherty, S.A., Center, S.A., Shaw, E.E. and Erb, H.A. (1991) Juvenile-onset polyarthritis syndrome in Akitas. *Journal of the American Veterinary Medical Association*, **198**, 849–856.

Drake, J.C. and Hime, J.M. (1967) Two syndromes in young dogs caused by *Toxoplasma gondii*. *Journal of Small Animal Practice*, **8**, 621–626.

Dubey, J.P. (1990) *Neospora caninum*: a look at a new *Toxoplasma*-like parasite of dogs and other animals. *Compendium on Continuing Education for the Practicing Veterinarian*, **12**, 653–663.

Duncan, I.D. and Griffiths, I.R. (1983) Myotonia in the dog. In: Kirk, R.W. (ed.) *Current Veterinary Therapy VIII*, p. 696. Philadelphia: WB Saunders.

Egger, E.L. and Freeman, L. (1985) Transarticular pinning and external splintage for treatment of congenital hyperextension of the stifle and tibiotarsal joint: a case report. *Journal of the American Animal Hospital Association*, **21**, 663–667.

Elkins, A.D., Morandi, M. and Zembo, M. (1993) Distraction osteogenesis in the dog using the Ilizarov external ring fixator. *Journal of the American Animal Hospital Association*, **29**, 419–426.

Fletch, S.M., Pinkerton, P.H. and Brueckner, P.J. (1975) The Alaskan malamute chondrodysplasia (dwarfism–anemia) syndrome *Journal of American Animal Hospital Association*, **11**, 353–361.

Fletch, S.M., Smart, M.E., Pennock, P.W. and Subden, R.E. (1973) Clinical and pathologic features of chondrodysplasia (dwarfism) in the Alaskan malamute. *Journal of the American Veterinary Medical Association*, **162**, 357–361.

Forell, E.B. and Schwarz, P.D. (1983) Use of external skeletal fixation for treatment of angular deformity secondary to premature distal ulnar physeal closure. *Journal of the American Animal Hospital Association*, **29**, 460–476.

Fowler, J.D., Presnell, K.R. and Holmberg, D.L. (1988) Scapulohumeral arthrodesis: results in seven dogs. *Journal of the American Animal Hospital Association*, **24**, 667–672.

Fox, M.W. (1964) Polyarthrodysplasia (congenital joint luxation) in the dog. *Journal of the American Veterinary Medical Association*, **145**, 1204–1205.

Fox, S.M., Burbidge, H.M., Bray, J.C. and Guerin, S.R. (1996) Ununited anconeal process: lag-screw fixation. *Journal of the American Animal Hospital Association*, **32**, 52–56.

Franczuszki, D. and Parkes, L.J. (1988) Glenoid excision as a treatment in chronic shoulder disabilities: surgical technique and clinical results. *Journal of the American Animal Hospital Association*, **24**, 637–643.

Gambardella, P.C. (1993) Legg–Calvé–Perthes disease in dogs. In: Bojrab, M.J. (ed.) *Disease Mechanisms in Small Animal Surgery*, pp. 804–807. Philadelphia: Lea & Febiger.

Gambardella, P.C., Osborne, C.A. and Stevens, J.B. (1975) Multiple cartilaginous exostoses in the dog. *Journal of the American Veterinary Medical Association*, **166**, 761–768.

Gee, B.R. and Doige, C.E. (1970) Multiple cartilaginous exostoses in a litter of dogs. *Journal of the American Veterinary Medical Association*, **156**, 53–59.

Gibson, K.L., Lewis, D.D. and Pechman, R.D. (1990) Use of external coaptation for the treatment of avascular necrosis of the femoral head in a dog. *Journal of the American Veterinary Medical Association*, **197**, 868–870.

Gibson, K.L., van Ee, R.T. and Pechman, R.D. (1991) Femoral capital physeal fractures in dogs: 34 cases (1979–1989). *Journal of the American Veterinary Medical Association*, **198**, 886–890.

Gilmore, D.R. (1984) Triceps tendon avulsion in the dog and cat. *Journal of the American Animal Hospital Association*, **20**, 239–242.

Gilson, S.D., Piermattei, D.L. and Schwarz, P.D. (1989) Treatment of humerolunar subluxation with a dynamic proximal ulnar osteotomy. A review of 13 cases. *Veterinary Surgery*, **18**, 114–122.

Goring, R.L. and Beale, B.S. (1990) Exposure of the medial and lateral trochlear ridges of the talus in the dog. Part II: Dorsolateral and plantarolateral surgical approaches to the lateral trochlear ridge. *Journal of the American Animal Hospital Association*, **26**, 19–24.

Goring, R.L. and Beale, B.S. (1993) Immune-mediated arthropathies. In: Bojrab, M.J. (ed.) *Disease Mechanisms in Small Animal Surgery*, pp. 742–757. Philadelphia: Lea & Febiger.

Greco, D.S., Feldman, E.C., Peterson, M.E., Turner, J.L., Hodges, C.M. and Shipman, L.W. (1991) Congenital hypothyroid dwarfism in a family of giant schnauzers. *Journal of Veterinary Internal Medicine*, **5**, 57–65.

Grøndalen, J. (1976) Metaphyseal osteopathy (hypertrophic osteodystrophy) in growing dogs. A clinical study. *Journal of Small Animal Practice*, **17**, 721–735.

Grøndalen, J., Sjaastad, O. and Teige, J. (1991) Enostosis (panosteitis) in three dogs suffering from hemophilia A. *Canine Practice*, **16**, 10–14.

Gurevitch, R. and Hohn, R.B. (1980) Surgical management of lateral luxation and subluxation of the canine radial head. *Veterinary Surgery*, **9**, 49–57.

Hall, D.S., Amann, J.F., Constantinescu, G.M. and Vogt, D.W. (1987) Anury in two Cairn terriers. *Journal of the American Veterinary Medical Association*, **191**, 1113–1115.

Hargis, A.M. and Mundell, A.C. (1992) Familial canine dermatomyositis. *Compendium on Continuing Education for the Practicing Veterinarian*, **14**, 855–864.

Haskins, M.E., Bingel, S.A., Northington, J.W. *et al.* (1983) Spinal cord compression and hindlimb paresis in cats with mucopolysaccharidosis VI. *Journal of the American Veterinary Medical Association*, **182**, 983–985.

Hauptman, J. and Butler, H.C. (1979) Effect of osteotomy of the greater trochanter with tension band fixation on femoral conformation in beagle dogs. *Veterinary Surgery*, **8**, 13–18.

Hayes, A.G., Boudrieau, R.J. and Hungerford, L.L. (1994) Frequency and distribution of medial and lateral patellar luxation in dogs: 124 cases (1982–1992). *Journal of the American Veterinary Medical Association*, **205**, 716–720.

Hazewinkel, H.A.W. (1993) Nutrition in orthopedics. In: Bojrab, M.J. (ed.) *Disease Mechanisms in Small Animal Surgery*, pp. 1119–1128. Philadelphia: Lea & Febiger.

Hazewinkel, H.A.W., Goedegebuure, S.A., Poulos, P.W. and Wolvekamp, W.T.C. (1985) Influences of chronic calcium excess on the skeletal development of growing great danes. *Journal of the American Animal Hospital Association*, **21**, 377–391.

Hedhammer, Å., Wu, F., Krook, L. *et al.* (1974) Overnutrition and skeletal disease. An experimental study in growing great danes. *Cornell Veterinarian*, **64**, 1–160.

Henry, W.B. (1984) Radiographic diagnosis and surgical management of fragmented medial coronoid process in dogs. *Journal of the American Veterinary Medical Association*, **184**, 799–805.

Heyman, S.J., Smith, G.K. and Cofone, M.A. (1993) Biomechanical study of the effect of coxofemoral positioning on passive hip joint laxity in dogs. *American Journal of Veterinary Research*, **54**, 210–215.

Hill, S.L., Shelton, G.D. and Lenehan, T.M. (1995) Myotonia in a cocker spaniel. *Journal of the American Animal Hospital Association*, **31**, 506–509.

Hohn, R.B., Craig, E.T. and Anderson, W.D. (1990) Treatment of shoulder joint luxations. In: Bojrab, M.J. (ed.) *Current Techniques in Small Animal Surgery*, pp. 740–748. Philadelphia: Lea & Febiger.

Hohn, R.B., Rosen, H., Bohning, R.H. and Brown, S.G. (1971) Surgical stabilization of recurrent shoulder luxation. *Veterinary Clinics of North America Small Animal Practice*, **1**, 537–548.

Houlton, J.E.F. and Meynink, S.E. (1989) Medial patellar luxation in the cat. *Journal of Small Animal Practice*, **30**, 349–352.

Huibregtse, B.A., Johnson, A.L., Muhlbauer, M.C. and Pijanowski, G.J. (1994) The effect of treatment of fragmented coronoid process on the development of osteoarthritis of the elbow. *Journal of the American Animal Hospital Association*, **30**, 190–195.

Huxtable, C.R. and Davis, P.E. (1976) The pathology of polyarthritis in young greyhounds. *Journal of Comparative Pathology*, **86**, 11–21.

Jacobson, L.S. and Kirberger, R.M. (1996) Canine multiple cartilaginous exostoses: unusual manifestations. A review of the literature. *Journal of the American Animal Hospital Association*, **32**, 45–51.

Jezyk, P.F. (1985) Constitutional disorders of the skeleton in dogs and cats. In: Newton, C.D. and Nunamaker, D.M. (eds) *Textbook of Small Animal Orthopaedics*, pp. 637–654. Philadelphia: JB Lippincott.

Johnson, A.L. (1995) Growth deformities. In: Olmstead, M.L. (ed.) *Small Animal Orthopedics*, pp. 293–309. St Louis: Mosby.

Johnson, K.A. (1981) Retardation of endochondral ossification at the distal ulnar growth plate in dogs. *Australian Veterinary Journal*, **57**, 474–478.

Johnson, S.G., Hulse, D.A., Vangundy, T.E. and Green, R.W. (1989) Corrective osteotomy for pes varus in the dachshund. *Veterinary Surgery*, **18**, 373–379.

Kallfelz, F.A. (1987) Skeletal and neuromuscular diseases. In: Lewis, L.D., Morris, M.L. and Hand, M.S. (eds) *Small Animal Clinical Nutrition III*, pp. 12-1–12-15. Topeka, KS: Mark Morris.

Kallfelz, F.A. and Dzanis, D.A. (1989) Overnutrition: an epidemic problem in pet animal practice? *Veterinary Clinics of North America Small Animal Practice*, **19**, 433–446.

Kaspar, L.V. and Lombard, L.S. (1963) Nutritional myodegeneration in a litter of beagles. *Journal of the American Veterinary Medical Association*, **143**, 284–288.

Kealy, R.D., Lawler, D.F., Monti, K.L. *et al.* (1993) Effects of dietary electrolyte balance on subluxation of the femoral head in growing dogs. *American Journal of Veterinary Research*, **54**, 555–562.

Kealy, R.D., Olsson, S.E., Monti, K.L. *et al.* (1992) Effects of limited food consumption on the incidence of hip dysplasia in growing dogs. *Journal of the American Veterinary Medical Association*, **201**, 857–863.

Keller, W.G. and Chambers, J.N. (1989) Antebrachial metacarpal arthrodesis for fusion of deranged carpal joints in two dogs. *Journal of the American Veterinary Medical Association*, **195**, 1382–1384.

Kene, R.O.C., Lee, R. and Bennett, D. (1982) The radiological features of congenital elbow luxation/subluxation in the dog. *Journal of Small Animal Practice*, **23**, 621–630.

Komtebedde, J. and Vasseur, P.B. (1993) Elbow luxation. In: Slatter, D. (ed.) *Textbook of Small Animal Surgery*, vol. 2, pp. 1729–1736. Philadelphia: WB Saunders.

Kornegay, J.N. (1984) Golden retriever muscular dystrophy. *Proceedings of the American College of Veterinary and Internal Medicine*, **2**, 470–472.

Kornegay, J.N., Gorgacz, E.J., Dawe, D.L. *et al.* (1980) Polymyositis in dogs. *Journal of the American Veterinary Medical Association*, **176**, 431–438.

Kramer, J.W., Hegreberg, C.A. and Hamilton, M.J. (1981) Inheritance of a neuromuscular disorder of labrador retriever dogs. *Journal of the American Veterinary Medical Association*, **179**, 380–381.

Krauser, K. (1989) Multiple enchondromatosis in the dog. *Veterinary Comparative Orthopedics and Traumatology*, **4**, 152–157.

Lantz, G.C. and Cantwell, H.D. (1986) Intermittent openmouth lower jaw locking in five dogs. *Journal of the American Veterinary Medical Association*, **188**, 1403–1405.

Lau, R.E. (1977) Inherited premature closure of the distal ulnar physis. *Journal of the American Animal Hospital Association*, **13**, 609–612.

Lees, G.E. and Sautter, J.H. (1979) Anemia and osteopetrosis in a dog. *Journal of the American Veterinary Medical Association*, **175**, 820–824.

Leighton, R.L. (1981). Muscle contractures in the limbs of dogs and cats. *Veterinary Surgery*, **10**, 132–135.

Lewis, D.D., McCarthy, R.J. and Pechman, R.D. (1992) Diagnosis of common developmental orthopedic conditions in canine pediatric patients. *Compendium on Continuing Education for the Practicing Veterinarian*, **14**, 287–301.

Lewis, D.D., Parker, R.B. and Hager, D.A. (1989) Fragmented medial coronoid process of the canine elbow. *Compendium on Continuing Education for the Practicing Veterinarian*, **11**, 703–715.

Lewis, R.E. and Van Sickle, D.C. (1970) Congenital hemimelia (agenesis) of the radius in a dog and a cat. *Journal of the American Veterinary Medical Association*, **156**, 1892–1897.

Llewellyn, H.R. (1976) Growth plate injuries – diagnosis, prognosis, and treatment. *Journal of the American Animal Hospital Association*, **12**, 77–82.

Lust, G., Williams, A.J., Burton-Wurster, N. *et al.* (1993) Joint laxity and its association with hip dysplasia in labrador retrievers. *American Journal of Veterinary Research*, **54**, 1990–1999.

MacDonald, J.M. and Matthiesen, D. (1991) Treatment of forelimb growth plate deformity in 11 dogs by radial dome osteotomy and external coaptation. *Veterinary Surgery*, **20**, 402–408.

MacPhearson, G.C. and Johnson, K.A. (1992) Radio-ulnar synostosis complicating partial mid-diaphyseal ulnar ostectomy in growing dogs. *Veterinary Comparative Orthopedics and Traumatology*, **5**, 26–30.

Malik, R. (1993) Hereditary myopathy of Devon rex cats. *Journal of Small Animal Practice*, **34**, 539–546.

Malik, R., Dowden, M., Davis, P.E. *et al.* (1995) Concurrent juvenile cellulitis and metaphyseal osteopathy: an atypical canine distemper virus syndrome? *Australian Veterinary Practitioner*, **25**, 62–67.

Mann, F.A., Tanger, C.H., Wagner-Mann, C. *et al.* (1987) A comparison of standard femoral head and neck excision and femoral head and neck excision using a biceps femoris muscle flap in the dog. *Veterinary Surgery*, **16**, 223–230.

Mason, T.A. and Baker, M.J. (1978) The surgical management of elbow joint deformity associated with premature growth plate closure in dogs. *Journal of Small Animal Practice*, **19**, 639–645.

Massat, B.J. and Vasseur, P.B. (1994) Clinical and radiographic results of total hip arthroplasty in dogs: 96 cases (1986–1992). *Journal of the American Veterinary Medical Association*, **205**, 448–454.

Matis, U., Krauser, K., Schwartz-Porsche, D. and Putzer-Brenig, A.V. (1989) Multiple enchondromatosis in the dog. *Veterinary Comparative Orthopedics and Traumatology*, **4**, 144–151.

Meyers, K.M. and Clemmons, R.M. (1983) Scotty cramp. In: Kirk, R.W. (ed.) *Current Veterinary Therapy VIII*, Philadelphia: WB Saunders.

Meyers, V.N., Jezyk, P.F., Aguirre, G.D. and Patterson, D.F. (1983) Short-limbed dwarfism and ocular defects in the Samoyed dog. *Journal of the American Veterinary Medical Association*, **183**, 975–979.

Miller, L.M., Lennon, V.A., Lambert, E.M. *et al.* (1983) Congenital myasthenia gravis in 13 smooth fox terriers. *Journal of the American Veterinary Medical Association*, **182**, 694–697.

Milton, J.L., Horne, R.D., Bartels, J.E. and Henderson, R.A. (1979) Congenital elbow luxation in the dog. *Journal of the American Veterinary Medical Association*, **175**, 572–582.

Milton, J.L. and Montgomery, R.D. (1987) Congenital elbow dislocations. *Veterinary Clinics of North America Small Animal Practice*, **17**, 873–888.

Montgomery, M. and Tomlinson, J. (1985) Two cases of ectrodyactyly and congenital elbow luxation in the dog. *Journal of the American Animal Hospital Association*, **21**, 781–785.

Montgomery, R.D., Hathcock, J.T., Milton, J.L. and Fitch, R.B. (1994) Osteochondritis dissecans of the canine tarsal joint. *Compendium on Continuing Education for the Practicing Veterinarian*, **16**, 835–845.

Montgomery, R.D., Long, I.R., Milton, J.L., DiPinto, M.N. and Hunt, J. (1989a) Comparison of aerobic culturettes, synovial membrane biopsy, and blood culture media in detection of canine bacterial arthritis. *Veterinary Surgery*, **18**, 300–303.

Montgomery, R.D., Milton, J.L., Henderson, R.A. and Hathcock, J.T. (1989b) Osteochondritis dissecans of the canine stifle. *Compendium on Continuing Education for the Practicing Veterinarian*, **11**, 1199–1205.

Montgomery, R.D., Milton, J.L., Hudson, J.A., Pernell, R.T. and Finn-Bodner, S.T. (1993) Medial congenital elbow luxation in a dog. *Veterinary Comparative Orthopedics and Traumatology*, **6**, 122–124.

Morgan, P.W. and Miller, C.W. (1994) Osteotomy for correction of premature growth plate closure in 24 dogs. *Veterinary Comparative Orthopedics and Traumatology*, **7**, 129–135.

Muir, P., Dubielzig, R.R. and Johnson, K.A. (1996a) Hypertrophic osteodystrophy and calvarial hyperostosis. *Compendium on Continuing Education for the Practicing Veterinarian*, **18**, 143–151.

Muir, P., Dubielzig, R.R. and Johnson, K.A. (1996b) Panosteitis. *Compendium on Continuing Education for the Practicing Veterinarian*, **18**, 29–33.

Newton, C.D. (1974) Surgical management of distal ulnar physeal growth disturbances in dogs. *Journal of the American Veterinary Medical Association*, **164**, 479–487.

Newton, C.D. and Bierly, D.N. (1989) Skeletal diseases. In: Ettinger, S.J. (ed.) *Textbook of Veterinary Internal Medicine*, vol. 2, pp. 2378–2399. Philadelphia: WB Saunders.

Newton, C.D., Nunamaker, D.M. and Dickinson, C.R. (1975) Surgical management of radial physeal growth disturbance in dogs. *Journal of the American Veterinary Medical Association*, **167**, 1011–1018.

Nunamaker, D.M. (1985) Osteomyelitis. In: Newton, C.D. and Nunamaker, D.M. (eds) *Textbook of Small Animal Orthopaedics*, pp. 499–510. Philadelphia: JB Lippincott.

O'Brien, S.E., Riedesel, E.A. and Miller, L.D. (1987) Osteopetrosis in an adult dog. *Journal of the American Animal Hospital Association*, **23**, 213–216.

O'Brien, T.R., Morgan, J.P. and Suter, P.F. (1971) Epiphyseal plate injury in the dog: a radiographic study of growth disturbance in the forelimb. *Journal of Small Animal Practice*, **12**, 19–36.

Olmstead, M.L. (1995a) The canine cemented modular total hip prosthesis. *Journal of the American Animal Hospital Association*, **31**, 109–124.

Olmstead, M.L. (1995b) Canine cemented total hip replacements: state of the art. *Journal of Small Animal Practice*, **36**, 395–399.

Olson, N.C., Brinker, W.O., Carrig, C.B. and Tvedten, H.W. (1981) Asynchronous growth of the canine radius and ulna: surgical correction following experimental premature closure of the distal radial physis. *Veterinary Surgery*, **10**, 125–131.

Padgett, G.A., Mostosky, U.V., Probst, C.W., Thomas, M.W. and Krecke, C.F. (1995) The inheritance of osteochondritis dissecans and fragmented coronoid process of the elbow joint. *Journal of the American Animal Hospital Association*, **31**, 327–330.

Pedersen, N.C., Wind, A., Morgan, J.P. and Pool, R.R. (1989) Joint diseases of dogs and cats. In: Ettinger, S.J. (ed.) *Textbook of Veterinary Internal Medicine*, vol. 2, pp. 2329–2377. Philadelphia: WB Saunders.

Pederson, N.C. (1968) Surgical correction of a congenital defect of the radius and ulna of a dog. *Journal of the American Veterinary Medical Association*, **153**, 1328–1331.

Pederson, N.C., Laliberte, L. and Ekman, S. (1983) A transient febrile 'limping' syndrome of kittens caused by two different strains of feline calicivirus. *Feline Practice*, **13**, 26–34.

Pernell, R.T., Cunstan, R.W. and DeCamp, C.E. (1992) Aneurysmal bone cyst in a six-month-old dog. *Journal of the American Veterinary Medical Association*, **201**, 1897–1899.

Person, M.W. (1989) Arthroscopic treatment of osteochondritis dissecans in the canine shoulder. *Veterinary Surgery*, **18**, 175–189.

Piermattei, D.L. (1993) *An Atlas of Surgical Approaches to the Bones and Joints of the Dog and Cat*. Philadelphia: WB Saunders.

Pool, R.R. and Leighton, R.L. (1969) Craniomandibular osteopathy in a dog. *Journal of the American Veterinary Medical Association*, **154**, 657–660.

Popovitch, C.A., Smith, G.K., Gregor, T.P. and Shofer, F.S. (1995) Comparison of susceptibility for hip dysplasia between rottweilers and German shepherd dogs. *Journal of the American Veterinary Medical Association*, **206**, 648–650.

Prata, R.G., Stoll, S.G. and Zaki, F.A. (1975) Spinal cord compression caused by osteocartilaginous exostoses of the spine in two dogs. *Journal of the American Veterinary Medical Association*, **166**, 371–375.

Presthues, J. and Nordstoza, K. (1989) Probable X-linked myopathy in a samoyed litter. *Proceedings of the European Society of Veterinary Neurology*, **10**, 52.

Probst, C.W., Flo, G.L., McLoughoin, M.A. and DeCamp, C.E. (1989) A simple medial approach to the canine elbow for treatment of fragmented coronoid process and osteochondritis dissecans. *Journal of the American Animal Hospital Association*, **25**, 331–334.

Prostredny, J.M., Toombs, J.P. and VanSickle, D.C. (1991) Effect of two muscle sling techniques on early morbidity after femoral head and neck excision in dogs. *Veterinary Surgery*, **20**, 298–305.

Puglisi, T.A., Tanger, C.H., Green, R.W., Mann, F.A., Mathey, W.S. and Shively, M.J. (1988) Stress radiography of the canine humeral joint. *Journal of the American Animal Hospital Association*, **24**, 235–240.

Read, R.A. (1994) Successful treatment of congenital shoulder luxation in a dog by closed pinning. *Veterinary Comparative Orthopedics and Traumatology*, **7**, 170–172.

Remedios, A.M., Basher, A.W.P., Runyon, C.L. and Fries, C.L. (1992) Medial patellar luxation in 16 large dogs. A retrospective study. *Veterinary Surgery*, **21**, 5–9.

Remedios, A.M., Clayton, H.M. and Skuba, E. (1994) Femoral head excision arthroplasty using the vascularised rectus femoris muscle sling. *Veterinary Comparative Orthopedics and Traumatology*, **7**, 82–87.

Remedios, A.M. and Fries, C.L. (1993) Implant complications in 20 triple pelvic osteotomies. *Veterinary Comparative Orthopedics and Traumatology*, **6**, 202–207.

Rettenmaier, J.L. and Constantinescu, G.M. (1991) Canine hip dysplasia. *Compendium on Continuing Education for the Practicing Veterinarian*, **13**, 643–653.

Richardson, E.F., Wey, P.D. and Hoffman, L.A. (1994) Surgical management of syndactyly in a dog. *Journal of the American Veterinary Medical Association*, **205**, 1149–1151.

Riser, W.H. (1993) Canine craniomandibular osteopathy. In: Bojrab, M.J. (ed.) *Disease Mechanisms in Small Animal Surgery*, pp. 892–899. Philadelphia: Lea & Febiger.

Riser, W.H. and Frankhauser, R. (1970) Osteopetrosis in the dog: a report of three cases. *Journal of the American Veterinary Radiology Society*, **11**, 29–34.

Riser, W.H., Haskins, M.E., Jezyk, P.F. and Patterson, D.F. (1980) Pseudoachondroplastic dysplasia in miniature poodles: clinical, radiologic, and pathologic findings. *Journal of the American Veterinary Medical Association*, **176**, 335–341.

Riser, W.H., Parkes, L.J., Thodes, W.H. and Shirer, J.F. (1969) Genu valgum: a stifle deformity of giant dogs. *Journal of the American Veterinary Radiology Society*, **10**, 28–37.

Riser, W.H. and Shirer, J.F. (1965) Normal and abnormal growth of the distal foreleg in large and giant dogs. *Journal of the American Veterinary Radiology Society*, **6**, 50–64.

Robins, G.M. and Read, R.A. (1993) Diseases of the sesamoid bones. In: Bojrab, M.J. (ed.) *Disease Mechanisms in Small Animal Surgery*, pp. 1094–1101. Philadelphia: Lea & Febiger.

Robinson, R. (1992) Spasticity in the Devon rex cat. *Veterinary Record*, **132**, 302.

Roy, R.G., Wallace, L.J. and Johnston, G.R. (1994) A retrospective long-term evaluation of ununited anconeal process excision on the canine elbow. *Veterinary Comparative Orthopedics and Traumatology*, **7**, 94–97.

Rudd, R.G., Whitehair, J.G. and Margolis, J.H. (1990) Results of management of osteochondritis dissecans of the humeral head in dogs: 44 cases (1982 to 1987) *Journal of the American Animal Hospital Association*, **26**, 173–178.

Santen, D.R., Payne, J.T., Pace, L.W., Kroll, R.A. and Johnson, G.C. (1991) Thoracolumbar vertebral osteochondroma in a young dog. *Journal of the American Veterinary Medical Association*, **199**, 1054–1056.

Schneck, G.W. (1974) Two cases of congenital malformation (peromelus ascelus and ectrodactyly) in cats. *Veterinary Medicine Small Animal Clinician*, **69**, 1025–1026.

Schrader, S.C. (1995) Joint diseases of the dog and cat. In: Olmstead, M.C. (ed.) *Small Animal Orthopedics*, pp. 437–471. St Louis: Mosby.

Schrader, S.C., Burk, R.L. and Liu, S.-K. (1983) Bone cysts in two dogs and a review of similar cystic bone lesions in the dog. *Journal of the American Veterinary Medical Association*, **182**, 490–495.

Schultz, V.A. and Watson, A.G. (1995) Lumbosacral transitional vertebra and thoracic limb malformations in a chihuahua puppy. *Journal of the American Animal Hospital Association*, **31**, 101–106.

Schulz, K.S., Payne, J.T. and Aronson, E. (1991) *Escherichia coli* bacteremia associated with hypertrophic osteodystrophy in a dog. *Journal of the American Veterinary Medical Association*, **199**, 1170–1173.

Seawright, A.A. and English, P.B. (1967) Hypervitaminosis A and deforming cervical spondylosis of the cat. *Journal of Comparative Pathology*, **77**, 29–39.

Shields Henney, L.H. and Gambardella, P.C. (1990) Partial ulnar ostectomy for treatment of premature closure of the proximal and distal radial physes in the dog. *Journal of the American Animal Hospital Association*, **26**, 183–188.

Shields Henney, L.H. and Gambardella, P.C. (1989) Premature closure of the ulnar physis in the dog: a retrospective clinical study. *Journal of the American Animal Hospital Association*, **25**, 573–581.

Shires, P.K., Hulse, D.A. and Kearney, M.T. (1985) Carpal hyperextension in two-month-old pups. *Journal of the American Veterinary Medical Association*, **186**, 49–52.

Shires, P.K., Nafe, L.A. and Hulse, D.A. (1983) Myotonia in a Staffordshire terrier. *Journal of the American Veterinary Medical Association*, **183**, 229–232.

Shiroma, J.T., Weisbrode, S.E., Biller, D.S. and Olmstead, M.L. (1993) Pathological fracture of an aneurysmal bone cyst in a lumbar vertebra of a dog. *Journal of the American Animal Hospital Association*, **29**, 434–437.

Sjöström, L., Kasström, H. and Källberg, M. (1995) Ununited anconeal process in the dog. Pathogenesis and treatment by osteotomy of the ulna. *Veterinary Orthopaedics and Comparative Traumatology*, **8**, 170–176.

Slater, M.R., Scarlett, J.M., Kaderly, R.E. and Bonnett, B.N. (1991) Breed, gender, and age as risk factors for canine osteochondritis dissecans. *Veterinary Comparative Orthopedics and Traumatology*, **4**, 100–106.

Slater, M.R., Scarlett, J.M., Donoghue, S. *et al.* (1992) Diet and exercise as potential risk factors for osteochondritis dissecans in dogs. *American Journal of Veterinary Research*, **53**, 2119–2124.

Slocum, B. and Devine, T. (1987) Pelvic osteotomy in the dog as treatment for hip dysplasia. *Seminars in Veterinary Medicine and Surgery (Small Animal)*, **2**, 107–116.

Smith, G.K., Biery, D.N. and Gregor, T.P. (1990) New concepts of coxofemoral joint stability and the development of a clinical stress-radiographic method for quantitating hip joint laxity in the dog. *Journal of the American Veterinary Medical Association*, **196**, 59–70.

Smith, G.K., Gregor, T.P., Rhodes, W.H. and Biery, D.N. (1993) Coxofemoral joint laxity from distraction radiography and its contemporaneous and prospective correlation with laxity, subjective score, and evidence of degenerative joint disease from conventional hip-extended radiography in dogs. *American Journal of Veterinary Research*, **54**, 1021–1042.

Smith, G.K., Popovitch, C.A., Gregor, T.P. and Shofer, F.S. (1995) Evaluation of risk factors for degenerative joint disease associated with hip dysplasia in dogs. *Journal of the American Veterinary Medical Association*, **206**, 642–647.

Smith, K.W. (1976) Achilles tendon surgery for correction of hyperextension of the hock joint. *Journal of the American Animal Hospital Association*, **12**, 848–849.

Smith, M.M. (1993) Orthopedic infections. In: Slatter, D. (ed.) *Textbook of Small Animal Surgery*, vol. 2, pp. 1685–1694. Philadelphia: WB Saunders.

Smith, M.M., Vasseur, P.B. and Morgan, J.P. (1985) Clinical evaluation of dogs after surgical and nonsurgical management of osteochondritis dissecans of the talus. *Journal of the American Veterinary Medical Association*, **187**, 31–35.

Sponenberg, D.P. and Bowling, A.T. (1985) Heritable syndrome of skeletal defects in a family of Australian shepherd dogs. *Journal of Heredity*, **76**, 393–394.

Stead, A.C., Camburn, M.A., Gunn, H.M. and Kirk, E.J. (1977) Congenital hindlimb rigidity in a dog. *Journal of Small Animal Practice*, **18**, 39–46.

Stevens, D.R. and Sande, R.D. (1974) An elbow dysplasia syndrome in the dog. *Journal of the American Veterinary Medical Association*, **165**, 1065–1069.

Teare, J.A., Krook, L., Kallfelz, F.A. and Hintz, H.F. (1979) Ascorbic acid deficiency and hypertrophic osteodystrophy in the dog: a rebuttal. *Cornell Veterinarian*, **69**, 384–401.

Thompson, K.G., Jones, L.P., Smylie, W.A. *et al.* (1984) Primary hyperparathyroidism in German shepherd dogs: a disorder of probable genetic origin. *Veterinary Pathology*, **21**, 370–376.

Tobias, T.A., Miyabayashi, T., Olmstead, M.L. and Hedrick, L.A. (1994) Surgical removal of fragmented medial coronoid process in the dog: comparative effects of surgical approach and age at time of surgery. *Journal of the American Animal Hospital Association*, **30**, 360–368.

Trevor, P.B., Stevenson, S., Carrig, C.B., Waldron, D.R. and Smith, M.M. (1992) Evaluation of biocompatible osteoconductive polymer as an orthopedic implant in dogs. *Journal of the American Veterinary Medical Association*, **200**, 1651–1660.

Turrel, J.M. and Pool, R.R. (1982) Primary bone tumors in the cat: a retrospective study of 15 cats and a literature review. *Journal of the American Veterinary Radiology Society*, **23**, 152–166.

van Bree, H. (1993) Comparison of the diagnostic accuracy of positive-contrast arthrography and arthrotomy in evaluation of osteochondrosis lesions in the scapulohumeral joint in dogs. *Journal of the American Veterinary Medical Association*, **203**, 84–88.

van Bree, H. (1994) Evaluation of subchondral lesion size in osteochondrosis of the scapulohumeral joint in dogs. *Journal of the American Veterinary Medical Association*, **204**, 1472–1474.

van Bree, H., Degryse, H., Van Ryssen, B., Ramon, F. and Desmidt, M. (1993) Pathologic correlations with magnetic resonance images of osteochondrosis lesions in canine shoulders. *Journal of the American Veterinary Medical Association*, **202**, 1099–1105.

van Ham, L.M.L., Desmidt, M., Tshamata, M., Hoorens, J.K. and Mattheeuws, D.R.G. (1993) Canine X-linked muscular dystrophy in Belgian Groenendailer shepherds. *Journal of the American Animal Hospital Association*, **29**, 570–574.

Van Ryssen, B. (1992) Arthroscopic evaluation of osteochondrosis lesions in the canine hock joint: a review of two cases. *Journal of the American Animal Hospital Association*, **28**, 295–299.

Van Ryssen, B., van Bree, H. and Simeons, P. (1993) Elbow arthroscopy in clinically normal dogs. *American Journal of Veterinary Research*, **54**, 191–198.

Van Vleet, J.F. (1975) Experimentally induced vitamin E-selenium deficiency in the growing dog. *Journal of the American Veterinary Medical Association*, **166**, 769–774.

Vandewater, A. and Olmstead, M.L. (1983) Premature closure of the distal radial physis in the dog. A review of 11 cases. *Veterinary Surgery*, **12**, 7–12.

Vasseur, P.B. (1983) Clinical results of surgical correction of shoulder luxation in dogs. *Journal of the American Veterinary Medical Association*, **182**, 503–505.

Vasseur, P.B. (1990) Arthrodesis for congenital luxation of the shoulder in a dog. *Journal of the American Veterinary Medical Association*, **197**, 501–503.

Vaughan, L.C. and France, C. (1986) Abnormalities of the volar and plantar sesamoid bones in Rottweilers. *Journal of Small Animal Practice*, **27**, 551–558.

Vaughan, L.C. and Jones, D.G.C. (1969) Congenital dislocation of the shoulder joint in the dog. *Journal of Small Animal Practice*, **10**, 1–3.

Vos, J.H., vander Linde-Sipman, J.S. and Goedegeburre, S.A. (1986) Dystrophy like myopathy in a cat. *Journal of Comparative Pathology*, **96**, 335–341.

Walker, T.L. and Prieur, W.D. (1987) Intertrochanteric femoral osteotomy. *Seminars in Veterinary Medicine and Surgery (Small Animal)*, **2**, 117–130.

Wallace, L.J. and Olmstead, M.L. (1995) Disabling conditions of the canine coxofemoral joint. In: Olmstead, M.L. (ed.) *Small Animal Orthopedics*, pp. 361–393. St Louis: Mosby.

Watson, A.D.J., Blair, R.C., Farrow, B.R.H., Baird, J.D. and Cooper, H.L. (1973) Hypertrophic osteodystrophy in the dog. *Australian Veterinary Journal*, **49**, 433–439.

Weinstein, M.J., Mongil, C.M., Rhodes, W.H. and Smith, G.K. (1995a) Orthopedic conditions of the rottweiler – part II. *Compendium on Continuing Education for the Practicing Veterinarian*, **17**, 925–939.

Weinstein, M.J., Mongil, C.M. and Smith, G.K. (1995b) Orthopedic conditions of the rottweiler – part I. *Compendium on Continuing Education for the Practicing Veterinarian*, **17**, 813–830.

Wentink, G.H., van der Linde-Sipman, J.S., Meijer, A.E.F.H. *et al.* (1972) Myopathy with a possible recessive X-linked inheritance in a litter of Irish terriers. *Veterinary Pathology*, **9**, 328–349.

Whitehair, J.G. and Rudd, R.G. (1990) Osteochondritis dissecans of the humeral head in dogs. *Compendium on Continuing Education for the Practicing Veterinarian*, **12**, 195–203.

Wilkens, B.E., McDonald, D.E. and Hulse, D.A. (1993) Utilization of a dynamic stifle flexion apparatus in preventing recurrence of quadriceps contracture: a clinical report. *Veterinary Comparative Orthopedics and Traumatology*, **6**, 219–223.

Wind, A.P. (1986) Elbow incongruity and developmental elbow diseases in the dog: part I. *Journal of the American Animal Hospital Association*, **22**, 711–724.

Wind, A.P. and Packard, M.E. (1986) Elbow incongruity and developmental elbow diseases in the dog: part II. *Journal of the American Animal Hospital Association*, **22**, 725–730.

Wisner, E.R., Berry, C.R., Morgan, J.P., Pool, R.R., Wind, A.P. and Vasseur, P.B. (1990) Osteochondrosis of the lateral trochlear ridge of the talus in seven Rottweiler dogs. *Veterinary Surgery*, **19**, 435–439.

Withrow, S.J. (1977) Temporary transarticular pinning. *Veterinary Medicine/Small Animal Clinician*, **72**, 1597–1602.

Woodard, J.C., Riser, W.H., Bloomberg, M.S., Gaskin, J.M. and Goring, R.L. (1991) Erosive polyarthritis in two greyhounds. *Journal of the American Veterinary Medical Association*, **198**, 873–876.

Yanoff, S.R., Hulse, D.A., Palmer, R.H. and Herron, M.R. (1992) Distraction osteogenesis using modified external fixation devices in five dogs. *Veterinary Surgery*, **21**, 480–487.

Zontine, W.J., Weitkamp, R.A. and Lippincott, C.L. (1989) Redefined type of elbow dysplasia involving calcified flexor tendons attached to the medial humeral epicondyle in three dogs. *Journal of the American Veterinary Medical Association*, **194**, 1082–1085.

Index

References to tables are followed by the letter 't'; references to figures are followed by the letter 'f'